Obesity: A Growing Concern

Volume I

Obesity: A Growing Concern
Volume I

Edited by **Carlyle Bennet**

FOSTER ACADEMICS

New Jersey

Published by Foster Academics,
61 Van Reypen Street,
Jersey City, NJ 07306, USA
www.fosteracademics.com

Obesity: A Growing Concern
Volume I
Edited by Carlyle Bennet

International Standard Book Number: 978-1-63242-300-9 (Hardback)

Printed in China.

Contents

Preface

This age's focus on body image is nothing short of dangerous for the human body. Images all around bombard us with what the media believes should be our body's weight, which is basically skinny, leaving the myriad body types and shapes that exist. But there is also a flip side to this media assault. Not everyone is leaning towards becoming an equivalent of a skeleton, but leaning the other way. Obesity is equally negative and harmful to one's body as starving oneself. The accumulation of body fat to the extent that there are dire effects on health is extremely bad for any kind of lifestyle and often drastically reduces a person's life expectancy. This has become in itself a disorder that restricts itself to hormonal imbalances. Mired in today's increasingly sedentary lifestyle and constant barrage of cheap and fattening foods, obesity needs to be looked at seriously. Considering the fact that there is some medical precedent with a genetic predisposition in some people to overeat, it can be beaten with exercise. The longer a person is overweight, the harder it becomes to lose it. Once a person is obese, one shouldn't just consider it a matter of vanity to lose weight but a matter of saving one's own life.

This book is an attempt to understand obesity as something to be overcome to have a healthy and long life and it brings together studies that work towards this. I would like to thank my family and friends for their support in this endeavour.

Editor

Prevalence and Trends of Adult Obesity in the US, 1999–2012

Ruopeng An

College of Applied Health Sciences, University of Illinois at Urbana-Champaign, George Huff Hall Room 2013, 1206 South 4th Street, Champaign, IL 61820, USA

Correspondence should be addressed to Ruopeng An; ran5@illinois.edu

Academic Editors: S. A. Lear and C. H. Wu

Aim. To provide national estimates of obesity among US adults aged 20 years and older in 2011-2012 and track its trends from 1999 to 2012. *Methods.* Measured weight/height from National Health and Nutrition Examination Survey 1999–2012 waves was used to calculate body mass index (BMI) and prevalence measures. Piecewise logistic regressions were conducted to test the differential trends before and after 2010. *Results.* In 2011-2012, the age-adjusted prevalence of overweight and obesity combined (BMI $\geq$ 25) was 71.1% (95% CI: 68.0%–74.2%) among men and 65.5% (61.8%–69.3%) among women, and the prevalence of obesity (BMI $\geq$ 30) was 33.3% (30.5%–36.2%) among men and 35.8% (32.3%–39.4%) among women. From 1990–2000 to 2009-2010, the prevalence of overweight and obesity combined, obesity, grades 2 and 3 obesity combined (BMI $\geq$ 35), and grade 3 obesity (BMI $\geq$ 40) increased by 7.2%, 17.8%, 17.6%, and 33.0%, respectively. Compared to 2009-2010, most gender- and race/ethnicity-specific prevalence measures remained unchanged or slightly decreased in 2011-2012. No significant difference in trends among prevalence measures was found before and after 2010. *Conclusions.* Concurrent evidence on the leveling off of obesity in the US is thin. Given its high prevalence and profound socioeconomic consequences, close monitoring of the trend is warranted.

1. Introduction

Obesity is a leading risk factor for many adverse health outcomes including type 2 diabetes, hypertension, dyslipidemia, coronary heart disease, and certain types of cancer [1]. The prevalence of adult obesity in the US had doubled from 1976–1980 to 1999-2000 [2]. In 2009 US ranked the highest in adult obesity prevalence among all countries in the Organization for Economic Cooperation and Development [3]. The estimated annual medical cost of obesity in the US totaled 147 billion US dollars in 2008 [4].

More recent data indicated a slowing down of the trend in adult obesity and even some leveling off in childhood obesity. Small but significant declines in the prevalence of obesity among low-income preschoolers aged 2–5 years were reported in 19 of 43 US states examined in the Pediatric Nutrition Surveillance System from 2008 to 2011 [5]. No significant change in the prevalence of adult obesity was found between 2003–2008 and 2009-2010 in the National Health and Nutrition Examination Survey (NHANES) [6]. The prevalence of morbid (i.e., grades 2 and 3) obesity was still increasing from 2005 to 2010, but its growth rate had slowed down as indicated in the Behavioral Risk Factor Surveillance System (BRFSS) [7].

Given the large disease burden of obesity and its high prevalence, it is crucial to continuously monitor the prevalence of obesity in the US. This study provides national estimates of obesity among US adults aged 20 years and older in 2011-2012 and tracks its trends from 1999 to 2012.

2. Methods

Study sample came from NHANES 1999-2000, 2001-2002, 2003-2004, 2005-2006, 2007-2008, 2009-2010, and 2011-2012 waves. NHANES is a program of studies designed to assess the health and nutritional status of adults and children and represents a multistage probability sample of the US civilian, noninstitutionalized population [8]. Participants' body weight and stature height were measured by digital scale and stadiometer in the NHANES mobile examination center [9]. Body mass index (BMI) is defined by weight

TABLE 1: Unweighted sample sizes and weighted percentages for adults aged 20 years and older: NHANES 2011-2012.

	All races/ethnicities	Non-Hispanic White	Non-Hispanic African American	Hispanic
Both genders	5,181 (100.00%)	1,899 (66.62%)	1,364 (11.48%)	1,037 (14.16%)
Male	2,585 (48.62%)	961 (35.32%)	662 (5.59%)	515 (7.74%)
Female	2,596 (51.38%)	938 (36.89%)	702 (6.85%)	522 (7.62%)

NHANES denotes National Health and Nutrition Examination Survey. Percentage is weighed using NHANES sampling weights to be representative of the US adult population in 2011-2012. The sum of sample sizes for non-Hispanic White, non-Hispanic African American, and Hispanic is not equal to the total sample size because of other races/ethnicities not shown in the table.

in kilograms divided by height in meters squared. Four prevalence measures were examined: overweight and obesity combined (BMI $\geq$ 25), obesity (BMI $\geq$ 30), grades 2 and 3 obesity combined (BMI $\geq$ 35), and grade 3 obesity (BMI $\geq$ 40). Age was adjusted by direct standardization to the year 2000 Census population using the age groups 20–39 years old, 40–59 years old, and 60 years and older. NHANES wave-specific sampling weight, sampling stratum, and primary sampling unit were taken into account in estimating prevalence in the population. Prevalence was estimated for both the overall population and subpopulations stratified by gender and race/ethnicity (i.e., non-Hispanic White, non-Hispanic African American, and Hispanic).

Piecewise logistic regressions were used to test the differential trends in adult obesity before and after 2010. The model has the following setup:

$$\begin{gathered}\operatorname{logit}(Y_i) = \beta_0 + \beta_1 X_i + \beta_2 (X_i - 2010) D_i + \epsilon_i, \\ D_i = \mathbf{1}\{X_i \geq 2010\}.\end{gathered} \tag{1}$$

In (1), Y_i is an indicator variable for overweight and obesity combined (BMI $\geq$ 25), obesity (BMI $\geq$ 30), grades 2 and 3 obesity combined (BMI $\geq$ 35), or grade 3 obesity (BMI $\geq$ 40); X_i a continuous variable taking the values of 2000, 2002, 2004, 2006, 2008, 2010, and 2012 for the NHANES waves 1999-2000, 2001-2002, 2003-2004, 2005-2006, 2007-2008, 2009-2010, and 2011-2012, respectively; D_i an indicator variable for $X_i \geq 2010$; and ϵ_i the error term. If the estimated coefficient β_2 is significantly different from zero (equivalent to the estimated odds ratio e^{β_2} to be significantly different from one), it indicates the trends of prevalence measures to be different before and after 2010. Piecewise logistic regressions were performed on the overall sample and on each gender and race/ethnicity group, controlling for age group (i.e., 20–39 years old, 40–59 years old, and 60 years and older) and accounting for survey design. All statistical analyses were performed in Stata 13.0 [10].

3. Results

In total, 5,560 adults aged 20 years and older participated in the NHANES 2011-2012 wave. Among them, 57 pregnant women and 322 individuals with missing values in body weight/height measures were excluded from the analyses. Table 1 reports unweighted sample sizes and weighted percentages of the total population. The effective sample size is 5,181, roughly equally split between genders. NHANES oversamples minorities: 1,364 non-Hispanic African Americans and 1,037 Hispanic were included besides non-Hispanic White.

Table 2 reports the estimated BMI and prevalence measures among US adults aged 20 years and older in 2011-2012. The age-adjusted mean BMI was 28.5 (95% CI: 28.0–29.0) among men and 28.8 (28.3–29.3) among women. Non-Hispanic African American women had the highest mean BMI of 32.3 (31.6–33.0) among all gender and race/ethnicity subgroups. The age-adjusted prevalence of overweight and obesity combined (BMI $\geq$ 25) was 71.1% (68.0%–74.2%) among men and 65.5% (61.8%–69.3%) among women, and the age-adjusted prevalence of obesity (BMI $\geq$ 30) was 33.3% (30.5%–36.2%) among men and 35.8% (32.3%–39.4%) among women. Among men, 11.8% (9.7%–13.9%) and 4.3% (2.2%–6.3%) were classified in grades 2 and 3 obesity combined (BMI $\geq$ 35) and grade 3 obesity (BMI $\geq$ 40), respectively, whereas among women, 16.7% (14.5%–8.9%) and 8.0% (6.6%–9.5%) were classified in grades 2 and 3 obesity combined and grade 3 obesity, respectively.

Substantial disparities in prevalence measures were present across genders and races/ethnicities. Women had higher prevalence of obesity, grades 2 and 3 obesity combined, and grade 3 obesity than men (although the differences were not always statistically significant) among all race/ethnicity groups. Non-Hispanic African American women had the highest prevalence of overweight and obesity combined (81.5%), obesity (56.4%), grades 2 and 3 obesity combined (28.7%), and grade 3 obesity (15.8%) among all gender and race/ethnicity groups, which were 29%, 73%, 92%, and 122% higher than among non-Hispanic White women, respectively.

Figure 1 shows the percentage change in prevalence measures among US adults of 20 years and older from 1999-2000 to 2011-2012 with 1999-2000 as the baseline. The age-adjusted prevalence of overweight and obesity combined (BMI $\geq$ 25), obesity (BMI $\geq$ 30), grades 2 and 3 obesity combined (BMI $\geq$ 35), and grade 3 obesity (BMI $\geq$ 40) in 2009-2010 were 7.2%, 17.8%, 17.6%, and 33.0% higher than in 1999-2000. Compared to 2009-2010, the prevalence measures slightly decreased in 2011-2012, but the reductions were not statistically significant at $P < 0.05$.

Figure 2 shows the gender- and race/ethnicity-specific trend in the age-adjusted prevalence of overweight and obesity combined (BMI $\geq$ 25), obesity (BMI $\geq$ 30), grades 2 and 3 obesity combined (BMI $\geq$ 35), and grade 3 obesity (BMI $\geq$ 40) among US adults aged 20 years and older from 1999-2000 to 2011-2012. Compared to 2009-2010, most gender-

TABLE 2: Age-adjusted BMI and prevalence of overweight and obesity combined (BMI ≥ 25), obesity (BMI ≥ 30), grades 2 and 3 obesity combined (BMI ≥ 35), and grade 3 obesity (BMI ≥ 40) among U.S. adults aged 20 years and older: NHANES 2011-2012.

	All races/ethnicities	Non-Hispanic White	Non-Hispanic African American	Hispanic
		BMI		
Both genders	28.67 (28.23–29.11)	28.36 (27.78–28.93)	30.83 (30.25–31.40)	29.58 (29.12–30.03)
Male	28.50 (28.04–28.95)	28.36 (27.85–28.88)	28.99 (28.45–29.54)	29.18 (28.68–29.67)
Female	28.84 (28.33–29.34)	28.35 (27.62–29.08)	32.33 (31.63–33.03)	29.94 (29.36–30.52)
		BMI ≥ 25 (%)		
Both genders	68.23 (65.07–71.39)	66.95 (63.07–70.83)	75.88 (72.36–79.40)	77.67 (74.20–81.13)
Male	71.11 (68.01–74.21)	71.11 (67.19–75.03)	69.08 (64.79–73.37)	78.51 (73.39–83.63)
Female	65.52 (61.78–69.27)	62.97 (57.97–67.98)	81.54 (77.81–85.27)	76.70 (73.16–80.23)
		BMI ≥ 30 (%)		
Both genders	34.63 (31.79–37.47)	32.36 (28.71–36.00)	47.63 (44.25–51.00)	42.05 (38.63–45.48)
Male	33.34 (30.51–36.17)	32.15 (29.32–34.97)	36.95 (33.13–40.77)	40.07 (35.65–44.49)
Female	35.81 (32.26–39.36)	32.55 (26.81–38.28)	56.38 (52.14–60.60)	43.73 (39.48–47.97)
		BMI ≥ 35 (%)		
Both genders	14.31 (12.52–16.11)	13.12 (10.64–15.60)	23.02 (20.70–25.35)	15.89 (13.47–18.30)
Male	11.80 (9.65–13.94)	11.19 (8.74–13.64)	16.03 (12.53–19.52)	11.56 (9.12–14.01)
Female	16.69 (14.48–18.91)	14.98 (11.76–18.21)	28.73 (25.66–31.80)	20.05 (16.80–23.30)
		BMI ≥ 40 (%)		
Both genders	6.19 (4.85–7.53)	5.41 (3.62–7.19)	11.76 (9.99–13.53)	5.67 (4.49–6.85)
Male	4.27 (2.23–6.32)	3.64 (1.12–6.16)	6.86 (5.17–8.54)	3.73 (2.54–4.91)
Female	8.04 (6.61–9.46)	7.13 (5.11–9.15)	15.84 (12.87–18.87)	7.49 (5.75–9.23)

BMI denotes body mass index defined by body weight in kilograms divided by height in meters squared. NHANES denotes National Health and Nutrition Examination Survey. Prevalence is weighed using NHANES sampling weights to be representative of the U.S. adult population in 2011-2012. Age is adjusted by direct standardization to the year 2000 Census population using the age groups 20–30 years old, 40–59 years old, and 60 years and older. 95% confidence interval is in parenthesis.

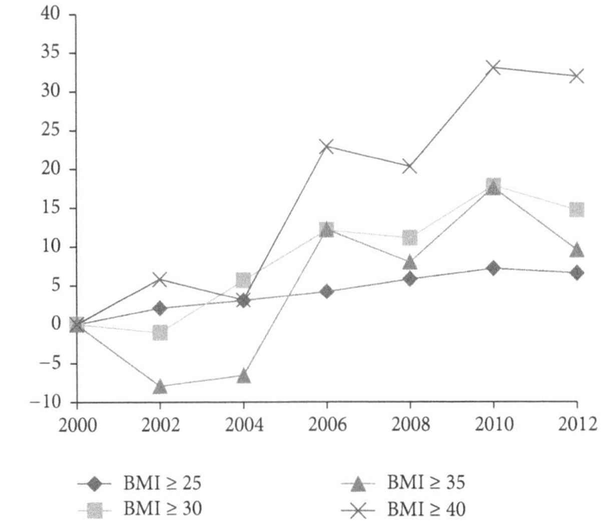

FIGURE 1: Percentage change in age-adjusted prevalence of overweight and obesity combined (BMI ≥ 25), obesity (BMI ≥ 30), grades 2 and 3 obesity combined (BMI ≥ 35), and grade 3 obesity (BMI ≥ 40) among US adults aged 20 years and older: NHANES 1999-2000 to 2011-2012 (NHANES 1999-2000 as baseline).

and race/ethnicity-specific prevalence measures remained unchanged or slightly decreased in 2011-2012, except for the prevalence of overweight and obesity combined among non-Hispanic White women, the prevalence of obesity among Hispanic men, and all 4 prevalence measures among Hispanic women which increased by 1.3 to 3.3 percentage points. None of the changes in gender- and race/ethnicity-specific prevalence measures (24 of them in total) between 2009-2010 and 2011-2012 were statistically significant at $P < 0.05$.

Table 3 reports the statistical tests for trends in obesity over the 14 years of survey cycles from 1999 to 2012 using piecewise logistic regressions. The coefficients are expressed as annualized odds ratios (ORs), denoting the estimated increase per year in the odds of a prevalence measure. A majority of the gender- and race/ethnicity-specific prevalence measures seemed to slightly increase over time (as indicated by the estimated $e^{\beta_1} > 1$). For example, the estimated OR for the prevalence of obesity (BMI ≥ 30) among Hispanic women is 1.03 (1.01–1.04), approximately equivalent to a yearly increase in obesity prevalence of 0.6 percentage points. Nearly all gender- and race/ethnicity-specific prevalence measures appeared to deviate downwards from the increasing trend (as indicated by the estimated $e^{\beta_2} < 1$) during 2010–2012, but those changes in trends were not statistically significant at $P < 0.05$.

4. Discussion

The obesity prevalence in the US increased substantially during the last few decades. The rate of increase appeared

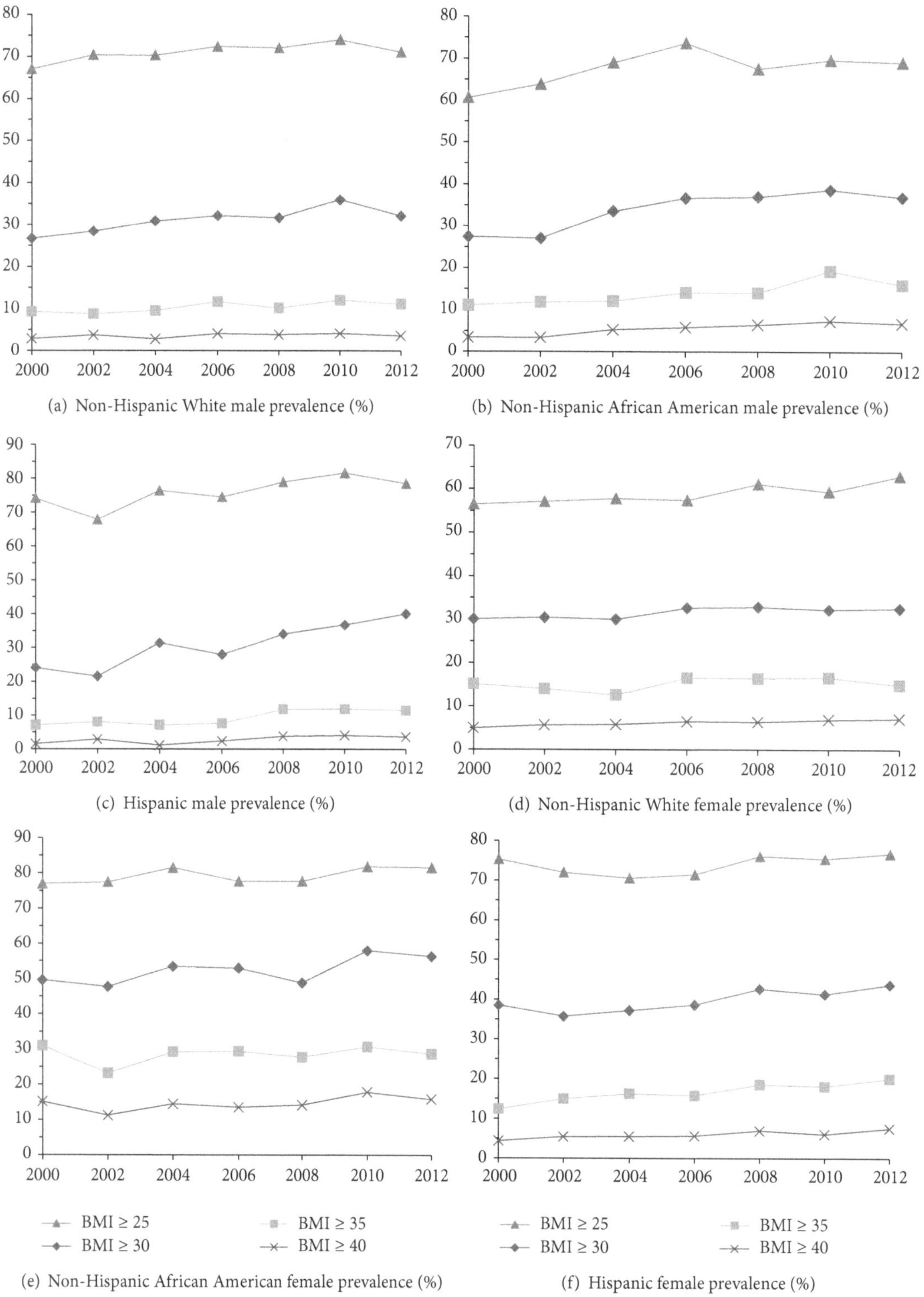

FIGURE 2: Gender- and race/ethnicity-specific trend in age-adjusted prevalence of overweight and obesity combined (BMI $\geq$ 25), obesity (BMI $\geq$ 30), grades 2 and 3 obesity combined (BMI $\geq$ 35), and grade 3 obesity (BMI $\geq$ 40) among US adults aged 20 years and older: NHANES 1999-2000 to 2011-2012.

to slow down since the 2000s and most recent data on childhood obesity even indicated some leveling off. Using a nationally representative sample, this study estimates the obesity prevalence among US adults aged 20 years and older in 2011-2012 and tracks its trends from 1999 to 2012. The main advantage of NHANES relative to other national health surveillance systems such as the BRFSS and the National Health Interview Survey (NHIS) is the objectively measured

TABLE 3: Estimated annual change in the odds of the prevalence of overweight and obesity combined (BMI ≥ 25), obesity (BMI ≥ 30), grades 2 and 3 obesity combined (BMI ≥ 35), and grade 3 obesity (BMI ≥ 40) among U.S. adults aged 20 years and older using piecewise logistic regressions: NHANES 1999-2000 to 2011-2012.

	All races/ethnicities		Non-Hispanic White		Non-Hispanic African American		Hispanic	
	e^{β_1}	e^{β_2}	e^{β_1}	e^{β_2}	e^{β_1}	e^{β_2}	e^{β_1}	e^{β_2}
BMI ≥ 25 (%)								
Both genders	1.020** (1.006–1.034)	0.972 (0.892–1.060)	1.021* (1.002–1.040)	0.981 (0.884–1.089)	1.032*** (1.015–1.049)	0.953 (0.849–1.069)	1.035** (1.011–1.059)	0.963 (0.845–1.098)
Male	1.030** (1.012–1.049)	0.902 (0.814–1.000)	1.029* (1.005–1.053)	0.905 (0.796–1.029)	1.041*** (1.021–1.063)	0.899 (0.794–1.018)	1.055** (1.022–1.089)	0.894 (0.732–1.092)
Female	1.012 (0.995–1.029)	1.033 (0.939–1.136)	1.016 (0.992–1.040)	1.042 (0.920–1.179)	1.020 (0.992–1.049)	1.021 (0.867–1.201)	1.013 (0.984–1.043)	1.045 (0.908–1.203)
BMI ≥ 30 (%)								
Both genders	1.027*** (1.013–1.040)	0.957 (0.889–1.030)	1.026** (1.009–1.043)	0.942 (0.855–1.039)	1.039** (1.017–1.061)	0.953 (0.857–1.060)	1.038** (1.014–1.061)	0.908 (0.822–1.002)
Male	1.040*** (1.022–1.058)	0.926 (0.847–1.013)	1.057*** (1.030–1.084)	0.892 (0.786–1.011)	1.060*** (1.028–1.093)	1.050 (0.903–1.221)	1.015 (0.995–1.034)	0.977 (0.847–1.127)
Female	1.015* (1.000–1.029)	0.986 (0.903–1.076)	1.027 (0.999–1.056)	1.001 (0.876–1.143)	1.019 (0.993–1.046)	1.007 (0.890–1.139)	1.026** (1.010–1.041)	0.942 (0.864–1.026)
BMI ≥ 35 (%)								
Both genders	1.034** (1.009–1.060)	0.953 (0.839–1.083)	1.028* (1.006–1.051)	0.941 (0.853–1.039)	1.054*** (1.031–1.078)	0.959 (0.857–1.072)	1.033* (1.002–1.064)	0.930 (0.796–1.085)
Male	1.020* (1.004–1.037)	0.933 (0.851–1.024)	1.062** (1.022–1.103)	0.907 (0.760–1.084)	1.063** (1.023–1.105)	0.948 (0.787–1.141)	1.023* (1.001–1.046)	0.921 (0.797–1.063)
Female	1.027** (1.007–1.048)	0.923 (0.817–1.044)	1.009 (0.983–1.036)	0.970 (0.859–1.095)	1.054*** (1.029–1.080)	0.952 (0.840–1.080)	1.031** (1.010–1.053)	0.972 (0.858–1.101)
BMI ≥ 40 (%)								
Both genders	1.031** (1.010–1.053)	0.972 (0.858–1.101)	1.034* (1.005–1.063)	0.950 (0.787–1.146)	1.045* (1.016–1.075)	0.928 (0.817–1.054)	1.066** (1.0165–1.118)	0.953 (0.801–1.132)
Male	1.038* (1.001–1.076)	0.958 (0.736–1.247)	1.034 (0.990–1.079)	0.912 (0.625–1.329)	1.088** (1.038–1.141)	0.876 (0.710–1.080)	1.092* (1.014–1.175)	0.892 (0.678–1.175)
Female	1.028* (1.005–1.051)	0.980 (0.873–1.100)	1.035* (1.003–1.068)	0.975 (0.818–1.162)	1.030 (0.996–1.065)	0.963 (0.822–1.129)	1.053* (1.003–1.105)	0.981 (0.811–1.186)

See (1) for model setup. Odds ratio and 95% confidence interval are reported. * $P < 0.05$, ** $P < 0.01$, and *** $P < 0.001$.

body weight and height, which eliminates self-report bias. However, the relatively small sample size of NHANES (about 5,000 in every two-year survey cycle, compared to about 0.4 million a year in BRFSS) limits the precision for population estimates. Unlike BRFSS or NHIS, NHANES is not suited for state-level estimates and between-state comparisons. Moreover, NHANES is a probability sample of the US civilian, noninstitutionalized population, excluding inmates of institutions (e.g., people in penal/mental facilities or homes for the aged, or on active duty in the Armed Forces).

The prevalence measures are based on BMI, a function of weight and height, rather than on body fatness. Although BMI has been found to be closely associated with percentage body fat measured by dual X-ray absorptiometry in the NHANES, these two measures are fundamentally different and their levels of agreement could be a function of gender, age, and race/ethnicity. For instance, percentage body fat was found to be more correlated with BMI in women than men [11]. The relation between percentage body fat and BMI in Hispanic American women differed from that of African American and European American women [12]. A thorough investigation on the differential relationship between BMI and body fatness across population groups and the long-term trend of obesity prevalence measured by percentage body fat is beyond the scope of this study but warranted in future research.

The growth rate of the obesity epidemic among US adults appears to have slowed down in 2000s, but it is still too early to conclude that it has already reached the plateau and begun to level off. Both Figures 1 and 2 showed some decline in the obesity prevalence measures in 2011-2012 compared to in 2009-2010, but none of the changes were statistically significant. This has also been indicated in the results of piecewise logistic regressions where the null hypotheses on the similarity in trends for prevalence measures before and after 2010 were not rejected.

In conclusion, concurrent evidence on the leveling off of the obesity epidemic in the US is thin and the trend is unclear and inconclusive at this time. Given the high prevalence of obesity and its profound socioeconomic consequences, close monitoring of the trend is warranted.

Conflict of Interests

There is no conflict of interests to declare.

References

[1] NIH, NHLBI Obesity Education Initiative, "Clinical Guidelines on the Identification, Evaluation, and Treatment of Overweight and Obesity in Adults, the Evidence Report," October 2013, http://www.nhlbi.nih.gov/guidelines/obesity/ob_gdlns.pdf.

[2] C. D. Fryar, M. D. Carroll, and C. L. Ogden, "Prevalence of overweight, obesity, and extreme obesity among adults: United States, trends 1960–1962 through 2009-2010," October 2013, http://www.cdc.gov/nchs/products/hestats.htm.

[3] OECD, "OECD Obesity Update 2012," October 2013, http://www.oecd.org/health/health-systems/theeconomicsofprevention.htm.

[4] E. A. Finkelstein, J. G. Trogdon, J. W. Cohen, and W. Dietz, "Annual medical spending attributable to obesity: payer-and service-specific estimates," *Health Affairs*, vol. 28, no. 5, pp. w822–w831, 2009.

[5] A. L. May, L. Pan, B. Sherry et al., "Vital signs: obesity among low-income, preschool-aged children-United States, 2008–2011," *Morbidity and Mortality Weekly Report*, vol. 62, no. 31, pp. 629–634, 2013.

[6] K. M. Flegal, D. Carroll, B. K. Kit, and C. L. Ogden, "Prevalence of obesity and trends in the distribution of body mass index among US adults, 1999-2010," *Journal of the American Medical Association*, vol. 307, no. 5, pp. 491–497, 2012.

[7] R. Sturm and A. Hattori, "Morbid obesity rates continue to rise rapidly in the United States," *International Journal of Obesity*, vol. 37, no. 6, pp. 889–891, 2013.

[8] CDC, "National Health and Nutrition Examination Survey," October 2013, http://www.cdc.gov/nchs/nhanes.htm.

[9] CDC, "National Health and Nutrition Examination Survey: Anthropometry Procedures Manual," October 2013, http://www.cdc.gov/nchs/data/nhanes/nhanes_11_12/Anthropometry_Procedures_Manual.pdf.

[10] StataCorp, *Stata Statistical Software: Release 13*, StataCorp, College Station, Tex, USA, 2013.

[11] K. M. Flegal, J. A. Shepherd, A. C. Looker et al., "Comparisons of percentage body fat, body mass index, waist circumference, and waist-stature ratio in adults," *American Journal of Clinical Nutrition*, vol. 89, no. 2, pp. 500–508, 2009.

[12] J. R. Fernández, M. Heo, S. B. Heymsfield et al., "Is percentage body fat differentially related to body mass index in Hispanic Americans, African Americans, and European Americans?" *American Journal of Clinical Nutrition*, vol. 77, no. 1, pp. 71–75, 2003.

2

Concurrent Associations between Physical Activity, Screen Time, and Sleep Duration with Childhood Obesity

Kelly R. Laurson,[1] Joey A. Lee,[1] Douglas A. Gentile,[2] David A. Walsh,[3] and Joey C. Eisenmann[4]

[1] *School of Kinesiology and Recreation, McCormick Hall, Illinois State University, Mailbox 5120, Normal, IL 61790, USA*
[2] *Department of Psychology, Iowa State University, Ames, IA 50011, USA*
[3] *Mind Positive Parenting, Minneapolis, MN 55406, USA*
[4] *Division of Sports and Cardiovascular Nutrition, Department of Radiology, Michigan State University, East Lansing, MI 48823, USA*

Correspondence should be addressed to Joey A. Lee; jalee3@ilstu.edu

Academic Editors: M. G. Matos and Z. Shi

Aim. To examine the simultaneous influence of physical activity, screen time, and sleep duration recommendations on the odds of childhood obesity (including overweight). *Methods.* Physical activity was assessed via pedometer and screen time, and sleep duration were assessed via survey in a cross sectional sample of 674 children (aged 7–12 years) from two Midwestern communities in the fall of 2005. Participants were cross tabulated into four groups depending on how many recommendations were being met (0, 1, 2, or all 3). Linear and logistic regression were used to examine the influence of physical activity, screen time and sleep duration on obesity and interactions among the three variables. *Results.* Children achieving all three recommendations simultaneously (9.2% of total sample) were the least likely to be obese. Approximately 16% of boys and 9% of girls achieving all recommendations were overweight or obese compared to 53% of boys and 42.5% of girls not achieving any. *Conclusions.* The odds of obesity increased in a graded manner for each recommendation which was not met. Meeting all three recommendations appears to have a protective effect against obesity. Continued efforts are warranted to promote healthy lifestyle behaviors that include meeting physical activity, screen time, and sleep duration recommendations concurrently.

1. Introduction

Physical activity (PA), screen time (ST; i.e., television/video games), and sleep (SLP) are modifiable lifestyle risk factors for childhood obesity [1]. Many cross sectional and prospective studies have shown these variables to be independently associated with obesity [2–7]. As such, these variables are frequently studied in childhood obesity and, along with diet, are the specific focus of a recent Institute of Medicine statement on childhood obesity prevention [8].

In an attempt to promote general well-being and prevent or treat obesity, these risk factors are associated with clinical and public health recommendations. These recommendations include limiting ST to ≤2 hours per day, achieving ≥60 minutes of moderate to vigorous PA per day [9] (equivalent to 13,000 and 11,000 steps per day for boys and girls, resp.) [10], and sleeping 10-11 hours per night for children aged 5–12 years [11].

Independently, the effect of PA, ST, or SLP on obesity is well established. However, few studies have focused on these risk factors concurrently. We have previously found that children failing to meet both PA and ST recommendations were 3 to 4 times more likely to be obese than children meeting both [12]. Vioque et al. [13] showed that self-reported PA, ST, and SLP were predictive of obesity in Spanish adults (aged 15+ years) in a logistic model. Ortega et al. [14] found that 9-10 and 15-16 year old youth reporting more sleep also tended to report more PA and less ST. Based on these findings, interactions seem to exist between the three variables. However, further research is critical to determine to what extent this effect modification impacts obesity risk. Therefore, the purpose of this study was to examine the interactions between ST, SLP, and PA and determine their simultaneous influence on overweight and obesity using the aforementioned recommendations. This study can highlight the influence modifiable lifestyle risk factors may have on childhood obesity.

2. Methods

2.1. Participants. Participants in the study were from a childhood obesity intervention known as SWITCH [15]. SWITCH was a community, family, and school based intervention that took place in two school districts in Lakeville, Minnesota, and Cedar Rapids, Iowa. These two school districts were approached due to the requirements of funding agencies and all 10 elementary schools in the districts participated. Data for the current analysis are cross sectional in nature and were collected prior to randomization into treatment or control groups in the fall of 2005. Further details about SWITCH sampling and methods can be found elsewhere [15, 16]. Before study initiation, risks and procedures were explained verbally and in writing to all participants and their primary caregivers. Written consent and assent were obtained from the primary caregiver and child, respectively, prior to data collection. The study protocol was approved by the University of Minnesota's Human Subjects Review Board and is in accordance with the Declaration of Helsinki.

A total of 1,360 of 2,113 school children from two Midwestern communities were elected to participate in the intervention (64% response rate). Due to missing anthropometric measures, SLP, or ST data, or exclusion due to PA monitoring criteria (see below), the final analytic sample was 674 children. The overall demographics of the analytic sample are similar to the school districts from which the children were enrolled [15, 16].

2.2. Anthropometry. Stature was measured with a stadiometer (Seca Road Rod; Seca, Hamburg, Germany). Body mass was measured with a strain gauge scale (Lifesource MD; Lifesource, Milpitas, CA, USA). The growth charts of the Centers for Disease Control and Prevention [17] were used to determine individual BMI z-score and percentile. Children were classified as normal weight (BMI percentile <85), overweight (≥85th to <95th percentile), or obese (≥95th percentile).

2.3. Habitual Physical Activity. PA was assessed by pedometer (Digiwalker SW-2000), which is a suitable PA measuring device [18]. Accuracy of each pedometer was verified before data collection and participants were given instructions on wearing the pedometer. Participants recorded the number of steps taken each day over a 7-day period. Pedometer data were considered valid if the participants wore the monitor for ≥10 hours/day over ≥4 days (including at least one weekend day). Previous research supports this approach for characterizing PA [19]. Boys and girls were classified as meeting PA recommendations [10], if they averaged at least 13,000 and 11,000 steps per day, respectively.

2.4. Screen Time. Children reported how much time they spent watching television across the day, from waking to lunch, lunch to dinner, and dinner to bedtime. These questions were asked for a typical school day and for a typical weekend day. From this, average weekly television time was calculated. This procedure was repeated to assess video game playing. Weekly television and video game time were summed to provide a weekly estimation of total ST. This methodology of assessing ST has been used successfully in children before [20, 21]. Participants were grouped according to the American Academy of Pediatrics recommendation of no more than 2 hours per day of ST [9].

2.5. Sleep Duration. Average SLP was assessed by self-report and calculated in a method similar to ST. Children were asked what time they woke in the morning and what time they go to bed at night on a typical school day and then for a typical weekend day. SLP was characterized using the National Sleep Foundation recommendation of ≥10 hours of sleep per night [11].

2.6. Statistical Analysis. Gender and age specific z-scores were calculated for PA, ST, and SLP. These z-scores were summed for each participant to provide a combined risk factor z-score (after multiplying the ST z-score by −1). The combined z-score characterizes the child's overall placement in the sample for all three lifestyle variables. Higher z-scores indicate more PA, longer SLP duration, and less ST relative to the sample.

Descriptive statistics were calculated and means were compared between normal weight and obese children using independent t-tests. Frequency of meeting the PA, ST, and SLP guidelines were calculated for each recommendation and for combinations of those recommendations (i.e., meeting 0, 1, 2, or 3) along with the prevalence of overweight/obesity. Logistic regression was used to model the odds of meeting the PA, ST, or SLP recommendations using the other two recommendations (i.e., to determine whether children meeting the ST recommendation are more or less likely to meet the PA or SLP recommendations).

Partial correlations (adjusting for age, height, leg length, and ethnicity) were used to identify potential relationships among the risk factors and BMI percentile. Hierarchal linear regression was conducted using all lifestyle variables as continuous variables to quantify associations with BMI percentile (controlling for age, height, leg length, and ethnicity). The hierarchal models included all possible two- and three-way interactions. Standardized beta coefficients (Stan. β) were used to characterize each behavior's utility to predict BMI percentile (where 0.5 is the 50th percentile) even though different scales of measurement were used.

Logistic regression was used to determine what influence meeting the recommendations had on the odds of obesity. Models were stratified by gender and conducted with each risk factor independently and then in one full model including all three behavioral recommendations. Finally, we compared the odds of obesity between children meeting all, two, one, or none of the recommendations, combining boys

TABLE 1: Descriptive statistics for boys and girls by weight status.

Variable	Boys		Girls	
	Normal weight (n = 206)	Overweight and obese (n = 97)	Normal weight (n = 245)	Overweight and obese (n = 126)
Age (years)	9.7 (0.9)	9.6 (0.9)	9.6 (0.9)	9.7 (1.0)
Height (cm)	137.6 (7.1)	140.6 (7.1)*	136.5 (7.9)	141.1 (8.0)*
Leg length (cm)	65.4 (4.5)	66.3 (4.3)	65.2 (4.7)	66.5 (5.1)*
Weight (kg)	31.6 (4.6)	42.8 (8.6)*	30.8 (5.2)	45.2 (9.7)*
BMI (kg/m^2)	16.6 (1.2)	21.5 (2.9)*	16.4 (1.5)	22.5 (3.0)*
Pedometer (steps/day)	13,382 (3,383)	11,647 (2,947)*	11,360 (2,461)	9,930 (2,550)*
Sleep duration (hours/day)	10.1 (1.0)	9.7 (1.0)*	10.3 (0.9)	10.1 (0.9)*
Screen time (hours/day)	4.2 (3.1)	5.4 (3.6)*	3.2 (2.3)	4.1 (2.9)*
Combined z-score	0.39 (1.7)	−0.83 (1.8)*	0.40 (1.6)	−0.78 (1.9)*

All values are mean SD.
*Overweight/obese significantly different from normal weight of same gender ($P < 0.05$).
Combined z-score = sum of age and gender specific z-scores from pedometer steps, sleep, and (inverse of) screen time.

TABLE 2: Percentage meeting physical activity, screen time, and sleep recommendations by overweight and obesity status.

Meeting recommendation	Boys (n = 303)			Girls (n = 371)			Full sample (n = 674)		
	Tot. (%)	Ov. (%)	Ob. (%)	Tot. (%)	Ov. (%)	Ob. (%)	Tot. (%)	Ov. (%)	Ob. (%)
Specific									
PA	42.2	13.3	7.0	45.0	17.4	8.4	43.8	15.6	7.8
ST	24.1	16.4	8.2	34.0	15.1	15.1	29.5	15.6	12.6
SLP	55.4	18.5	6.5	69.3	18.7	12.5	63.1	18.6	10.1
General									
Meet all	6.3	15.8	0.0	11.6	7.0	2.3	9.2	9.7	1.6
Meet 2 of 3	29.7	14.4	3.3	35.8	22.6	10.5	33.1	19.3	7.6
Meet 1 of 3	43.6	18.9	15.2	41.8	17.4	21.9	42.6	18.1	18.8
Meet none	20.5	30.6	22.3	10.8	12.5	30.0	15.1	23.5	25.5

Specific groups are not exclusive; youth may be represented in multiple groups.
Tot. (%) = percentage of total sample meeting the recommendation.
Ov. (%) = prevalence of overweight within group.
Ob. (%) = prevalence of obesity within group.

and girls into one model and controlling for gender. Adequate fit and variance accounted for by the logistic models were determined using the Hosmer-Lemeshow test of goodness of fit and the Nagelkerke pseudo r^2. All data analyses were conducted using SPSS version 18 (Chicago, IL, USA).

3. Results

Descriptive statistics are provided in Table 1. One-third of the sample was overweight or obese, and these youth were taller (boys $t = -3.49$, $P = 0.001$; girls $t = -5.26$, $P < 0.001$), less active (boys $t = 4.34$, $P < 0.001$; girls $t = 5.24$, $P < 0.001$), engaged in more ST (boys $t = -2.92$, $P = 0.004$; girls $t = -3.01$, $P = 0.001$), and slept less (boys $t = 3.07$, $P = 0.002$; girls $t = 2.69$, $P = 0.008$) than normal weight children. Additionally, normal weight youth had a mean combined z-score in the upper half of the sample, compared to obese children with a mean combined z-score in the lower half (boys $t = 5.75$, $P < 0.001$; girls $t = 6.26$, $P < 0.001$). These differences were consistent for boys and girls excluding leg length, where normal weight girls had shorter legs ($t = -2.55$; $P = 0.011$).

Table 2 shows the percentage of children that met the PA, ST, and SLP recommendations with the prevalence of overweight/obesity in each group. The bottom panel of Table 2 shows the percentage of children meeting all, two, one, or none of the recommendations. About 75% of youth met one or two of the three recommendations, with approximately 10% meeting all three and 15% meeting none. Of the 62 children meeting all three recommendations, 1 was obese (1.6%) and 6 were overweight (9.7%). In contrast, the prevalence of obesity in children not meeting any recommendations was approximately 26% with another 24% being overweight.

The correlation matrices examining the associations between BMI percentile and lifestyle variables are in Table 3. The strength of most correlations were low to moderate (e.g., $r = 0.1$–0.6). PA was significantly associated with BMI percentile in girls but not boys. Conversely, ST and SLP were significantly correlated to BMI percentile in boys, but not girls. The combined z-score showed the strongest correlation with BMI percentile ($r = -0.23$ in both boys and girls). Weak, inverse associations were found between SLP and PA and SLP and ST.

TABLE 3: Correlations between body mass index percentile and behavioral risk factors.

Variables	Girls (n = 371)				
	BMI percentile	Physical activity	Sleep duration	Screen time	Combined z-score
Boys (n = 303)					
BMI percentile	1	−0.22*	−0.10	0.10	−0.23*
Pedometer steps	−0.11	1	−0.13*	−0.04	0.51*
Sleep duration	−0.18*	−0.14*	1	−0.20*	0.60*
Screen time	0.12*	−0.06	−0.19*	1	−0.68*
Combined z-Score	−0.23*	0.51*	0.58*	−0.70*	1

*Statistically significant ($P < 0.05$).
Correlations adjusted for age, height, leg length, and ethnicity.
Combined z-score = sum of age and gender specific z-scores from pedometer steps, sleep, and (inverse of) screen time.

Results from logistic regression show that boys meeting the ST recommendation were 2.2 times more likely to also be meeting the SLP recommendation (1.2–3.8, P = 0.008). The results were similar for girls, where those meeting the ST recommendation were 2.0 times more likely to also be meeting the SLP recommendation (1.2–3.3, P = 0.007). Girls meeting the PA guidelines were 0.6 times less likely to also be meeting the SLP guidelines (0.4–0.9, P = 0.017) than girls not meeting the PA threshold.

For the hierarchal linear regression, all interactions (PA × ST, PA × SLP, ST × SLP, and PA × ST × SLP) were initially included but did not yield any significant predictors of BMI percentile. Therefore, none of the two- or three-way interactions were used in the final model. Results of the regression indicated that, when PA, ST, and SLP were entered within the same model, both PA and SLP were the strongest predictors of BMI percentile. ST had no significant association with BMI percentile in either the boys' or girls' model (both $P > 0.05$). Specifically for boys, the standardized beta coefficients indicated that SLP (Stan. $\beta = -0.172$) was a better predictor of BMI percentile than PA (Stan. $\beta = -0.119$). However, the opposite was true for girls where the standardized β for SLP was −0.101 and the standardized β for PA was twice as large at −0.202.

Results of the logistic models predicting obesity are in Table 4. Generally, children failing to meet the PA and SLP recommendations were more likely to be obese than children that complied with the recommendations. However, when considered independently in the univariate models, the screen time recommendation alone was not a significant predictor of weight status in either boys or girls, and sleep duration was not a significant predictor for girls. However, all other logistic models had adequate fit when predicting weight status. When modeling all three recommendations concurrently, it appears that not meeting the PA recommendation is the strongest predictor of obesity. Girls and boys not meeting the PA recommendation were approximately 2.5 and 3 times more likely to be obese than children meeting the recommendations, respectively. Boys not getting the recommended amount of sleep were about 2.5 times more likely to be obese, but this association was not statistically significant for girls. In all, compared to children that met the three recommendations, those that failed one, two, and all three of the recommendations were approximately 2.5, 4.5, and 8.0 times more likely to be obese, respectively.

4. Discussion

The present study considered the concurrent influence of PA, ST, and SLP recommendations on childhood obesity. The main finding was that children meeting no risk factor recommendations were eight times more likely to be obese than those meeting all of the recommendations. The odds of obesity increased with each additional risk factor not being met. These variables appear to exert a synergistic effect on the odds of obesity when examined concurrently. For example, 50% of the children failing all three recommendations were overweight or obese, while only 11.3% of the children achieving all of the risk factors were overweight or obese. These results demonstrate the utility of these risk factor guidelines in respect to childhood obesity as well as quantify the impact of failing to meet multiple cutpoints simultaneously.

Few studies have examined the effects PA, ST, and SLP have on childhood obesity simultaneously. Martinez-Gomez et al. [22] found a positive association between the number of risk factors (PA, ST, SLP, and diet) and markers of adiposity in Spanish adolescents. Vioque et al. [13] found that obese Spanish adults spent more time watching TV and less time sleeping and were less active than nonobese individuals. They also found that television viewing time is a more important risk factor than PA in predicting obesity. In contrast, we found PA to be the most important risk factor for obesity. A potential reason for the disparity is that PA was assessed using different methodology. The strength of the association between physical activity and adiposity may depend on the method of measurement [23].

We found that children who spent more time sleeping spent less time being physically active. In contrast, Ortega et al. [14] found that youth who spent more time sleeping also tended to be more active. A potential reason for the inconsistency between studies might be due to differences in the methods that SLP and PA were quantified. Both studies assessed SLP via self-report, but Ortega et al. quantified sleep using categorical responses, while the current study had participants report sleep time as a continuous variable. Providing participants with categories to report sleep time restricts

TABLE 4: Odds ratios for obesity using recommended guidelines for physical activity, screen time, and sleep.

Risk factor	Univariate model			Full model[a]		
	OR	95% CI	Nagelkerke r^2	OR	95% CI	Nagelkerke r^2
Specific[b]						
Boys failing to meet						
Physical activity	2.7	(1.6, 4.5)	0.065	3.1	(1.7, 5.5)	0.281
Screen time	1.5	(0.9, 2.9)	0.011	1.4	(0.7, 2.7)	—
Sleep	2.1	(1.3, 3.4)	0.039	2.4	(1.4, 4.3)	—
Girls failing to meet						
Physical activity	1.9	(1.3, 3.1)	0.034	2.5	(1.5, 4.2)	0.325
Screen time	1.3	(0.8, 2.1)	0.005	1.1	(0.7, 1.9)	—
Sleep	1.5	(0.9, 2.4)	0.011	1.6	(0.9, 2.8)	—
General						
Boys and girls						
Meeting all	Ref.	—	0.066	Ref.	—	0.291
Meeting 2 of 3	2.9	(1.3, 6.7)	—	2.6	(1.1, 6.5)	—
Meeting 1 of 3	4.6	(2.0, 10.5)	—	4.7	(1.9, 11.3)	—
Meeting none	7.6	(3.1, 18.1)	—	8.2	(3.2, 21.2)	—

[a]Adjusted specific models (boys $n = 303$; girls $n = 371$) controlling for age, height, leg length, ethnicity, and other risk factors (physical activity, sleep, and/or screen time). Adjusted general model ($n = 674$) controlling for age, height, leg length, ethnicity, and gender.

[b]Referent groups (OR = 1.0) are children meeting the specific recommendation.

responses and may desensitize the impact of SLP. Also, Ortega et al. used weekday SLP, disregarding weekend sleep (though they did include weekend PA in the analysis). We calculated a weighted average of weekday and weekend SLP. Measuring weekend SLP may provide a more accurate estimate of overall SLP, especially when covarying for weekend PA. Since PA was objectively measured in the current study, it would make sense that children that wore the pedometer longer during the day would record more steps. Considering this, we used strict exclusion criteria (≥4 days with >10 hours/day of wear time) in hopes of decreasing any potential influence.

Unique aspects of the current study are the analytical design and specific attention to the interactions of PA, SLP, and ST. The study simultaneously examined three lifestyle risk factors for childhood obesity using established recommendations. As shown, the variables are correlated to some degree, making joint analyses of the variables critical to understanding their combined influence on childhood obesity. Further, we chose to focus on PA, SLP, and ST guidelines that practitioners use in the field. Therefore, the results provide practical and empirical evidence for clinicians, researchers, and policy makers.

Limitations of the study should be noted. Given the cross sectional design, it is not possible to determine whether not meeting current recommendations is the cause or outcome of obesity. Another limitation is the use of self-reporting for ST and SLP. Objective measurement was not feasible. However, both ST and SLP values reported here are comparable to national estimates [24, 25]. Finally, not all children in the school districts chose to participate in the intervention, which could lead to bias. However, when comparing the demographics of the analytic sample to those of the school districts the children were enrolled, there were no significant differences, indicating that the potential for bias is low.

5. Conclusion

Meeting the recommendations for PA, ST, and SLP appears to exert a robust protective effect from obesity. Compared to those meeting all three recommendations, children that failed to achieve any one, two, or all three were approximately 2.5, 4.5, and 8.0 times more likely to be obese, respectively. Only 1 of the 62 (1.6%) children meeting all three recommendations was obese. Continued efforts are warranted to promote healthy lifestyle behaviors that include meeting recommendations for physical activity, screen time, and sleep. Interventions should promote action for healthy levels of PA, ST, and SLP, instead of attempting to target them individually.

Conflict of Interests

The authors have no conflict of interests to report and they have no financial relationships relevant to this paper to disclose. In Lakeville, Minnesota SWITCH was sponsored by Medica Foundation, Healthy and Active America Foundation, and Fairview Health Services. In Cedar Rapids, Iowa SWITCH was sponsored by Cargill and the Healthy and Active America Foundation. SWITCH is a trademark of Iowa State University.

References

[1] J. C. Han, D. A. Lawlor, and S. Y. Kimm, "Childhood obesity," *The Lancet*, vol. 375, no. 9727, pp. 1737–1748, 2010.

[2] J. F. Bell and F. J. Zimmerman, "Shortened nighttime sleep duration in early life and subsequent childhood obesity," *Archives of Pediatrics and Adolescent Medicine*, vol. 164, no. 9, pp. 840–845, 2010.

[3] A. Must and S. M. Parisi, "Sedentary behavior and sleep: paradoxical effects in association with childhood obesity," *International Journal of Obesity*, vol. 33, supplement 1, pp. S82–S86, 2009.

[4] K. L. Rennie, J. C. K. Wells, T. A. McCaffrey, and M. B. Livingstone, "The effect of physical activity on body fatness in children and adolescents," *Proceedings of the Nutrition Society*, vol. 65, no. 4, pp. 393–402, 2006.

[5] M. Sekine, T. Yamagami, K. Handa et al., "A dose-response relationship between short sleeping hours and childhood obesity: results of the Toyama birth cohort study," *Child*, vol. 28, no. 2, pp. 163–170, 2002.

[6] S. B. Sisson, T. S. Church, C. K. Martin et al., "Profiles of sedentary behavior in children and adolescents: the US National Health and Nutrition Examination Survey, 2001–2006," *International Journal of Pediatric Obesity*, vol. 4, no. 4, pp. 353–359, 2009.

[7] K. D. M. Wittmeier, R. C. Mollard, and D. J. Kriellaars, "Physical activity intensity and risk of overweight and adiposity in children," *Obesity*, vol. 16, no. 2, pp. 415–420, 2008.

[8] S. Mcguire, "Institute of Medicine, Early Childhood Obesity Prevention Policies. Washington, DC: The National Academies Press," *Advances in Nutrition*, vol. 3, no. 1, pp. 56–57, 2012.

[9] S. E. Barlow, "Expert committee recommendations regarding the prevention, assessment, and treatment of child and adolescent overweight and obesity: summary report," *Pediatrics*, vol. 120, supplement 4, pp. S164–S192, 2007.

[10] Council on Sports Medicine and Fitness and Council on School Health, "Active healthy living: prevention of childhood obesity through increased physical activity," *Pediatrics*, vol. 117, no. 5, pp. 1834–1842, 2006.

[11] National Sleep Foundation, "Children and sleep—information on sleep health and safety," 2011, http://www.sleepfoundation.org/article/sleep-topics/children-and-sleep.

[12] K. R. Laurson, J. C. Eisenmann, G. J. Welk, E. E. Wickel, D. A. Gentile, and D. A. Walsh, "Combined influence of physical activity and screen time recommendations on childhood overweight," *Journal of Pediatrics*, vol. 153, no. 2, pp. 209–214, 2008.

[13] J. Vioque, A. Torres, and J. Quiles, "Time spent watching television, sleep duration and obesity in adults living in Valencia, Spain," *International Journal of Obesity and Related Metabolic Disorders*, vol. 24, no. 12, pp. 1683–1688, 2000.

[14] F. B. Ortega, J. R. Ruiz, I. Labayen et al., "Sleep duration and activity levels in Estonian and Swedish children and adolescents," *European Journal of Applied Physiology*, vol. 111, no. 10, pp. 2615–2623, 2011.

[15] J. C. Eisenmann, D. A. Gentile, G. J. Welk et al., "SWITCH: rationale, design, and implementation of a community, school, and family-based intervention to modify behaviors related to childhood obesity," *BMC Public Health*, vol. 8, article 223, 2008.

[16] D. A. Gentile, G. Welk, J. C. Eisenmann et al., "Evaluation of a multiple ecological level child obesity prevention program: switch what you do, view, and chew," *BMC Medicine*, vol. 7, article 49, 2009.

[17] C. L. Ogden, R. J. Kuczmarski, K. M. Flegal et al., "Centers for Disease Control and Prevention 2000 growth charts for the United States: improvements to the 1977 National Center for Health Statistics version," *Pediatrics*, vol. 109, no. 1, pp. 45–60, 2002.

[18] S. E. Crouter, P. L. Schneider, M. Karabulut, and D. R. Bassett Jr., "Validity of 10 electronic pedometers for measuring steps, distance, and energy cost," *Medicine and Science in Sports and Exercise*, vol. 35, no. 8, pp. 1455–1460, 2003.

[19] S. G. Trost, R. R. Pate, P. S. Freedson, J. F. Sallis, and W. C. Taylor, "Using objective physical activity measures with youth: how many days of monitoring are needed?" *Medicine and Science in Sports and Exercise*, vol. 32, no. 2, pp. 426–431, 2000.

[20] C. A. Anderson, D. A. Gentile, and K. E. Buckley, *Violent Video Game Effects on Children and Adolescents Theory, Research, and Public Policy*, Oxford University Press, New York, NY, USA, 2007.

[21] D. A. Gentile, S. Coyne, and D. A. Walsh, "Media violence, physical aggression, and relational aggression in school age children: a short-term longitudinal study," *Aggressive Behavior*, vol. 37, no. 2, pp. 193–206, 2011.

[22] D. Martinez-Gomez, L. A. Moreno, J. Romeo et al., "Combined influence of lifestyle risk factors on body fat in Spanish adolescents—the AVENA study," *Obesity Facts*, vol. 4, no. 2, pp. 105–111, 2011.

[23] A. V. Rowlands, D. K. Ingledew, and R. G. Eston, "The effect of type of physical activity measure on the relationship between body fatness and habitual physical activity in children: a meta-analysis," *Annals of Human Biology*, vol. 27, no. 5, pp. 479–497, 2000.

[24] V. Rideout, D. Roberts, and U. Foehr, *Generation M2: Media in the Lives of 8- to 18-Year Olds*, Kaiser Family Foundation, Menlo Park, Calif, USA, 2010.

[25] E. K. Snell, E. K. Adam, and G. J. Duncan, "Sleep and the body mass index and overweight status of children and adolescents," *Child Development*, vol. 78, no. 1, pp. 309–323, 2007.

3

Body Adiposity Index: Its Relevance and Validity in Assessing Body Fatness of Adults

Shilpi Gupta and Satwanti Kapoor

Obesity Research Unit, Physiological Anthropology Laboratory, Department of Anthropology, University of Delhi, New Delhi 110007, India

Academic Editors: M. M. Al-Nozha, D. Micic, E. Rodríguez, and D. Tekin

Background. One of the limitations of body mass index is its accuracy to assess body fatness. To address this limitation, a new index, body adiposity index, has been developed. However its validity needs to ascertained. *Objective.* Our aim was to investigate sex-specific relationship between BAI, BMI, and percent body fat in an endogamous population of Delhi, India. *Method.* Data was collected from 578 adults on bodyweight, height, skinfold thicknesses, hip circumference, waist circumference, and systolic and diastolic blood pressure. Pearson's correlations were calculated for BAI and BMI with PBF. Differences in the correlation coefficients were examined using Fisher's z tests. Receiver operating characteristic analysis was used to compare the predictive validity and to determine optimal cut-off values. Odds ratios were calculated to assess the risk of having hypertension using the proposed cut-off points. *Results.* The correlations of PBF with BMI (men: $r = 0.83$; women: $r = 0.71$) were stronger than those with BAI (men: $r = 0.66$; women: $r = 0.58$). In men, the sensitivity and specificity of BAI to predict hypertension were higher than other anthropometric markers but lower than BMI. In women, the sensitivity of BAI was higher than BMI and WC. *Conclusions.* BAI can be used as an additional marker for screening population; however its validity needs to be demonstrated on other populations too.

1. Introduction

The body mass index (BMI) is a heuristic proxy for human body fat based on an individual's weight and height. It was invented by Adolphe Quetelet between 1830 and 1850 [1]; since then it has been used to assess body fat. BMI is a fascinating anthropometric index because it meets the first four requirements for an ideal method, that is, (1) initial cost, (2) training of the operator, (3) maintenance and operating costs, and (4) precision [2]. The two instruments (scale and anthropometer) that are required are inexpensive, require minimal training to use, and are virtually maintenance-free; repeat values can be obtained with good precision and with no fear of exposure hazard. It has been shown to correlate significantly with other measures of adiposity too [3].

A graded classification of overweight and obesity using BMI classification provides valuable information about increasing body fatness. It allows meaningful inter- and intrapopulation comparison of body weight and identifies individuals or groups at risk of morbidity and mortality, thus paving the way for the identification of priorities in intervention at an individual or community level and for evaluating the effectiveness of such interventions. However, the accuracy of BMI in assessing the body fatness of an individual remains debated. Although BMI has been widely used as a surrogate measure of adiposity, it is a measure of excess weight relative to height, rather than excess body fat. It does not distinguish between fat mass and lean body mass. Besides the distribution of fat over the body is not captured. There is accumulating evidence that excess visceral fat increases the risk of chronic metabolic disorders such as cardiovascular disease and stroke [4]. Thus other adiposity measures like waist circumference, waist-to-hip ratio (WHR), and skinfold thickness supplement information regarding body fatness in addition to BMI.

Recently, Bergman et al. [5] have introduced a new index of adiposity, namely, body adiposity index (BAI), to counter the limitation of BMI. They reported stronger correlations of BAI with percentage body fat (PBF) determined by dual-energy X-ray absorptiometry (DEXA) than that of BMI. Although BAI was reported as a better predictor of PBF, however, certain questions need to be addressed before accepting it as a new measure of body adiposity. The index was developed in samples of Mexican-American and black individuals. It needs to be validated on other populations too. Further sexual dimorphism has not been taken into account. As mentioned by Schulze and Stefan [6], cut-offs of body fat in relation to type 2 diabetes, cardiovascular morbidity, and mortality need to be constructed.

In the present study, the validity of BAI has been investigated in North Indian population. In addition, the sex-specific relationship between BAI and PBF was examined. Cut-off of PBF estimated by BAI was also constructed. Furthermore, odds of hypertension were also computed with the derived cut-offs of BAI.

2. Materials and Methods

2.1. Subjects. Cross-sectional study was conducted on Aggarwal Baniyas, an endogamous caste group of Delhi. Data was collected during 2008-2009 by a household survey on 578 adult Aggarwal Baniyas (271 men, 307 women) aged 30 years upwards. Nonresponse rate for all the variables of interest was 2.6% for men and 4.9% for women in all cases. Final analysis was performed on the data of 264 men and 292 women with complete information. Information was collected during household visits using a schedule that included information on body weight, height, skinfold thicknesses, hip circumference, waist circumference, and systolic and diastolic blood pressure. Written informed consent was obtained from all participants and the protocol of the study was approved by the ethical committee of the Department of Anthropology, Faculty of Sciences, University of Delhi, India.

2.2. Measurements. Body weight was measured by using spring balance to the nearest 500 g, stature with the help of anthropometer to the nearest mm. Waist circumference and hip circumference were measured with a nonstretchable steel tape to the nearest 0.1 cm. The anthropometric measurements were taken according to the standardized techniques described by Weiner and Lourie [7]. Measurements were conducted by trained personnel and all instruments were calibrated once weekly. As an indicator of fatness, body mass index was calculated as weight in kg divided by stature in meter square. BAI was calculated as hip circumference in centimeters divided by height in meters to the 1.5 power minus 18. The biceps, triceps, suprailiac and subscapular skinfold thicknesses of the subjects were measured with Holtain skinfold calipers which exerted a constant pressure of 10 gm/mm^2 over the contact surface. Published equations of Durnin and Womersley [8] were used to calculate BF% using skinfolds.

Blood pressure (BP) was measured using manual (mercury) sphygmomanometer. The subject was asked to sit relaxed on a chair with her/his arm supported comfortably at the vertical level. The pressure cuff was applied closely to the upper arm; the cuff was rapidly inflated until the artery was completely occluded. The stethoscope was then placed lightly over the brachial artery and the mercury column was allowed to fall at the rate of 2 mmHg per second. The systolic blood pressure was determined by the appearance of Korotkoff sound. After recording the systolic blood pressure, the mercury column was allowed to fall further till the sound ceased to be tapping in quality, became fully muffled, and finally disappeared. The level where it disappeared was taken as diastolic blood pressure. Three consecutive readings were taken for each measurement and their mean was taken as the final reading.

2.3. Statistical Analysis. Results have been described by summary statistics such as mean and standard deviation. Sex-specific partial Pearson correlations were calculated for BAI and BMI with PBF separately. For total percentage body fat, differences in the correlation coefficients for BAI versus BMI were examined using z-tests after applying Fisher z-transformation [9, 10]. Receiver operating characteristic (ROC) analysis was used to compare the predictive validity and to determine optimal cut-off values [11–13]. Area under the curve (AUC) was also measured to determine the diagnostic power of a test and to describe the probability that a test would correctly identify subjects with the disorder. Optimal cut-off values of BAI were measured by calculating the sensitivity and specificity of the anthropometric measurements at various cut-off points of BMI.

The accuracy of BAI, BMI, WC, and WHtR in detecting hypertension was examined by calculating sensitivity, specificity, and positive and negative predictive values (PPVs and NPVs) [14]. Odds ratios were calculated to assess the risk of having hypertension using the proposed cut-off points.

3. Results

The basic characters of our study have been published previously [15]. In brief, the mean age of males was 43.4 yr (SD ± 5.3) and that of females was 38.7 yr (SD ± 4.9). The prevalence of obesity was 42.7% in women and 21.2% in men. The prevalence of prehypertension was 48.7% and 45.6% among males and females, respectively. The percentage of hypertensive males and females was 21.6% and 7.4%, respectively.

While the correlations of BMI and BAI with PBF in both men (BMI: $r = 0.83$; BAI: $r = 0.66$) and women (BMI: $r = 0.71$; BAI: $r = 0.58$) were statistically significant, the correlations of PBF with BMI (men: $r = 0.83$; women: $r = 0.71$) were stronger than those with BAI (men: $r = 0.66$; women: $r = 0.58$) among both men and women (Table 1). The correlations between anthropometric indices and PBF were consistently lower for women compared with men. However when both sexes were taken together, the correlations of BAI with percentage body fat (0.80, $P < 0.001$) were better than BMI (0.70, $P < 0.001$). The regression model for BAI explained 66.4% of the variance in fat percentage in men and 57.7% in women, whereas the corresponding regression

Table 1: Mean and standard deviation of BAI, BMI, and PBF and the correlations between these variables.

	Mean (SD)			r (95% CI)[1]		
	BAI	BMI	PBF	BAI and PBF	BMI and PBF	P value[2]
Men	27.6 (3.8)	26.1 (4.3)	29.0 (5.9)	0.66	0.83	4.36 (0.001)
Women	39.2 (6.4)	29.4 (4.8)	40.7 (3.7)	0.58	0.71	2.68 (0.05)
Total	33.8 (7.9)	27.9 (4.8)	35.8 (6.6)	0.80 3.52 (0.001)[3]	0.70 1.66 (0.09)[3]	4.02 (0.001)

[1]All correlations are statistically significant at $P < 0.001$.
[2]Comparing the correlations of BMI and BAI with Fat%.
[3]Comparing the correlations of BMI and BAI with Fat% across gender.
BAI: body adiposity index; BMI: body mass index; PBF: percentage body fat.

Table 2: The areas under ROC curve (AUC), optimal cut-off values, and sensitivities and specificities of BAI associated with BMI and hypertension.

	BMI				BP			
	AUC (95% CI)[1]	Cut-off	Sens (%)	Spec (%)	AUC (95% CI)[1]	Cut-off	Sens (%)	Spec (%)
Men								
By our own criteria	0.93 (0.90, 0.96)	25.6	88.4	92.6	0.70 (0.62–0.77)	25.3	83.7	54.0
By WHO criteria	0.90 (0.86, 0.94)	27.2	77.6	91.7				
Women								
By our own criteria	0.93 (0.92, 0.97)	37.7	91.2	85.5	0.62 (0.55–0.68)	37.7	91.2	85.5
By WHO criteria	0.94 (0.90, 0.96)	36.4	74.3	100.0				

[1]All values are statistically significant at $P < 0.001$.
BAI: body adiposity index; BMI: body mass index; BP: blood pressure; AUC: area under curve; CI: confidence interval; Sens: sensitivity; Spec: specificity; WHO: World Health Organization.

model for BMI explained 82.8% variance in men and 70.7% in women (Figure 1).

ROC curve analysis of BAI with BMI and BP is summarized in Table 2. The results of the AUC analysis were significantly different from what was expected by chance ($P < 0.001$). The values of AUC ranged from 0.90 to 0.94 for BMI while for BP they were 0.62 in women and 0.70 in men. The cut-off points of BAI were determined as the point of intersection of the curves for sensitivity and specificity. The BAI cut-off values corresponding to WHO-based BMI's cut-off were 27.2 in men and 36.4 in women, whereas BAI cut-offs based on derived population-based BMI cut-off values were 25.6 in men and 37.7 in women. BAI cut-offs based on BP risk were 25.3 in men and 37.7 in women.

The sensitivity and specificity of BAI to predict hypertension are presented in Table 3. Sensitivity and specificity of various anthropometric markers, that is, BMI, WC, WHR, and WHtR to predict hypertension have already been published [16]. In men, the sensitivity and specificity of BAI were higher than WC, WHR, and WHtR but lower than BMI. In women, the sensitivity of BAI was higher than BMI and WC.

Logistic regression analysis was performed to see if the determined cut-off points of BAI independently reflected the increased risk of having hypertension (Table 4). Odds of systolic and diastolic blood pressure on BAI were significant in both men and women; however, the odds were found to be higher in males than in females. The logistic regression analysis of other anthropometric markers for hypertension by optimal cut-offs has already been published [16]. In men, odds of hypertension on BAI were lower than other anthropometric markers while in women, they were higher for other anthropometric markers.

4. Discussion

We examined the validity of BAI to reflect PBF for adult men and women as compared to other anthropometric markers in an endogamous population of North India. Further sex-specific cut-off of BAI was determined based on BMI as well as BP.

In the present study, body fat appears to be more correlated with BMI than with BAI. The regression model including BMI explained greater variance in fat percentage as compared to BAI. We also demonstrated sex-specific differences in correlations between BAI and total percentage body fat. In contrast to Bergman et al.'s study [5], in the present study the relationships between percentage fat and BAI for males and females lie on very different linear representations. As expected, males are localized on the lower end of the curve, because males tend to have a lower adiposity compared to females, this is also reflected in a lower value of mean BAI for men.

Although BMI appeared to be equivalently correlated to PBF in both men and women, BAI was more strongly correlated with PBF in men than in women indicating that BAI predicts PBF among males quite well. As BAI is based on hip circumference, the finding is counterintuitive to the general assumption that hip circumference might be more informative compared to waist circumference to predict PBF among women than men [17]. The lower correlations for

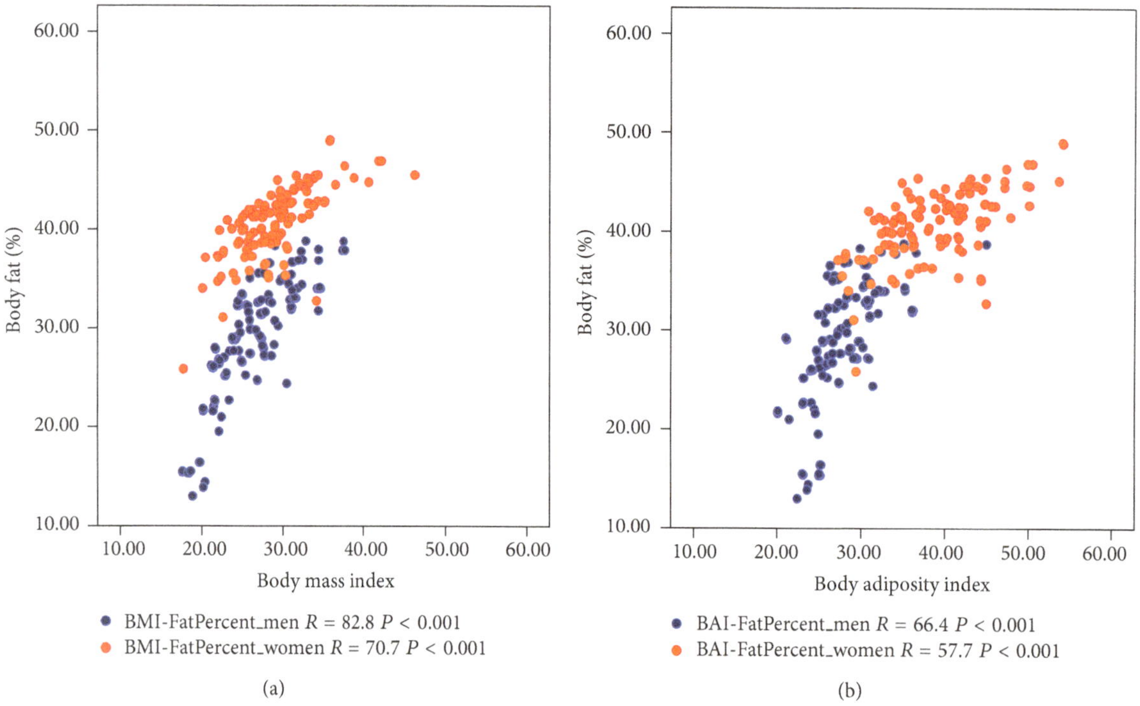

FIGURE 1: Relationship between percentage body fat versus body adiposity index and body Mass index. The lines indicate the linear relationships between the 2 variables.

TABLE 3: Diagnostic accuracy of BAI to detect blood pressure by different cut-off points.

	AUC	Sensitivity (%)	Specificity (%)	Positive PV	Negative PV
Men					
BAI (optimal-25.6)	0.70	79.47	56.58	82.06	53.75
BAI (WHO-27.2)		57.89	72.37	83.97	40.74
Women					
BAI (optimal-37.7)	0.62	67.68	56.34	64.16	60.15
BAI (WHO-36.4)		71.95	47.88	61.96	59.65

BAI: body adiposity index; AUC: area under curve; PV: positive predictive; WHO: world health organization.

TABLE 4: Odds ratios of hypertension in obese subjects determined by the cut-off points of BAI.

	SBP			DBP			SBP or DBP		
	ORs	95% CI	*P*	ORs	95% CI	*P*	ORs	95% CI	*P*
Women									
BAI (optimal)	2.70	1.70–4.31	0.001	3.94	2.40–6.45	0.001	3.28	1.95–5.51	0.001
BAI (WHO)	2.36	1.47–3.79	0.001	3.39	2.07–5.54	0.001	2.99	1.79–4.99	0.001
Men									
BAI (optimal)	5.32	2.98–9.49	0.001	3.33	1.72–6.63	0.001	4.23	1.85–9.67	0.001
BAI (WHO)	3.60	2.02–6.43	0.001	3.82	1.84–7.90	0.001	4.02	1.56–10.35	0.001

women may be related to differences in the distribution of fat between sexes and aging—women tend to have a more peripheral than central fat distribution in early adulthood [18], yet gain central fat with increasing age [19]. However, different correlations of BAI for males versus females reflect the well-established difference in body composition between males and females [20].

Though the correlation of BMI with PBF was higher than BAI, sensitivity and specificity of BAI to predict hypertension were better than BMI as well as other anthropometric markers, except for BMI defined by our cut-off [16]. A BMI value of >30 kg/m^2 has high specificity but poor sensitivity for diagnosing hypertension; as a result, it may miss many patients with true excess adiposity. In addition, WHtR overestimates substantially the prevalence of hypertension in the present population, especially in women. Sensitivity and specificity of WHR were found to be equally poor in both sexes [16].

In Bergman's study, percentage fat was positively correlated with hip circumference and negatively correlated with height; however, this might not be the case in other populations. In the present study, although the correlation of PBF with hip circumference was stronger than weight, the correlation with height was not negative (not shown in data). Furthermore although measuring hip circumference is easier in difficult terrain, calculation of BAI is comparatively tedious in the field.

We acknowledge potential limitations inherent in our study. There were a relatively small number of subjects included in the study; therefore, the findings may not be generalizable to other populations, and our analyses may have been underpowered. Further absence of direct measurement of PBF by refined instrument such as DEXA and Bioelectrical Impedance (BI) could also limit our findings. In conclusion, although the correlation of BMI is better than BAI, the sensitivity and specificity of BAI are similar to, if not better than, BMI. BAI can be used as an additional marker in addition to BMI for screening population; however its validity needs to be demonstrated on other populations too, before accepting it as a new marker for body fat measurement to predict cardiovascular and other health risks.

Conflict of Interests

The authors declare that there is no conflict of interests regarding the publication of this paper.

Acknowledgments

The authors extend their gratitude to all their participants without whose cooperation, this data could not have been known. They also acknowledge the support of the Department of Anthropology, University of Delhi, India, for providing them with the infrastructure for conducting their study. Financial assistance to Shilpi Gupta from the Indian Council of Medical Research (ICMR) is greatly acknowledged.

References

[1] G. Eknoyan, "Adolphe Quetelet (1796–1874)—the average man and indices of obesity," *Nephrology Dialysis Transplantation*, vol. 23, no. 1, pp. 47–51, 2008.

[2] J. S. Garrow and J. Webster, "Quetelet's index (W/H^2) as a measure of fatness," *International Journal of Obesity*, vol. 9, no. 2, pp. 147–153, 1985.

[3] S. Kapoor, P. Bhasin, and M. Dhall, "Reproductive characteristics and socio-demographic factors as predictors of general and regional obesity among adult women," *Indian Journal of Physical Anthropology and Human Genetics*, vol. 29, no. 1-2, pp. 1–19, 2010.

[4] H.-M. Lakka, D. E. Laaksonen, T. A. Lakka et al., "The metabolic syndrome and total and cardiovascular disease mortality in middle-aged men," *Journal of the American Medical Association*, vol. 288, no. 21, pp. 2709–2716, 2002.

[5] R. N. Bergman, D. Stefanovski, T. A. Buchanan et al., "A better index of body adiposity," *Obesity*, vol. 19, no. 5, pp. 1083-1089, 2011.

[6] M. B. Schulze and N. Stefan, "The body adiposity index and the sexual dimorphism in body fat," *Obesity*, vol. 19, no. 9, p. 1729, 2011.

[7] J. S. Weiner and J. A. Lourie, *Human Biology—A Guide of Field Methods*, IBP Handbook No. 9, Blackwell Scientific, Oxford, UK, 1969.

[8] J. V. G. A. Durnin and J. Womersley, "Body fat assessed from total body density and its estimation from skinfold thickness: measurements on 481 men and women aged from 16 to 72 years," *British Journal of Nutrition*, vol. 32, no. 1, pp. 77–97, 1974.

[9] G. Ramseyer, "Testing the difference between dependent correlations using the Fisher Z," *The Journal of Experimental Education*, vol. 47, pp. 307–310, 1979.

[10] X.-L. Meng, R. Rosenthal, and D. B. Rubin, "Comparing correlated correlation coefficients," *Psychological Bulletin*, vol. 111, no. 1, pp. 172–175, 1992.

[11] J. A. Swets, "The relative operating characteristic in psychology," *Science*, vol. 182, no. 4116, pp. 990–1000, 1973.

[12] C. E. Metz, "Basic principles of ROC analysis," *Seminars in Nuclear Medicine*, vol. 8, no. 4, pp. 283–298, 1978.

[13] Y. T. Van der Schouw, A. L. M. Verbeek, and J. H. J. Ruijs, "ROC curves for the initial assessment of new diagnostic tests," *Family Practice*, vol. 9, no. 4, pp. 506–511, 1992.

[14] D. Altman, *Practical Statistics for Medical Researchers*, Chapman& Hall/CRC, Boca Raton, Fla, USA, 2nd edition, 1992.

[15] S. Gupta and S. Kapoor, "Sex differences in blood pressure levels and its association with obesity indices: who is at greater risk," *Ethnicity and Disease*, vol. 20, no. 4, pp. 370–375, 2010.

[16] S. Gupta and S. Kapoor, "Optimal cut-off values of anthropometric markers to predict hypertension in north indian population," *Journal of Community Health*, vol. 37, no. 2, pp. 441–447, 2012.

[17] K. M. Flegal, J. A. Shepherd, A. C. Looker et al., "Comparisons of percentage body fat, body mass index, waist circumference, and waist-stature ratio in adults," *American Journal of Clinical Nutrition*, vol. 89, no. 2, pp. 500–508, 2009.

[18] P. Arner, "Regional adipocity in man," *Journal of Endocrinology*, vol. 155, no. 2, pp. 191–192, 1997.

[19] J. C. K. Wells, T. J. Cole, and P. Treleaven, "Age-variability in body shape associated with excess weight: the UK national sizing survey," *Obesity*, vol. 16, no. 2, pp. 435–441, 2008.

[20] C. Li, E. S. Ford, G. Zhao, L. S. Balluz, and W. H. Giles, "Estimates of body composition with dual-energy X-ray absorptiometry in adults," *American Journal of Clinical Nutrition*, vol. 90, no. 6, pp. 1457–1465, 2009.

Appetite Sensations, Appetite Signaling Proteins, and Glucose in Obese Adolescents with Subclinical Binge Eating Disorder

Kristi B. Adamo,[1,2,3] Shanna L. Wilson,[1] Zachary M. Ferraro,[1] Stasia Hadjiyannakis,[1,3,4] Éric Doucet,[2] and Gary S. Goldfield[1,2,5]

[1] *Healthy Active Living and Obesity Research Group, Children's Hospital of Eastern Ontario Research Institute, 401 Smyth Road, Ottawa, ON, Canada K1H 8L1*
[2] *School of Human Kinetics, Faculty of Health Sciences, University of Ottawa, Ottawa, ON, Canada K1N 6N5*
[3] *Department of Pediatrics, Faculty of Medicine, University of Ottawa, Ottawa, ON, Canada K1N 6N5*
[4] *Division of Endocrinology, Children's Hospital of Eastern Ontario, Ottawa, ON, Canada K1H 8L1*
[5] *School of Psychology, Faculty of Social Sciences, University of Ottawa, Ottawa, ON, Canada K1N 6N5*

Correspondence should be addressed to Kristi B. Adamo; kadamo@cheo.on.ca

Academic Editors: A. Erkner, D. Micic, and C. Schmidt

Objective. This study aimed to investigate potential differences in appetite sensations, ghrelin, peptide YY, and glucose and their relationship with energy and macronutrient intake in obese adolescents with subclinical binge eating disorder. *Methods.* Fifteen obese adolescents (six and nine individuals with and without subclinical binge eating disorder, resp.) qualified for this study. Visual analog scales and Three-Factor Eating Questionnaires were used to assess eating behaviours. Circulating ghrelin, peptide YY, and glucose were measured after fasting and at multiple time points postprandially following a standardized breakfast meal. Energy and macronutrient intake were measured with an *ad libitum* lunch buffet. *Results.* Emotional eating scores were significantly higher in obese adolescents with subclinical binge eating disorder. Hunger levels rose and satiety levels fell significantly over the course of the monitoring period but there was no difference between the two groups. Obese adolescents with subclinical binge eating disorder did not have significantly different levels of appetite signaling proteins or glucose. Obese adolescents with subclinical binge eating disorder had a nonsignificantly higher energy and macronutrient intake. *Conclusions.* A significant difference between the two groups in terms of their emotional eating scores highlights the important role that psychological factors play in relation to eating behaviours.

1. Introduction

Health complications associated with obesity are a major public health concern, especially in the adolescent population who may carry adipose-related disease risk (i.e., type 2 diabetes, cardiovascular disease) forward into adulthood [1]. Of particular interest in adolescents is the presence and severity of eating disorders and the potential associations with obesity. Binge eating disorder (BED) is a psychiatric (eating) disorder characterized by the rapid intake of large quantities of food in a short period of time, relative to what most people eat in a similar time frame [2]. There is also an associated sense of loss of control (LOC), a lack of compensatory behavior characteristic of bulimia nervosa, and the presence of clinically significant distress [2]. This disorder affects 1–5% of adults [3], and 2% of children and adolescents [4]. At least 30% of obese children presenting to obesity management clinics have subclinical binge eating disorder or full-fledged BED [5], which contribute to obesity onset and maintenance [6]. However, it can often be difficult to diagnose individuals with binge eating disorder due to the stringent criteria and ambiguous notion of what constitutes a large amount of food. In a study of 105 children (6–13 years of age) with no full-fledged BED diagnosis, 30% of study participants noted the presence of one LOC episode during their lifetime [7]. Individuals with subclinical binge eating disorder (BE) do not present with all criteria required for a full BED diagnosis and thus it is pertinent to study these adolescents in regard to appetite regulation and control of food intake [8].

Hunger and satiety cues are paramount in regulating food intake in the general population but are also especially critical for individuals with BE who experience LOC over their eating. In a study of obese women with and without BED, there was a significant difference in satiety levels at the end of a meal but no change in hunger or satiety over the meal duration nor was there a difference in hunger and satiety ratings after adjusting for the amount of food consumed [9]. Mirch et al. found no significant differences in hunger and satiety in overweight children prior to access to an *ad libitum* lunch following a standardized breakfast [10]. However, they identified that the children with BE were satiated for a shorter time period following the standardized breakfast and had a higher energy intake at the buffet [10].

Ghrelin, a hunger-signaling protein, is low in adult obesity [11], and, similarly, obese children have significantly lower levels than those with normal weight [12]. Monteleone et al. found no difference in ghrelin levels between the two groups of obese women (with and without BED) at a single fasting time point [13]. However, Geliebter et al. found that obese women with BED, as compared to nonbinge eating controls, had lower levels of fasting ghrelin and significantly lower concentrations over time [14].

Inconsistent evidence to date on the effects of obesity on peptide YY (PYY), a satiety-signaling protein, underscores the need for further investigation in both adult and adolescent populations [15–18]. In regard to binge eating, Geliebter et al. found no differences in PYY levels in a study of obese women with and without BED following a liquid mixed meal [19].

The glucostatic theory of food control postulates that decreases in circulating glucose signals hunger as well as the initiation of the next meal and this theory has received partial support from animal models as well as human trials [20, 21]. It has been further confirmed that satiety is related to rapid changes in blood glucose and ghrelin concentrations [22]. However, glucose concentrations were not significantly different between obese women separated into three different groups (nonbinge eating control, subclinical BED, and BED) when measured at a single time point or over time [14].

The aim of this study was to determine potential differences between adolescents with and without BE by investigating appetite sensations as well as fasting and postprandial responses of appetite signaling proteins and glucose. Our secondary outcome was to determine the relationship between these factors and energy and macronutrient intake in obese adolescents with BE. We hypothesized that obese adolescents with BE would report less postprandial satiety and greater hunger following the standardized breakfast. We also hypothesized that obese adolescents with BE would have a lower suppression of ghrelin following a standardized breakfast and a smaller increase in PYY. Finally, we hypothesized that appetite sensations, appetite signaling proteins, and glucose may be related to increased energy and macronutrient intake in obese adolescents with BE during an *ad libitum* lunch buffet, either individually or as a combination of the different factors.

2. Materials and Methods

2.1. Participants. Participants were recruited specifically for this study through the pediatric endocrinology clinic at the Children's Hospital of Eastern Ontario (CHEO). Approval was obtained from the CHEO Research Ethics Board prior to study initiation with informed assent/consent was obtained from the adolescents and their parents prior to participation. Body weight was assessed using a balance beam scale and height was assessed using a SECA stadiometer. Obesity was defined as having a BMI $\geq$ 95th percentile based on age and sex [23]. Body composition was measured using foot-to-foot bioelectrical impedance analysis using the Tanita TBF-310. Waist measurements were taken according to standard measurement procedures. The females included in this study were postmenarchal and the males were postpubertal according to Tanner Stage 4 and serum testosterone levels. Participants were excluded if they had type 2 diabetes or were taking medications and/or supplements (e.g., metformin) that could have an effect on body composition or appetite. Participants were classified as having BE if they self-reported binge eating at least once per week in the last three months as assessed by the Eating Disorder Diagnostic Scale, such that this group could be considered to have a subclinical form of BED [24]. Control participants had no history of regular binge eating episodes (<5 episodes in their lifetime and none in the past 3 months).

2.2. Protocol. Participants arrived at the laboratory following an overnight fast and a blood sample was drawn. Participants were then provided with a 571 kcal standardized breakfast with a fixed macronutrient content (50% CHO, 35% FAT, and 15% PRO) and were instructed to consume the meal within 20 minutes. Blood measurements were taken postprandially at 15, 30, 60, 90, 120, and 240 minutes. At the end of four-hour monitoring period, participants were asked to complete an 18-item Three-Factor Eating Questionnaire (TFEQ-18), which consists of three categories of eating behaviours (cognitive restraint, uncontrolled eating, and emotional eating) [25] and is a modified version of the original TFEQ questionnaire [26]. Immediately following the last blood draw, participants were provided with an *ad libitum* preweighted buffet lunch, in privacy, and instructed to eat as much as they wanted in 45 minutes. Hunger and satiety were assessed using 150 mm visual analog scales (VAS) at fasting, at blood sampling time points, and immediately after the *ad libitum* lunch buffet [27]. Energy and macronutrient intake were measured based on the remaining food from the buffet and was analyzed using the ESHA Food Processor SQL dietary analyses software (ESHA Research, USA), using the 2007 Canadian Nutrient File.

2.3. Assays. Blood samples were collected in vacutainers containing EDTA and protease inhibitor aprotinin. The protease inhibitor dipeptidyl peptidase-IV (DPP-IV) was also added to the total PYY sample. All of the samples were kept on ice and centrifuged within 30 minutes of collection. Total PYY was analyzed using ELISA (Millipore, USA, Cat

Table 1: Participant characteristics of the study population.

	Obese adolescents without BE ($n = 9$)	Obese adolescents with BE ($n = 6$)
Age (years)	13.7 ± 0.7	14.5 ± 0.8
Sex	6 M/3 F	1 M/5 F
Weight (kg)	99.8 ± 7.7	104.3 ± 6.8
Height (cm)	165.6 ± 3.0	164.7 ± 3.5
BMI (kg/m^2)	35.9 ± 2.2	38.5 ± 3.0
Waist circumference (cm)	112.9 ± 3.6	118.0 ± 5.2
Fat mass (kg)	41.9 ± 7.0	53.7 ± 7.8
Fat %	41.8 ± 3.8	50.8 ± 4.2
Fasting VAS hunger[a] (mm)	65.6 ± 12.1	87.2 ± 12.1
Fasting VAS full[a] (mm)	30.5 ± 11.6	28.2 ± 11.6
Fasting ghrelin[b] (pg/mL)	178.2 ± 20.3	202.0 ± 22.2
Fasting PYY[b] (pg/mL)	74.9 ± 16.0	104.6 ± 17.5
Fasting glucose[b] (mmol/L)	4.9 ± 0.3	4.9 ± 0.3

BE: subclinical binge eating disorder; BMI: body mass index; VAS: visual analog scale; PYY: peptide YY.
Effect size: fasting hunger ($d = 0.799$), fasting satiety ($d = 0.089$), ghrelin ($d = 0.479$), and PYY ($d = 0.758$).
[a]$n = 6$ (non-BE) after adjusting for sex and body fat mass.
[b]$n = 7$ (non-BE) after adjusting for sex and body fat mass.

number EZHPPYT66K; Intra-assay CV [16.7%]; Interassay CV [22.1%]). Total ghrelin was also measured using ELISA (Millipore, USA, Cat number EZGRT-89K; Intra-assay CV [15.1%]; Interassay CV [17.5%]). All ELISA samples were done in duplicate. Glucose was measured using the Cholestech LDX system (Alere, USA).

2.4. Statistical Analysis. Analysis of covariance (ANCOVA) and chi-squared tests (categorical variables) were used to analyze potential differences in participant characteristics, baseline appetite sensations and appetite signaling proteins, and buffet lunch characteristics. Four-hour area under the curve (AUC), using the trapezoidal method, was calculated for the temporal hunger and satiety VAS responses (range = 15 to 240 minutes), interpolating for any missing questionnaire time points [28]. Linear mixed models (LMM) were utilized to assess potential longitudinal differences in appetite sensations, appetite signaling proteins, and glucose. These models defined group as the independent factor with time as the repeated measure and utilized a first-order autoregressive (AR1) covariance matrix. Partial correlations were calculated at the end of the monitoring period between appetite sensations and energy/macronutrient intake with appetite signaling proteins, glucose, and TFEQ factors. All performed correlations were assessed using a significance threshold defined by a Bonferroni-adjusted P value. All analyses were adjusted for sex and fat mass (kg). Results are presented as mean ± standard error mean (SEM). Significance was set at a threshold value of $P < 0.05$, unless otherwise stated. All analyses were performed using SPSS 20.0 (IBM, USA).

3. Results

In total, 23 participants consented to participate in the study. However, four participants were unable to complete the study because of difficulties with the blood draw procedures, fainting, or other illness. Additionally, one participant was deemed ineligible after the fact due to an error in BMI calculation and three participants were excluded due to medication changes between recruitment and assessment. Overall, 15 adolescents from 11 to 17 years of age participated in this study with 6 individuals classified as having BE and 9 in the control group without BE.

Participant characteristics, including demographics and baseline measures of appetite sensations, appetite signaling proteins, and glucose, were not significantly different between obese adolescents with and without BE (Table 1). A significant rise in hunger ($P < 0.001$) and decrease in satiety ($P < 0.001$) occurred after the standardized breakfast (Figure 1). Obese adolescents with BE had nonsignificant lower overall satiety scores (47 ± 7 versus 63 ± 6, $P = 0.07$) using the LMM, and there was no difference in hunger scores (Figure 1, Table 2) using the LMM or the 4 hr AUC. Glucose levels slowly decreased after the standardized breakfast ($P < 0.001$) but there was no change in ghrelin or PYY concentrations following the meal. Overall concentrations of glucose, ghrelin, and PYY across the monitoring period did not significantly differ between the two groups (Figure 2).

As shown in Table 3, obese adolescents with BE had higher emotional eating scores (TFEQ-18) as compared to the control group (9.09 ± 0.65 versus 5.07 ± 0.60; $P = 0.002$). While higher cognitive restraint and uncontrolled eating score were present in obese adolescents with BE, they did not significantly differ between the groups.

As for energy intake at the *ad libitum* lunch buffet, the obese adolescents with BE consumed more total calories (+357.2 kcal), protein (+10.9 g), carbohydrates (+37.00 g), and fat (+18.46 g), albeit not statistically significant (Table 4).

We did not observe any significant correlations between energy/macronutrient intake with appetite sensations, appetite signaling proteins, glucose, or TFEQ categories.

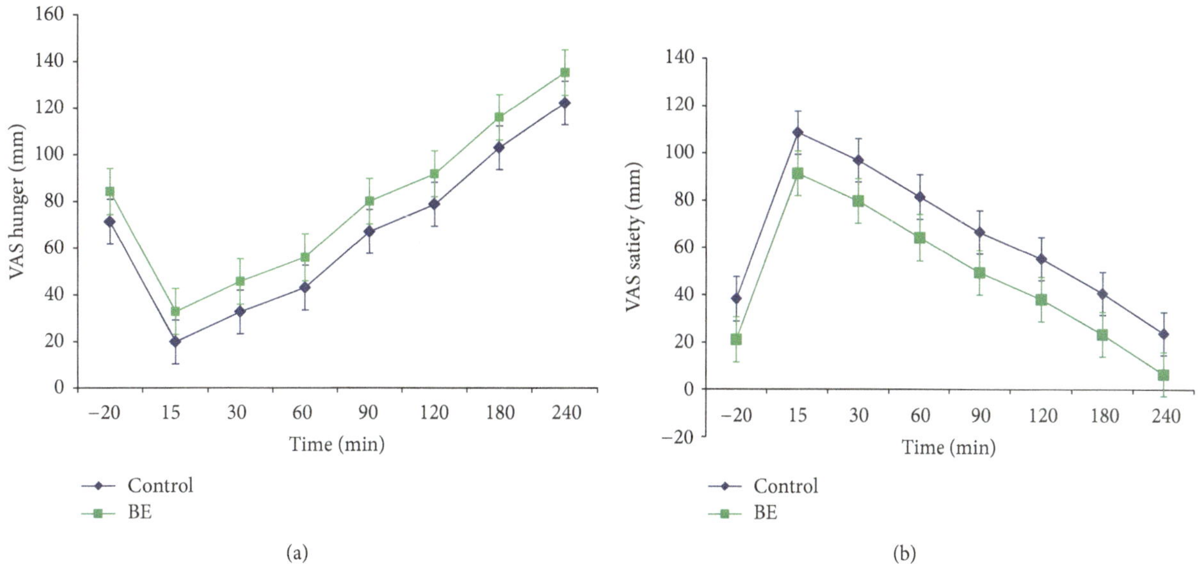

FIGURE 1: VAS hunger and satiety in obese adolescents with and without BE. Temporal changes in hunger and satiety during a four-hour monitoring period following a standardized, mixed breakfast. Error bars represent ±1 SEM. VAS: visual analog scale; BE: subclinical binge eating disorder.

TABLE 2: Measures of appetite sensations over the course of the entire study protocol (15–240 minutes) prior to the *ad libitum* lunch buffet, using 4 hr VAS AUC (mm × min).

	Obese adolescents without BE ($n = 7$)	Obese adolescents with BE ($n = 6$)
Hunger	17079.64 ± 1804.19	21096.26 ± 1969.96
Satiety	13693.39 ± 2049.18	7983.124 ± 2237.46

BE: subclinical binge eating disorder; VAS: visual analog scale; AUC: area under the curve.
Effect size: hunger ($d = 0.910$); satiety ($d = 1.139$).

Similarly, appetite sensations (hunger and satiety) were not significantly correlated with appetite signaling proteins, glucose, or TFEQ categories in this cohort.

4. Discussion

We aimed to examine potential differences in appetite sensations, appetite signaling proteins, and glucose and their relationship with energy and macronutrient intake in obese adolescents with and without BE. There were no differences in hunger and satiety between obese adolescents with and without BE, albeit there was a nonsignificant trend towards impaired satiety in the BE group. Mirch et al. found no significant differences in the ratings of appetite sensations (hunger and satiety) in overweight children with and without BE prior to access to an *ad libitum* lunch following a standardized breakfast [10]. However, they found that children with BE had a shorter time spent satiated following a standardized breakfast with higher energy intake at the *ad libitum* lunch buffet [10]. This conflicts with Tanofsky-Kraff et al. who found that adolescents with LOC, regardless of BMI, did not have a higher energy intake at normal or binging meals as compared to the control group without LOC, with the exception of overweight and obese girls with LOC who had a higher energy intake during their binge meal [29]. Therefore, obese adolescents with BE may be hungrier or less satiated later in the study protocol for a given caloric intake even if they demonstrate similar initial hunger and satiety which may lead to overconsumption at a subsequent meal.

Obese adolescents with BE had significantly higher emotional eating scores when compared to the control group. This highlights the psychological aspect of the eating disorder in which negative emotions may be associated with eating as assessed by TFEQ questions such as "when I feel anxious, I find myself eating" or "when I feel blue, I often overeat". Obese adolescence (10–16 years of age) with LOC had significantly more emotional and external eating behaviours as compared to a control group with no LOC [30]. There may also be a potential difference between these groups in uncontrolled eating as is evidenced by higher disinhibition scores in the obese individuals with BE, nonsignificant differences between the groups but a very large effect size ($d = 1.056$). This aligns with previous research demonstrating that overweight children with BE have a higher disinhibition score as compared to a control group [10]. Thus, obese adolescents with BE may exhibit a greater LOC or emotional eating at meal time which could potentially lead to increased energy intake over the course of the day.

In contrast to our initial expectations, postprandial response analyses showed no significant difference in ghrelin over time or between the two groups. Our results are in line with Monteleone et al. but contrast with Geliebter et al. [13, 14]. There were no temporal or group differences in PYY consistent with Geliebter et al. [19] but unexpected as it was originally postulated that there would be a smaller increase in

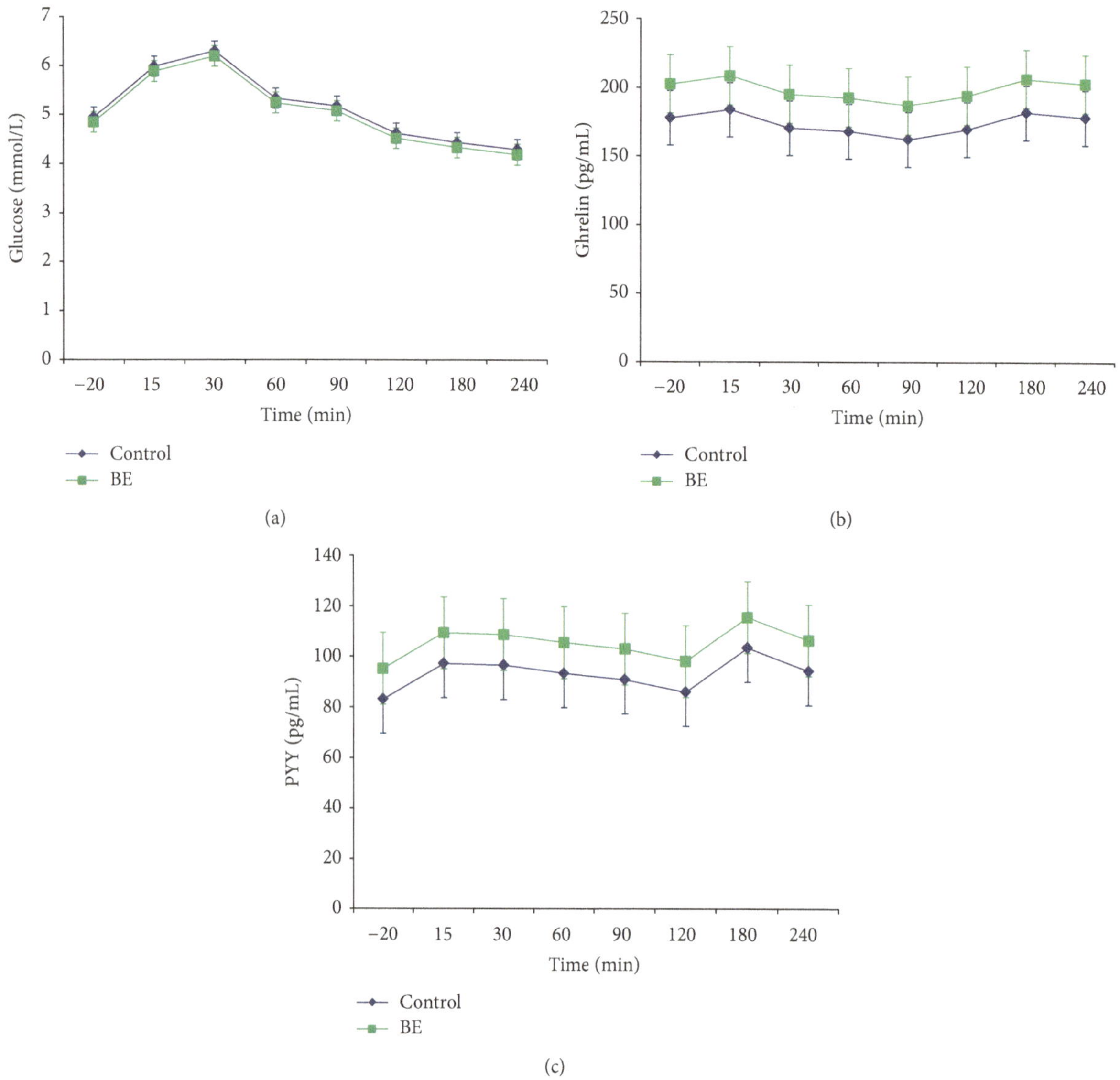

FIGURE 2: Glucose, ghrelin, and PYY in obese adolescents with and without BE. Temporal changes in glucose, ghrelin, and PYY during a four-hour monitoring period following a standardized, mixed breakfast. Error bars represent ±1 SEM. PYY: peptide YY; BE: subclinical binge eating disorder.

TABLE 3: Three-Factor Eating Questionnaire responses after the standardized breakfast at 240 minutes postprandially.

	Obese adolescents without BE (n = 7)	Obese adolescents with BE (n = 6)	P value
Restraint[a]	12.33 ± 1.11	13.28 ± 1.21	0.60
Uncontrolled Eating[b]	17.68 ± 2.46	24.04 ± 2.69	0.14
Emotional eating[c]	5.07 ± 0.60	9.09 ± 0.65	0.002*

BE: subclinical binge eating disorder; [a]range of score (6–24); [b]range of score (9–36); [c]range of score (3–12).
Effect size: restraint (d = 0.350); uncontrolled eating (d = 1.056); emotional eating (d = 2.750).
*Significant difference at $P < 0.05$.

PYY in obese adolescents with BE. As expected, postprandial response analyses showed a significant difference in glucose levels over time but with no difference between the two groups which is consistent with Geliebter et al. [14].

We acknowledge several limitations to our study. Given that many of the effect sizes obtained were moderate to large, an increased sample size may have provided the power to detect statistically significant differences and minimized the chance of type II error [31]. Moreover, using additional endocrine markers such as leptin, glucagon-like peptide-1, or cholecystokinin could provide a more comprehensive picture of appetite regulation in obese adolescents with BE. The fixed

TABLE 4: Nutrient intake profile at the "*ad libitum*" lunch buffet.

	Obese adolescents without BE ($n = 7$)	Obese adolescents with BE ($n = 6$)
Calories (kcal)	975.50 ± 164.7	1332.7 ± 179.8
Protein (g)	32.4 ± 4.6	42.4 ± 4.9
Protein (%)	13.2 ± 1.8	13.6 ± 2.0
Carbohydrates (g)	116.8 ± 19.8	153.8 ± 21.6
Carbohydrates (%)	47.1 ± 2.9	44.1 ± 3.2
Fat (g)	46.0 ± 9.6	64.5 ± 10.5
Fat (%)	39.6 ± 2.6	42.3 ± 2.9

BE: subclinical binge eating disorder.
Effect size: calories (kcal) ($d = 0.862$); protein (g) ($d = 0.899$); carbohydrates (g) ($d = 0.764$).

macronutrient breakfast was selected to study its effects on secretion of endocrine signaling proteins between the two different groups and was given to all subjects regardless of differences in body composition. As secretion is related to the quantity of the ingested nutrients, initial adjustment for body composition was not performed to prevent confounding of this effect. It has also been shown that obese individuals with full BED have a larger stomach capacity while obese individuals with subclinical forms of BED tend to have stomach capacities similar to nonbinging obese individuals [32]. Differences in stomach capacity may affect energy intake as Geliebter et al. has previously shown that stomach capacity is correlated with test meal intake [33]. It may also affect concentrations of signaling proteins as increased gastric capacity in obese individuals with full-fledged BED resulted in decreased fasting ghrelin levels [32]. The lack of significant differences in signaling proteins between the two groups may be somewhat influenced by the subjectivity of self-reported diagnoses and the subject's potential anatomical similarities to the control group. Therefore, a continuum scale of obese adolescents with full-fledged BED and subclinical BED as compared to a control group is needed to fully understand the spectrum of disordered eating behaviours associated with binge eating disorder [34]. Additional research has also proposed investigating LOC in children (6–12 years of age) as opposed to BE or BED due to the efficacy of LOC in identifying disordered eating in children [35].

5. Conclusions

Appetite sensations (hunger and satiety) did not differ between obese adolescents with and without BE. Lack of differences in appetite signaling proteins and glucose suggests that this may not be the best mechanism to investigate regarding etiology of the disorder. A significant difference between the two groups in terms of their emotional eating TFEQ cues highlights the importance that psychological factors play in relation to eating behaviour. This relevant finding could be used as a target in clinical practice to ensure control of these internal cues in obese adolescents with BE. The release of the new *Diagnostic and Statistical Manual for Mental Disorders: Fifth Edition* saw the inclusion of BED as an accepted eating disorder with a refined definition as it was previously only listed as a potential diagnostic category requiring further investigation. Overall, this highlights the importance of subclinical and full-fledged BED and need for further investigation regarding the psychological and metabolic effects of the binging and LOC episodes on obese adolescents.

Conflict of Interests

The authors declare that there is no conflict of interests regarding the publication of this paper.

Acknowledgments

The authors would like to acknowledge the CHEO Research Institute (Internal Grant) and the Canada Foundation of Innovation (Leader's Opportunity Fund) for supporting this research. They would also like to acknowledge Kerry Hamilton for her efforts in setting up the study protocol, Kristine deJesus for her contributions to recruitment and coordination, and Maria Psihogios, Dr. Cici Zhu, and Hanna Imad for their assistance with the trial. They would also like to thank Dr. Nina Fowler for performing the ELISA work, Kimberly Grattan for her help with the glucose assays, and Dr. Nick Barrowman for his consultation on statistical analysis.

References

[1] D. P. Guh, W. Zhang, N. Bansback, Z. Amarsi, C. L. Birmingham, and A. H. Anis, "The incidence of co-morbidities related to obesity and overweight: a systematic review and meta-analysis," *BMC Public Health*, vol. 9, article 88, 2009.

[2] American Psychiatric Association, *Diagnostic and Statistical Manual of Mental Disorders*, American Psychiatric Association, Washington, DC, USA, 4th edition, 1994.

[3] D. E. Smith, M. D. Marcus, C. E. Lewis, M. Fitzgibbon, and P. Schreiner, "Prevalence of binge eating disorder, obesity, and depression in a biracial cohort of young adults," *Annals of Behavioral Medicine*, vol. 20, no. 3, pp. 227–232, 1998.

[4] M. D. Marcus and M. Kalarchian, "Binge eating in children and adolescents," *International Journal of Eating Disorders*, vol. 34, supplement 1, pp. S47–S57, 2003.

[5] V. Decaluwe, C. Braet, and C. G. Fairburn, "Binge eating in obese children and adolescents," *International Journal of Eating Disorders*, vol. 33, no. 1, pp. 78–84, 2003.

[6] A. E. Field, S. B. Austin, C. B. Taylor et al., "Relation between dieting and weight change among preadolescents and adolescents," *Pediatrics*, vol. 112, no. 4, pp. 900–906, 2003.

[7] M. Tanofsky-Kraff, D. Faden, S. Z. Yanovski, D. E. Wilfley, and J. A. Yanovski, "The perceived onset of dieting and loss of control eating behaviors in overweight children," *International Journal of Eating Disorders*, vol. 38, no. 2, pp. 112–122, 2005.

[8] M. M. Antony, W. G. Johnson, R. E. Carr-Nangle, and J. L. Abel, "Psychopathology correlates of binge eating and binge eating disorder," *Comprehensive Psychiatry*, vol. 35, no. 5, pp. 386–392, 1994.

[9] F. Samuels, E. J. Zimmerli, M. J. Devlin, H. R. Kissileff, and B. T. Walsh, "The development of hunger and fullness during a laboratory meal in patients with binge eating disorder,"

International Journal of Eating Disorders, vol. 42, no. 2, pp. 125–129, 2009.

[10] M. C. Mirch, J. R. McDuffie, S. Z. Yanovski et al., "Effects of binge eating on satiation, satiety, and energy intake of overweight children," *The American Journal of Clinical Nutrition*, vol. 84, no. 4, pp. 732–738, 2006.

[11] T. McLaughlin, F. Abbasi, C. Lamendola, R. S. Frayo, and D. E. Cummings, "Plasma ghrelin concentrations are decreased in insulin-resistant obese adults relative to equally obese insulin-sensitive contrls," *The Journal of Clinical Endocrinology & Metabolism*, vol. 89, no. 4, pp. 1630–1635, 2004.

[12] L. Soriano-Guillen, V. Barrios, G. Martos, J. A. Chowen, A. Campos-Barros, and J. Argente, "Effect of oral glucose administration on ghrelin levels in obese children," *European Journal of Endocrinology*, vol. 151, no. 1, pp. 119–121, 2004.

[13] P. Monteleone, M. Fabrazzo, A. Tortorella, V. Martiadis, C. Serritella, and M. Maj, "Circulating ghrelin is decreased in non-obese and obese women with binge eating disorder as well as in obese non-binge eating women, but not in patients with bulimia nervosa," *Psychoneuroendocrinology*, vol. 30, no. 3, pp. 243–250, 2005.

[14] A. Geliebter, M. E. Gluck, and S. A. Hashim, "Plasma ghrelin concentrations are lower in binge-eating disorder," *The Journal of Nutrition*, vol. 135, no. 5, pp. 1326–1330, 2005.

[15] R. L. Batterham, M. A. Cohen, S. M. Ellis et al., "Inhibition of food intake in obese subjects by peptide YY_{3-36}," *The New England Journal of Medicine*, vol. 349, no. 10, pp. 941–948, 2003.

[16] P. T. Pfluger, J. Kampe, T. R. Castaneda et al., "Effect of human body weight changes on circulating levels of peptide YY and peptide YY_{3-36}," *The Journal of Clinical Endocrinology & Metabolism*, vol. 92, no. 2, pp. 583–588, 2007.

[17] C. L. Roth, P. J. Enriori, K. Harz, J. Woelfle, M. A. Cowley, and T. Reinehr, "Peptide YY is a regulator of energy homeostasis in obese children before and after weight loss," *The Journal of Clinical Endocrinology & Metabolism*, vol. 90, no. 12, pp. 6386–6391, 2005.

[18] S. Stock, P. Leichner, A. C. Wong et al., "Ghrelin, peptide YY, glucose-dependent insulinotropic polypeptide, and hunger responses to a mixed meal in anorexic, obese, and control female adolescents," *The Journal of Clinical Endocrinology & Metabolism*, vol. 90, no. 4, pp. 2161–2168, 2005.

[19] A. Geliebter, S. A. Hashim, and M. E. Gluck, "Appetite-related gut peptides, ghrelin, PYY, and GLP-1 in obese women with and without binge eating disorder (BED)," *Physiology & Behavior*, vol. 94, no. 5, pp. 696–699, 2008.

[20] J. Mayer, "Glucostatic mechanism of regulation of food intake," *The New England Journal of Medicine*, vol. 249, no. 1, pp. 13–16, 1953.

[21] L. A. Campfield and F. J. Smith, "Blood glucose dynamics and control of meal initiation: a pattern detection and recognition theory," *Physiological Reviews*, vol. 83, no. 1, pp. 25–58, 2003.

[22] C. de Graaf, W. A. Blom, P. A. M. Smeets, A. Stafleu, and H. F. J. Hendriks, "Biomarkers of satiation and satiety," *The American Journal of Clinical Nutrition*, vol. 79, no. 6, pp. 946–961, 2004.

[23] CDC growth chart data, http://www.cdc.gov/growthcharts/.

[24] E. Stice, C. F. Telch, and S. L. Rizvi, "Development and validation of the Eating Disorder Diagnostic Scale: a brief self-report measure of anorexia, bulimia, and binge-eating disorder," *Psychological Assessment*, vol. 12, no. 2, pp. 123–131, 2000.

[25] J. Karlsson, L.-O. Persson, L. Sjöström, and M. Sullivan, "Psychometric properties and factor structure of the Three-Factor Eating Questionnaire (TFEQ) in obese men and women. Results from the Swedish Obese Subjects (SOS) study," *International Journal of Obesity*, vol. 24, no. 12, pp. 1715–1725, 2000.

[26] A. J. Stunkard and S. Messick, "The three-factor eating questionnaire to measure dietary restraint, disinhibition and hunger," *Journal of Psychosomatic Research*, vol. 29, no. 1, pp. 71–83, 1985.

[27] P. J. Rogers and J. E. Blundell, "Effect of anorexic drugs on food intake and the micro-structure of eating in human subjects," *Psychopharmacology*, vol. 66, no. 2, pp. 159–165, 1979.

[28] E. Doucet, S. St-Pierre, N. Alméras, and A. Tremblay, "Relation between appetite ratings before and after a standard meal and estimates of daily energy intake in obese and reduced obese individuals," *Appetite*, vol. 40, no. 2, pp. 137–143, 2003.

[29] M. Tanofsky-Kraff, J. R. McDuffie, S. Z. Yanovski et al., "Laboratory assessment of the food intake of children and adolescents with loss of control eating," *The American Journal of Clinical Nutrition*, vol. 89, no. 3, pp. 738–745, 2009.

[30] L. Goossens, C. Braet, and V. Decaluwé, "Loss of control over eating in obese youngsters," *Behaviour Research and Therapy*, vol. 45, no. 1, pp. 1–9, 2007.

[31] J. Cohen, *Statistical Power Analysis For the Behavioural Sciences*, Lawerence Erlbaum, Hillside, NJ, USA, 1988.

[32] A. Geliebter, E. K. Yahav, M. E. Gluck, and S. A. Hashim, "Gastric capacity, test meal intake, and appetitive hormones in binge eating disorder," *Physiology & Behavior*, vol. 81, no. 5, pp. 735–740, 2004.

[33] A. Geliebter, P. M. Melton, R. S. McCray, D. R. Gallagher, D. Gage, and S. A. Hashim, "Gastric capacity, gastric emptying, and test-meal intake in normal and bulimic women," *The American Journal of Clinical Nutrition*, vol. 56, no. 4, pp. 656–661, 1992.

[34] A. B. Goldschmidt, M. Jones, J. L. Manwaring et al., "The clinical significance of loss of control over eating in overweight adolescents," *International Journal of Eating Disorders*, vol. 41, no. 2, pp. 153–158, 2008.

[35] M. Tanofsky-Kraff, M. D. Marcus, S. Z. Yanovski, and J. A. Yanovski, "Loss of control eating disorder in children age 12 years and younger: proposed research criteria," *Eating Behaviors*, vol. 9, no. 3, pp. 360–365, 2008.

The Work behind Weight-Loss Surgery: A Qualitative Analysis of Food Intake after the First Two Years Post-Op

Angela A. Geraci, Ardith Brunt, and Cindy Marihart

Department of Health Nutrition and Exercise Sciences, North Dakota State University, 351 EML, Box 6050, Fargo, ND 58108-6050, USA

Correspondence should be addressed to Angela A. Geraci; angela.geraci@my.ndsu.edu

Academic Editors: F. J. Elgar, J. J. Gleysteen, and H. Gordish-Dressman

Purpose. Obesity has reached epidemic proportions in the U.S. and has nearly doubled worldwide since 1980. Bariatric surgery is on the rise, but little focus has been placed on the psychosocial impacts of surgery. The purpose of this study was to explore experiences of patients who have undergone bariatric surgery at least two years before to gain an understanding of the successes and challenges they have faced since surgery. *Methods.* This study used a phenomenological approach, to investigate the meaning and essence of bariatric patients with food after surgery. Semi-structured interviews were conducted on a sample of nine participants who had undergone surgery at least two years prior. *Findings.* Two main themes regarding food intake emerged from the data: (a) food after the first year post-surgery and (b) bariatric surgery is not a magic pill. Upon further analysis, food after the first year post-surgery had four subthemes emerge: diet adherence after the first year post-surgery, food intolerances, amount of food, and tendencies toward coping with food do not magically disappear. *Conclusion.* Findings revealed that post-operative diet and exercise adherence becomes increasingly difficult as weight loss slows. Many participants find that only after the first year after surgery the work really begins.

1. Introduction/Purpose

Obesity is now a global public health issue and has nearly doubled worldwide since 1980 [1]. Global obesity estimates from 2008 reported that 35% of adults over the age of 20 were overweight and 11% were considered obese [1]. In addition, obesity rates continue to rise and remain epidemic in the United Sates, as well. More than two-thirds of American adults (68.8%) are considered overweight or obese and more than one-third (35.7%) of adults are obese, constituting more than 78 million American men and women [2]. Individuals who are considered morbidly, or clinically severely, obese (those with BMI of 35 in addition to documented health problems or those with a BMI over 40) are considered potential candidates for bariatric surgery [3].

Individuals elect to undergo bariatric surgery hoping to achieve long-term weight loss and to improve obesity-related comorbid conditions [4]. In 2008, nearly 350,000 bariatric procedures were performed globally [5], with an estimated 220,000 in the United States alone [6].

However, questions still arise on long-term success and its effect on weight loss maintenance and prevention of the return of lifestyle diseases [4, 7]. Previous research indicated that, about a year and a half to two years after bariatric surgery, weight loss from surgery stops and a significant number of individuals begin to regain the weight they had lost [8]. This is when support is needed most; nevertheless, many longitudinal follow-up bariatric surgery studies are short-termed and incomplete [4].

Bariatric surgery is a life-changing procedure that requires a lifelong commitment from the individual. Most research on bariatric surgery primarily focuses on health-related outcomes. Limited research exists examining personal and psychosocial experiences, including satisfaction

Table 1: Open-ended interview questions.

(1) How has bariatric surgery affected your quality of life now that you are 2+ years post-op?
(2) What is different for you now than after the first year post-op?
(3) How has bariatric surgery impacted your health? (both positively and negatively)
(4) How has bariatric surgery impacted your emotional health?
(5) How has bariatric surgery impacted your personal relationships?
(6) How has weight-loss surgery (WLS) affected your nutritional intake?
(7) What types of WLS support groups or online communities do you participate in, if any? Why or why not?
(8) What are the things only people who have had WLS know about that most outsiders would not?
(9) What are the cultural/social implications you have experienced since having WLS?
(10) Tell me about your personal satisfaction with bariatric surgery.

with weight loss and challenges patients experience following the first year after bariatric surgery. Using a qualitative approach to explore the meaning of the bariatric experience and sharing it with others provides an opportunity for future patients, families of patients, and healthcare providers to gain an understanding of what it is like to undergo a bariatric procedure and to live with the persistent change that accompanies it, after the first two years post-surgery and beyond. This study sought to answer the question: what is the experience of bariatric patients who are at least two years post-surgery?

2. Participants and Methods

This study used a qualitative research design, guided by a phenomenological approach, to investigate and describe the meaning and essence of experience of patients at least two years after bariatric surgery [9, 10]. Phenomenological studies are primarily open-ended, searching for themes of meaning in participants' lives [10]. Research is conducted through in-depth interviews. The researcher seeks to understand the deep meaning of a person's experience and how one describes this experience [11]. Exploring the lived experience of patients at least two years after bariatric surgery provided a deeper understanding and awareness of the impact of weight-loss surgery. Through the use of interview questions as a guide, semistructured interviews were conducted (Table 1).

2.1. Participants. The method of in-depth, phenomenological interviews applied to a sample of participants who have all experienced similar social conditions gives power to the stories of relatively few participants [10], such as life experience. The researchers used purposeful convenience sampling, which enabled relatively easy access to participants [9]. By contacting participants who were acquainted with the researchers and met inclusion criteria for this study, the researcher was able to conduct semistructured interviews with nine bariatric surgery patients at least two years post-surgery. Criteria for inclusion was set so that the participants who were at least two years after operation and over the age of 18 were recruited through email/telephone regardless of gender, age, surgery type, ethnicity, or socioeconomic status.

The study sample included nine women who ranged from 27 to 57 years of age ($M = 42$). Seven participants had the vertical sleeve gastrectomy (VSG) surgery and 2 had the Roux en Y gastric bypass (RNYB). Self-identified ethnicities of participants were Caucasian ($n = 5$), Hispanic ($n = 2$), and African-American ($n = 2$). Participants ranged from two to seven years after operation ($M = 3$) (Table 2). Weight before surgery following the preoperative diet ranged from 199 pounds to 298 pounds ($M = 247.4$). Initial weight loss after surgery ranged from 58 pounds to 116 pounds ($M = 88$). Weight gain after reaching plateau ranged from none to 48 pounds ($M = 8.7$) (Table 3).

Data analysis included the use of field notes, audiotapes, a reflexive journal, and peer debriefing. Each audiotaped interview was transcribed verbatim and field notes were taken during each interview. After transcription, each interview was printed for clarity. Post-it notes of various colors aided in identifying themes. The first transcript reading helped develop the coding categories, and then the second reading was conducted to start formal coding in a systematic way using colored post-it notes to group related data [9]. The second transcript aided in identifying new categories of information and the two lists were merged into one list, which then represented the final codebook. The transcript of the third interview was compared to the previous code list to see if new categories emerged and this process continued comparing each subsequent transcript for coding categories. Themes were eventually developed into a written description of the participants' experience with bariatric surgery to answer the research question. Quotes from the participants provided a rich, thick description of their experience [11].

2.2. Reflexive Researchers' Statement. The researchers personal experience as bariatric patients included preconceived beliefs that bariatric surgery should be for obese individuals who had failed attempts at losing weight through traditional methods with diet and exercise and who need an additional weight-loss tool to aid in achieving a healthy body weight. Being part of the weight-loss surgery community comes with a very "pro-surgery" mentality that the researchers acknowledged. To focus on the participants' experience after bariatric surgery, the researchers were required to bracket those beliefs. Hays and Wood [10] define bracketing as setting aside any assumptions made in everyday life and expressed the need for the researcher to reserve all prejudgments of their experience and rely on intuition and imagination to obtain the picture of the experience.

2.3. Trustworthiness. Establishing trustworthiness of the findings was utilized by engaging in peer debriefing of instrument protocol and through prolonged discussions of the research project with peers. Researcher reflexivity was

TABLE 2: Participant demographics.

Name	Age	Ethnicity	Marital status	Time since surgery	Surgery type
P1	54	Caucasian	Divorced	7 yrs. 5 mo.	RNYB
P2	30	Caucasian	Married	2 yrs. 11 mo.	VSG
P3	45	Hispanic	Married	2 yrs. 4 mo.	VSG
P4	27	Caucasian	Married	2 yrs. 5 mo.	VSG
P5	56	Caucasian	Married	3 yrs.	VSG
P6	57	Caucasian	Divorced	2 yrs. 7 mo.	VSG
P7	31	African-American	Single	2 yrs. 5 mo.	VSG
P8	34	Hispanic	Divorced	2 yrs. 9 mo.	RNYB
P9	45	African-American	Divorced	2 yrs. 5 mo.	VSG

TABLE 3: Self-reported participants presurgery and current anthropometrics.

Name	Day of surgery weight (pounds)	Day of surgery BMI*	Lowest weight achieved (pounds)	Postsurgery weight-loss (pounds)	Current weight (pounds)	Current BMI*
P1	289	49.6	176	113	184	31.6
P2	220	43	162	58	210	41
P3	199	36.4	139	60	139	25
P4	235	36.8	154	81	164	27.7
P5	210	38.4	140	70	145	26.5
P6	243	40.4	128	115	133	22.1
P7	298	48.1	184	114	184	29.7
P8	283	47.1	172	111	175	28.2
P9	240	39.9	170	70	170	28.3

*Note. Body Mass Index (BMI) Formula: weight (lb.)/[height (in.)]^2 × 703.

engaged by keeping a journal and field notes, and simultaneous data collection and analysis, which involved collecting and analyzing data simultaneously [9].

3. Findings

Review of the data, including individual interviews and field notes, was conducted to analyze and identify themes of the participants' experience with food after bariatric surgery. Two main themes emerged from the data: (a) food after the first year post-op and (b) bariatric surgery is not a magic pill.

3.1. Food after the First Year Post-Op. The overarching theme of viewing weight-loss as work after the first year emerged from the data as participants described the mounting difficulty of adhering to the recommended post-op diet once the first year had passed. In addition, tendencies towards using food as comfort and emotional eating were still a struggle that many participants experienced.

> ...I know I have to keep staying on top of it, it's just that I'm sick of protein, I'm sick of water, I'm sick of working out, I'm just sick of it. I just want eat normal sometimes, but I know I just need to suck it up and deal with it. Finding that balance after the first year...it's so important. [P7]

3.1.1. Diet Adherence after the First Year Post-Op. The recommended diet after bariatric surgery varies among surgeons and across different bariatric surgeries, but there are some commonalities that all participants experienced. Generally agreed upon nutritional guidelines are that supplemental minerals and vitamins should be taken daily, small bites of food should be chewed thoroughly before swallowing, liquids should be either ingested well before meals or at least 30 minutes afterwards, and at least 60 grams of proteins should be preferentially eaten before fats and carbohydrates [12–15].

> Consuming the right food and the vitamins and doing the right thing with food exist on a continuum...it's not a matter of being all right or all wrong or all good or all bad...every day you're striving to make the best choices you can in that moment. [P3]

> In the second year, I noticed I had to be very careful about what I ate and I had to really focus on my vitamins every day and make sure to get my protein and water in every day...the first year, you did not really have to think much and you'd still lose weight. Now I have to focus and pay attention to what I put in my mouth... [P9]

> I am more aware of what I'm eating now because my intake is so small, you really have to pay

> attention to what you're putting in your body. It's quality now, I'm going for the filet minion [sic] before the ground hamburger. [P7]

3.1.2. Food Intolerances. Potential long-term dietary complications include dumping syndrome (e.g., sweating, weakness, hypoglycemia, vomiting, diarrhea, and nausea) related to eating foods high in concentrated sugar or fat [16, 17]. All participants expressed problems with dumping syndrome and/or intolerances to various foods, namely, refined carbohydrates and sugar. It should be noted that food intolerances vary with surgery type. Most participants talked about food intolerances, especially to sugar.

> I think the one good thing is that I cannot eat a huge amount of sweets without being nauseated...I can eat a little that's more cracker-ish or cookies...but, like, big bakery pastries or pies, or a big hunk of cake or something, well, that's not going to work very well so I try to avoid it. [P1]

> Besides sweets, I have problems with all white carbs like rice, bread, and pasta. It makes me feel woozy. [P9]

3.1.3. Amount of Food. All participants discussed the amount of food they were able to consume in some way, noting reduced intake even years after surgery compared to presurgery amounts.

> As far as eating...I can eat many more calories at one time than I used to be able to eat when recently post-op. [P3]

> You do have more hunger, though you still cannot eat like you used to...and I have a bit more of a desire to eat than I did the first year...I'm still restricted in how much I can eat and eat about 3 ounces of dense protein and 1 ounce of vegetables and 1 ounce of starch for a meal. [P6]

3.1.4. Tendencies towards Coping with Food Do Not Just Magically Disappear. Many participants were identified as still grappling with food as a means to cope and it can be a challenge to find new ways to channel emotions without turning to food [18, 19]. Participants also identified that it was easier to manage the food cravings after surgery as well as the "head hunger" which involves not having physical hunger but the desire to eat anyway.

> I'm realizing now that there is a real emotional and physical effect that different foods have on your body. For example, the effect that sugar might have on your emotions or energy level, the way alcohol affects your body almost immediately post-op...these things are intensified. [P3]

> I still have those gnawing cravings from time to time and I just find it easier to say you do not need it right now, you can wait. It's not like before where I had to have the food otherwise I was gonna die. [P6]

> If I'm going to have something bad like sugar or something, I make sure I have protein first so I'm full, then it's not such a big deal. I try not to tell myself "no" on anything because the minute I say "no," then I start have mental issues with it. [P5]

> There are certain times where I think. Damn. I'm feeling depressed today and I wish I could just go eat a couple of pieces of cheesecake and that would only make me happy temporarily...I've tried to self-sabotage and I'm glad I get sick. It kind of conditioned me to not do that anymore...like, "hey, this is bad for you. Do not do it." [P4]

3.2. Bariatric Surgery Is Not a Magic Pill. This theme was common across all participants and it deserves to be noted that many patients who passed the first two years of surgery realize (e.g., by experiencing weight regain) that bariatric surgery is intended to be used only as a "tool" to aid in weight loss or to reduce physical hunger. All participants offered words of advice and/or caution to those considering bariatric surgery.

> I think that the surgery is not a fix all...it is a tool to help you achieve weight loss, but it is only a tool. It is not the end to all answers. It helps you with the amount you can eat and can definitely help you lose weight but if you still do not pick the right [food] choices to eat and exercise, it's still not going to do you any good in the long term. [P2]

> Weight loss is not something that's going to happen on its own. I mean, everybody has this misconception that you have surgery and then get magically skinny and that's not how it works. You still have to put in the work and your everything into this every day. [P4]

> I think people have it in their heads that you go into surgery and have it done and come out instantly thin. They do not realize that you cannot eat and drink at the same time or you can only eat 3 ounces of food at once...nobody talks about all that and all the working out and that you've been gutted like a fish, they just think you're instantly skinny within a month...I do not know why people think it's so easy...it's harder actually. It's life-long. [P7]

4. Discussion

Experience of participants was profiled in an attempt to share their qualities through thick description. The experience of all participants' lives after bariatric surgery provided a glimpse of what role food now plays after the first two years after operation.

Food was still considered a huge part of life, though limited in quantity, even years after bariatric surgery. Participants discussed not consuming their recommended daily intake of protein and not taking their vitamins. Low iron, B12, and vitamin D were consequences of poor supplementation. Participants compared food cravings to addictions to alcohol or drugs and there was still grief felt in regard to being unable to enjoy the same meals socially and with family as before surgery. Participants adjusted to changes in diet in different ways, and some were more successful than others, though many still fight the urges to use food to cope in certain situations. In addition, many participants experienced food intolerances and/or dumping syndrome. Many found eating a simple food such as a cracker (carbs) or any refined sugar may make them become unpleasantly ill.

Having bariatric surgery is a lifelong decision that requires follow-up care. These patients face medical and psychosocial challenges that require continuing care for years after surgery, and the hard work begins post-surgery [20]. It is also pointed out that not much has been written on the topic of follow-up care, but rather the focus has been on who is a good candidate for surgery rather than what patients go through after the procedure [20].

A qualitative study using phenomenological approach was used for this study in order to gain a better understanding of the experience of participants who were at least two years after bariatric surgery. The use of semistructured interviews allowed the participants to express their feelings and experience of life after bariatric surgery which many follow-up surveys lack and may expand the knowledge base from the participants own lived encounters with bariatric surgery. The themes around food generated from the data collected in this study provided a glimpse of life once the magic of the first year has passed and the reality of the surgery had set in. Additional emerging themes from this study to be analyzed include the role of social support and perceptions of self and society.

While obesity threatens to explode into a reverberating pandemic, there is a need to understand and support those individuals who have made the decision to have bariatric surgery. Studies such as this can offer health care professionals needed insight and information to be supportive and provide the care necessary to this vulnerable population. One participant who has struggled more than two years post-surgery with weight regain, and who stands apart from the others in current postoperative BMI (Table 3), summed up the lifelong impact of diet for the bariatric patient.

> It's lifelong and a lifestyle change... I mean you cannot have your stomach cut out and then think you can eat crap food like you did before. I noticed that it is very easy to eat junk food like chips and soda...these foods go down easily...also if you drink your calories...you'll gain the weight back. There are ways to eat around bariatric surgery. I just think that if you want long-term success with bariatric surgery then it's a complete lifestyle change and it's not a temporary thing, I know that now. You cannot lose all the weight and then think you can go back to unhealthy eating like you did before surgery. You need to learn how to eat from the start of the journey.

Conflict of Interests

The authors declare that there is no conflict of interests.

Acknowledgment

This research was not supported by any participating grant or foundation. The North Dakota State University Institutional Review Board accepted approval for this study.

References

[1] World Health Organization (WHO), "Overweight and obesity," 2013, http://www.who.int/gho/ncd/risk_factors/overweight/en/index.html.

[2] K. M. Flegal, D. Carroll, B. K. Kit, and C. L. Ogden, "Prevalence of obesity and trends in the distribution of body mass index among US adults, 1999–2010," *The Journal of the American Medical Association*, vol. 307, no. 5, pp. 491–497, 2012.

[3] National Institutes of Health, "Obesity," 2012, http://www.nlm.nih.gov/medlineplus/obesity.html.

[4] H. Buchwald, Y. Avidor, E. Braunwald et al., "Bariatric surgery: a systematic review and meta-analysis," *The Journal of the American Medical Association*, vol. 292, no. 14, pp. 1724–1728, 2004.

[5] H. Buchwald and D. M. Oien, "Metabolic/bariatric surgery worldwide 2008," *Obesity Surgery*, vol. 19, no. 12, pp. 1605–1611, 2009.

[6] American Society for Metabolic and Bariatric Surgery, "Benefits of bariatric surgery," 2013.

[7] R. H. Freire, M. C. Borges, J. I. Alvarez-Leite, and M. I. T. D. Correia, "Food quality, physical activity, and nutritional follow-up as determinant of weight regain after Roux-en-Y gastric bypass," *Nutrition*, vol. 28, no. 1, pp. 53–58, 2012.

[8] S. H. Niego, M. D. Kofman, J. J. Weiss, and A. Geliebter, "Binge eating in the bariatric surgery population: a review of the literature," *International Journal of Eating Disorders*, vol. 40, no. 4, pp. 349–359, 2007.

[9] D. G. Hays and A. A. Singh, *Qualitative Inquiry in Clinical and Educational Settings*, The Guilford Press, New York, NY, USA, 2011.

[10] D. G. Hays and C. Wood, "Infusing qualitative traditions in counseling research designs," *Journal of Counseling and Development*, vol. 89, no. 3, pp. 288–295, 2011.

[11] G. B. Rossman and S. F. Rallis, *Learning in the Field*, Sage, Thousand Oaks, Calif, USA, 2003.

[12] M. M. McMahon, M. G. Sarr, M. M. Clark et al., "Clinical management after bariatric surgery: value of a multidisciplinary approach," *Mayo Clinic Proceedings*, vol. 81, no. 10, supplement, pp. S34–S45, 2006.

[13] L. Rickers and C. McSherry, "Bariatric surgery: nutritional considerations for patients," *Nursing Standard*, vol. 26, no. 49, pp. 41–48, 2012.

[14] L. E. Bocchieri, M. Meana, and B. L. Fisher, "A review of psychosocial outcomes of surgery for morbid obesity," *Journal of Psychosomatic Research*, vol. 52, no. 3, pp. 155–165, 2002.

[15] R. J. Presutti, R. S. Gorman, and J. M. Swain, "Primary care perspective on bariatric surgery," *Mayo Clinic Proceedings*, vol. 79, no. 9, pp. 1158–1166, 2004.

[16] L. Dalcanale, C. P. M. S. Oliveira, J. Faintuch et al., "Long-term nutritional outcome after gastric bypass," *Obesity Surgery*, vol. 20, no. 2, pp. 181–187, 2010.

[17] V. G. Villagra, "A primer on bariatric surgery: treatment of last resort for morbid obesity," *Disease Management*, vol. 7, supplement 1, pp. S23–S30, 2004.

[18] J. Ogden, S. Avenell, and G. Ellis, "Negotiating control: patients' experiences of unsuccessful weight-loss surgery," *Psychology and Health*, vol. 26, no. 7, pp. 949–964, 2011.

[19] L. E. Bocchieri, M. Meana, and B. L. Fisher, "Perceived psychosocial outcomes of gastric bypass surgery: a qualitative study," *Obesity Surgery*, vol. 12, no. 6, pp. 781–788, 2002.

[20] V. S. Elliott, "Bariatric surgery patients need care for a lifetime," 2004, http://www.ama-assn.org/amednews/2004/06/28/hlsa0628.htm.

6

Lifestyle Risk Factors of General and Abdominal Obesity in Students of the School of Medicine and Health Science of the University of Development Studies, Tamale, Ghana

Victor Mogre,[1] Rauf Nyaba,[2] and Samuel Aleyira[2]

[1] *Department of Human Biology, School of Medicine and Health Sciences, University for Development Studies, P.O. Box TL 1883, Tamale, Ghana*

[2] *Department of Allied Health Sciences, School of Medicine and Health Sciences, University for Development Studies, P.O. Box TL 1883, Tamale, Ghana*

Correspondence should be addressed to Victor Mogre; mogrevictor@yahoo.com

Academic Editors: C. A. Gibson and D. Tekin

This study evaluated the prevalence of general and abdominal obesity among students of the University for Development Studies, School of Medicine and Health Sciences (UDS-SMHS), Tamale, Ghana. Also, lifestyle risk factors for the two obesity indices were investigated. This study was conducted among a sample of 646 students. Anthropometric measures of weight, height, and waist circumference were appropriately assessed. The prevalence of general and abdominal obesity was 1.9% and 4.2%, respectively. Risk factors of general obesity were being female (crude OR = 6.9, 95% CI = 1.85–25.80, $P = 0.0021$), engaging in light PA (OR = 12.45, 95% CI = 2.96–52.41, $P = 0.0006$), being aged 28–37 years (OR = 5.37, 95% CI = 1.39–20.68, $P = 0.0329$), nonintake of coffee (OR = 4.1, 95% CI = 1.10–15.28, $P = 0.0357$), being married (OR = 5.7, 95% CI = 1.48–22.02, $P = 0.0286$), and being abdominally obese (OR = 02.7, 95% CI = 25.61–11.60, $P < 0.0001$). Risk factors for abdominal obesity were being female, being married, having general obesity, and nonintake of coffee. Abdominal obesity was more prevalent than general obesity. Risk factors included being female, married, and generally obese and nonintake of coffee.

1. Introduction

Obesity has become a disease of public health concern for both developed and developing countries. Globally, obesity has been estimated to be the fifth leading cause of mortality [1]. The World Health Organization [2] estimates that 1.1 billion adults living in both developed and developing countries are overweight in which 300 million of them are obese. The prevalence of obesity in the USA has increased from 12.0% to 19.8% [3, 4] and half of its adult population are now overweight or obese [5]. An obesity prevalence of 10% has been reported in West Africa [6] and specifically 18% in the Republic of Benin [6]. In Ghana, a study conducted by Mogre et al. [7] in Tamale, Ghana, reported the prevalence of central obesity to be 31.2% among civil servants. Several studies have revealed that the prevalence of obesity in Ghana and other sub-Saharan African countries is increasing especially among women [7–9].

This growing epidemic is not only found in adults but also among children and young adults. The prevalence of obesity among school-aged children has more than tripled since the 1970s [10]. Several studies have demonstrated the childhood roots of adult obesity [11, 12]. Studies have reported a rising prevalence of childhood obesity in Ghana and other sub-Saharan countries [13–15]. However, there is limited data regarding obesity in the young adult group in Ghana. The few studies available used only BMI to assess the nutritional status of students studying various health related programs, a target group of particular interest as they are the future health care providers. The use of waist circumference (WC) in conjunction with BMI to assess abdominal and general obesity has not been extensively examined, particularly among Ghanaian students studying health related programs.

Both general and abdominal obesity are associated with increased risk of morbidity and mortality [16]. Abdominal obesity is a predisposing factor of cardiovascular diseases (CVDs), the main cause of obesity-related deaths. Traditionally, BMI has been chosen as an indicator to measure body size and composition and to diagnose underweight and overweight. Alternative measures such as WC, waist-to-hip ratio, and waist-to-height ratio that reflect abdominal adiposity have been suggested as being superior to BMI in predicting CVD risk. WC has been shown to be strongly predictive of all-cause mortality in young and middle-aged adults compared to older people and those with low BMI and could replace waist-to-hip ratio and BMI as a single risk factor for all-cause mortality [17].

The development of both general and abdominal obesity has been associated with potentially modifiable lifestyle factors such as physical inactivity, smoking, and alcohol consumption [18–20].

The aim of this cross-sectional study was to assess the prevalence of general and abdominal obesity among students studying health related programs in the University for Development Studies, School of Medicine and Health Sciences (UDS-SMHS), Tamale, Ghana. In addition, we investigated the effect of the lifestyle risk factors (age, gender, marital status, physical activity (PA), smoking, and alcohol and coffee consumption) on the two obesity indices (BMI and WC).

2. Methods

2.1. Participants. This cross-sectional study was executed between January and July 2013 among students studying health related academic programs in the University for Development Studies, School of Medicine and Health Sciences, (UDS-SMHS) Tamale, Ghana. From an eligible student population of 1809, a proportionate random sample of 646 (35.7% response rate) students that included more students from larger departments was selected to participate in the study with the help of a random number statistical table. Participants who were pregnant or had recent child births were excluded from the study. Demographic and sociocultural variables such as age, smoking status, and alcohol and coffee intake were also assessed. Participation in the study was voluntary and informed consent was obtained from each participant. The Ethics Committee of the University for Development Studies, School of Medicine and Health Sciences, Ghana, approved the study.

2.2. Anthropometric Variables. Anthropometric variables of waist circumference (WC), weight, and height were measured without shoes and with light clothing by trained personnel. WC was measured midway between the inferior angle of the ribs and the suprailiac crest [16]. During the measurement, participants stood in an upright position, with arms relaxed at the side, feet evenly spread apart, and body weight evenly distributed in accordance with the WHO expert consultation report on waist circumference and waist-hip ratio [16]. Abdominal obesity was determined as a waist circumference >102 cm in men and >88 cm in women according to the World Health Organization cutoff points and risk of metabolic complications for waist circumference [16]. Weight was measured to the nearest 0.1 kg using a UNICEF electronic scale manufactured by SECA. Prior to use, all scales were calibrated with a standard weight. Two measurements were taken and, if there were differences by a margin of more than 0.5 kg, a third measurement was taken and the mean of the closest two measurements was recorded. Height was measured to nearest 0.5 cm using a wall-mounted microtoise. Two measurements were made and compared and, if the measurements differed by more than 0.5 cm, a third measurement was taken and the mean of the closest two measurements was recorded. Body mass index (BMI) was calculated as BMI (kg/m^2) = weight (kg)/[height (m^2)]. General overweight and obesity were defined using the current World Health Organization definitions: underweight: BMI < 18.5 kg/m^2, normal weight: BMI 18.5–24.9 kg/m^2, overweight (preobese): BMI 25–29.9 kg/m^2, and obese: BMI > 30 kg/m^2 [21].

2.3. Physical Activity Level. The Global Physical Activity Questionnaire (GPAQ) was used to measure the level of physical activity of the participants [22]. The GPAQ consists of 16 questions about physical activity level in a typical week. The frequency and duration of time spent doing physical activity are measured in 3 domains: activity at work, travel to and from places, and recreational activities.

The GPAQ was used due to its standardization, easiness to administer, relative unobtrusiveness, and inexpensiveness. Its reliability and validity have been found to be 0.67–0.81 and 0.54, respectively [23]. Without modifications, the questionnaire was fully adapted for the study. However, to suit the Ghanaian context, local examples of types and intensity of activities were used. The GPAQ analysis protocol for the collection of all data and processing was followed [22]. All activity durations were converted into minutes. Energy expenditure, measured in metabolic equivalents (MET), was estimated using duration, intensity, and frequency of physical activities performed within 7 days. MET is the ratio of specific physical activity metabolic rates to the resting metabolic rate (1 MET = the energy cost of sitting quietly and was equivalent to a caloric consumption of 1 kcal/kg/hour). A MET-minute showed the total activity volume on a weekly basis and was calculated by multiplying time spent on each activity during a week by the MET values of each level of activity. Using the compendium of physical activities [24], MET values for various levels of activities were established. MET values of 4 and 8 were set for moderate-intensity (transport-related walking or cycling) and vigorous-intensity physical activity, respectively. Total MET/minutes/week was computed by the sum of all moderate- to vigorous-intensity physical activities performed at work, transport, and recreation. Based on the total MET/minutes/week, subjects were classified into light, moderate, and vigorous physical activity (PA) intensity as defined by the GPAQ analysis framework [22].

Vigorous. A participant is found within any of the following categories: vigorous-intensity activity on at least three days achieving at least 1,500 MET-minutes/weeks OR seven or more days of any combination of walking, moderate, or vigorous-intensity activities achieving at least 3,000 MET-minutes per week.

Moderate. A participant is not achieving the criteria for the high category but either of the following three criteria: (a) 3 or more days of vigorous-intensity activities of at least 20 minutes per day OR (b) 5 or more days of moderate-intensity activities and/or walking of at least 30 minutes per day OR (c) 5 or more days of any combination of walking, moderate-, or vigorous-intensity activities accumulating at least 600 MET-minutes/week.

Light. Participant's reported activity is lower than the categories outlined above or no activity is reported at all.

2.4. Statistical Analysis. The results were expressed as proportion and compared using Fischer's exact test or χ^2 for trend analysis as appropriate. A level of $P < 0.05$ was considered as statistically significant. GraphPad Prism version 5.00 (GraphPad Software, San Diego, California, USA, http://www.graphpad.com/) for Windows was used for statistical analysis.

3. Results

The general characteristics of the participants stratified by gender are recorded in Table 1. The mean age of the participating students was 23.06 ± 2.77 years. Significantly, male students (23.52 ± 2.83) were older than female students (22.03 ± 2.33). Only 1.1% of the students were smokers, 13.2% drank alcohol, and 57.1% drank coffee. More male (n = 29) students than female (n = 9) students were married. However, the differences were not significant when marital status of the students was stratified by gender using Fisher's exact test.

The mean BMI of the students was 21.79 ± 3.10 Kg/m^2. The prevalence of general overweight and obesity was 9.3% and 1.9%, respectively. Whereas more male students (n = 404) than female students (n = 138) had normal weight, more female students than male students had general overweight (n = 42 versus n = 18) and obesity (n = 9 versus n = 3). The differences were significant when BMI status was stratified by gender using Fisher's exact test.

The prevalence of abdominal obesity was 4.2% (males: 0.7%, females: 11.9%, $P < 0.0001$).

In general, 14.7% engaged in light physical activity (PA) (males: 8.3%, females: 28.9%), 48.8% in moderate PA (males: 44.0%, females: 59.2%), and 36.5% in vigorous PA (males: 47.6%, females: 11.9%). The differences were significant when PA intensity was stratified by gender using Fisher's exact test.

BMI and WC statuses were stratified by age using Chi-square for trend analysis and presented in Table 2. The prevalence of general overweight and obesity was 10.0% and 1.8%, respectively, in students aged 18–24 years, 4.8% and 2.4% in those aged 25–31 years, and 30.0% and 0.0% in those aged 32–28 years. The differences were not significant when BMI status was stratified by age category using Chi-square for trend analysis.

The prevalence of abdominal obesity was 3.5% in students aged 18–24 years, 4.8% in those aged 25–31 years, and 0.0% in those aged 32–38 years.

Using Chi-square for trend analysis, PA intensity was stratified by BMI and WC and presented in Figure 1. About 14.0% of normal weight students engaged in light PA, 47.4% in moderate PA, and 39.1% in vigorous PA. Generally, the prevalence of normal weight increased with an increase in PA intensity. Significantly, 85.0% of overweight students engaged in either light or moderate activity compared to 15.0% of them engaging in vigorous activity (P = 0.0014). The prevalence of obesity decreased significantly with an increase in PA intensity. Out of the 27 abdominally obese students, 22.2% participated in light PA, 44.4% in moderate PA, and 33.3% in vigorous PA. However, the differences were not significant when abdominal obesity was stratified by PA intensity using Chi-square for trend analysis.

The effect of different factors on the risk of developing obesity is recorded in Table 3. The factors that increased general obesity as determined by univariate analysis were being female, engaging in light PA, being aged 28–37 years, nonintake of coffee, being married, and being abdominally obese.

Table 4 shows the effect of lifestyle factors on the risk of developing abdominal obesity. Female students were several-fold at risk of developing abdominal obesity. Other lifestyle factors that increased the risk of developing abdominal obesity were nonintake of coffee, being married, and having general obesity.

4. Discussion

The current study brings to light the occurrence of general obesity and abdominal obesity and their associated risk factors coexisting with underweight among young adults in a developing country undergoing nutrition transition. It presents the problem of the double burden of malnutrition that requires a comprehensive approach to curb it. Results of this study emphasized the need for adopting a health policy to assess and control obesity and its risk factors among young adults in Ghana. University students provide an enormous opportunity for health authorities to design targeted programs to help curb the rising prevalence of obesity in older adults.

In the current study, the prevalence of general overweight and obesity was found to be 9.3% and 1.9%, respectively. Our findings concur with the 11.4% and 2.0% prevalence of overweight and obesity, respectively, among medical students in Delhi [25] and 10.4% prevalence of overweight among university students in Malaysia [26]. The prevalence of obesity in this study can be said to be among the lowest in literature in Sub-Saharan Africa and other countries. A study among university students living in halls of residence of the Nsukka campus of the University of Nigeria showed that 21.0% of the participants were obese [27]. Another study in 2008 among students of a Nigerian university found 23.9% and 3.4% of the study participants being overweight and obese, respectively [28]. In

Variable	Total (n = 646)	Male (n = 445)	Female (n = 201)	P value
Mean ± SD (age)	23.06 ± 2.77	23.52 ± 2.83	22.03 ± 2.33	<0.0001
Smoking				
Yes	7 (1.1%)	7 (1.3%)	0 (0.0%)	0.1055
No	639 (98.9%)	438 (98.4%)	201 (100.0%)	
Drinks alcohol				
Yes	85 (13.2%)	70 (15.7%)	15 (7.5%)	0.8805
No	561 (86.8%)	375 (84.3%)	186 (92.5%)	
Drinks coffee				
Yes	369 (57.1%)	260 (58.4%)	109 (54.2%)	0.3451
No	277 (42.9%)	185 (41.6%)	92 (45.8%)	
Married				
Yes	38 (5.9%)	29 (6.5%)	9 (4.2%)	0.3689
No	608 (94.1%)	416 (93.4%)	192 (90.6%)	
BMI status				
Underweight	32 (5.0%)	20 (4.5%)	12 (6.0%)	0.4367
Normal weight	542 (83.9%)	404 (90.8%)	138 (68.7%)	<0.0001
Overweight	60 (9.3%)	18 (4.0%)	42 (20.9%)	<0.0001
Obesity	12 (1.9%)	3 (0.7%)	9 (4.5%)	0.0021
Mean ± SD (BMI)	**21.79 ± 3.10**	**21.32 ± 2.33**	**22.84 ± 4.15**	<0.0001
Abdominal obesity				
Yes	27 (4.2%)	3 (0.7%)	24 (11.9%)	<0.0001
No	619 (95.8%)	442 (99.3%)	177 (88.1%)	
Mean ± SD	**77.36 ± 6.45**	**76.32 ± 4.79**	**79.65 ± 8.74**	<0.0001
Physical activity				
Light	95 (14.7%)	37 (8.3%)	58 (28.9%)	<0.0001
Moderate	315 (48.8%)	196 (44.0%)	119 (59.2%)	0.0005
Vigorous	236 (36.5%)	212 (47.6%)	24 (11.9%)	<0.0001

Data are presented as proportion and compared using Fischer's exact test.

TABLE 2: BMI status and abdominal obesity stratified by age.

Variable	18–24 (n = 510)	25–31 (n = 126)	32–38 (n = 10)	Chi-square	P value
BMI status					
Underweight	28 (5.5%)	4 (3.2%)	0 (0.0%)	1.67	0.1965
Normal weight	422 (82.7%)	113 (89.7%)	7 (70.0%)	1.13	0.2879
Overweight	51 (10.0%)	6 (4.8%)	3 (30.0%)	0.22	0.6411
Obesity	9 (1.8%)	3 (2.4%)	0 (0.0%)	0.03	0.8533
Abdominal obesity					
Yes	18 (3.5%)	6 (4.8%)	0 (0.0%)	0.07	0.7918
No	492 (96.5%)	120 (95.2%)	10 (100.0%)	—	—

Data was presented as proportion and analyzed using Chi-square for trend.

Malaysia, Gopalakrishnan et al. [29] found the prevalence of overweight and obesity to be 14.8% and 21.1% among medical students.

The prevalence of abdominal obesity measured by WC was found to be 4.2% and higher than the prevalence of general obesity. This corresponds with the findings of Hazizi et al. [26] among university students in which the prevalence of abdominal obesity was found to be 17.2% as determined by WC and 3.4% as determined by BMI. WC is more sensitive than BMI. Waist circumference correlates more closely with

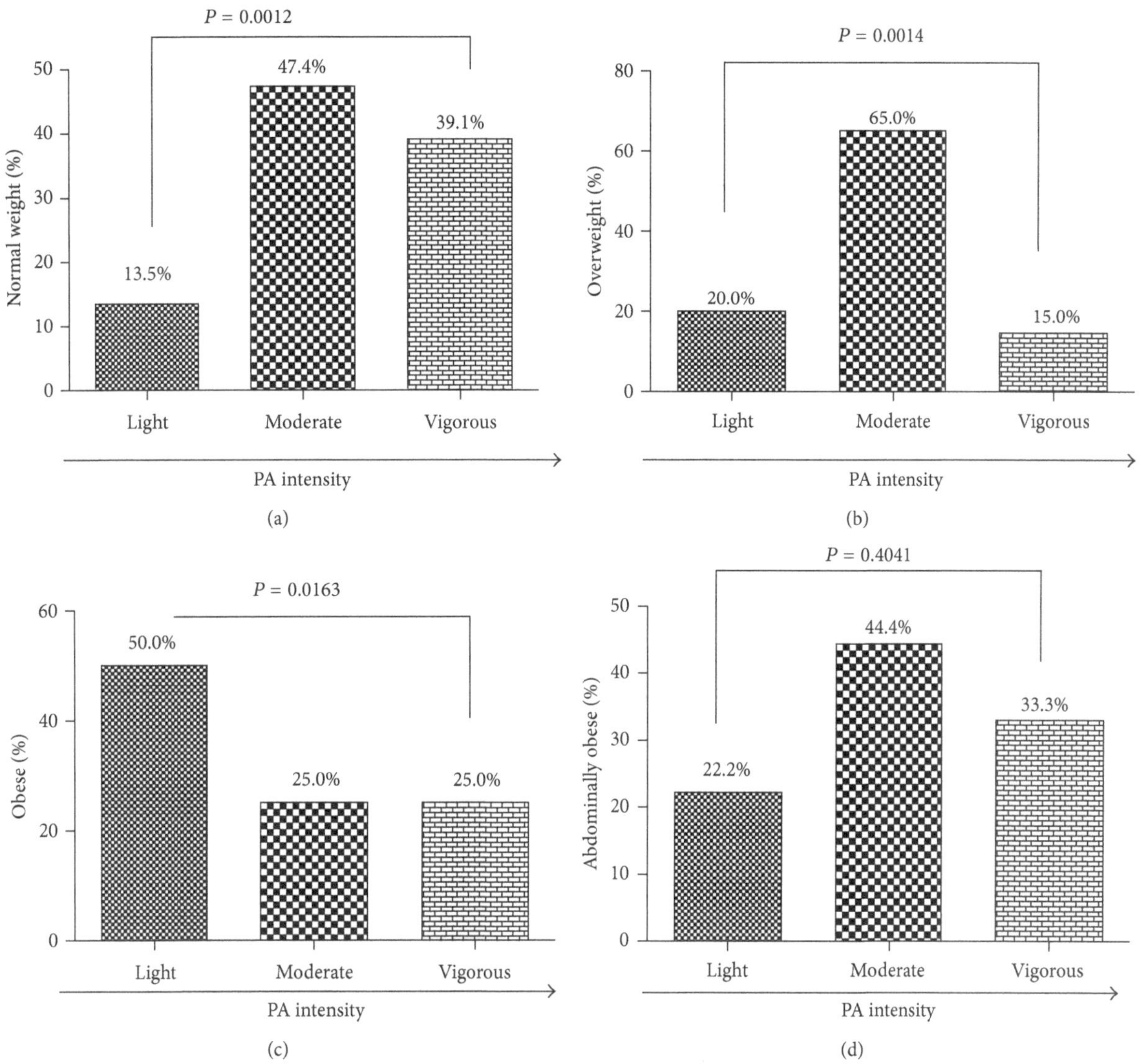

FIGURE 1: Association between PA intensity and normal weight (a), PA intensity and overweight (b), PA intensity and obesity (c), and PA intensity and abdominal obesity (d). Data was presented as proportion and analyzed using Chi-square for trend.

abdominal adipose tissue than BMI [16]. It is much easier and more accurate to measure WC than to measure weight and height [16]. In addition WC is a strong predictor of all-cause mortality in young and middle-aged adults compared to older people and those with low BMI [17]. Measures of abdominal obesity have also been shown to be better than BMI as predictors of CVD risk, although combining BMI with these measures may improve their discriminatory capability [30]. This suggests that relying on only BMI might underestimate the proportion of obese students and those at risk of developing CVDs and diabetes.

Generally, studies in older Ghanaians had a higher prevalence of obesity than seen in this study [19, 31, 32]. The implication of this finding is that efforts at addressing general and abdominal obesity in the adult population should commence at younger ages. This will help to address chronic diseases such as CVDs and diabetes. University students could be appropriate targets for such interventions.

The prevalence of both general and abdominal obesity was significantly higher in female than in male students. Using univariate analysis female students were severalfold at risk of developing general and abdominal obesity. This concurs with several studies conducted among young and older adults in Sub-Saharan Africa [19, 27, 28, 31, 33, 34]. This could be due to the fact that more females than males significantly participated in light PA. Findings of the current study showed that participants who engaged in light PA were severalfold at risk of becoming obese as determined by BMI. The higher prevalence of general and abdominal obesity in female students could also be as a result of the notion that being obese is considered as a sign of well-being in Africa. A study among university students in Nigeria showed that most subjects believed that being obese gives respect and is a sign of living well [35].

Interestingly, nondrinkers of coffee were at 4.1 and 4.2 times at risk of developing general and abdominal obesity

TABLE 3: Risk factors for general obesity using univariate analysis.

Variable	n/N^*	Rate of obesity	OR (95% CI)	P value
Gender				
Male	3/445	0.7%	6.9 (1.85–25.80)	0.0021
Female	9/201	4.5%	Ref	Ref
Physical activity				
Light	6/37	16.2%	Ref	Ref
Moderate	3/196	1.5%	12.45 (2.96–52.41)	0.0006
Vigorous	3/212	1.4%	13.48 (3.21–56.72)	0.0004
Age				
18–27	9/605	1.5%	5.4 (1.39–20.68)	0.0329
28–37	3/41	7.3%	Ref	Ref
Smoking				
Yes	0/7	0.0%	Ref	Ref
No	12/639	1.9%	3.3 (0.18–61.91)	1
Alcohol consumption				
Yes	0/85	0.0%	Ref	Ref
No	12/561	2.1%	0.3 (0.02–4.39)	0.3825
Drinks coffee				
Yes	3/369	0.8%	4.1 (1.10–15.28)	0.0357
No	9/277	3.2%	Ref	Ref
Marital status				
Yes	3/38	7.9%	Ref	Ref
No	9/608	1.5%	5.7 (1.48–22.02)	0.0286
Abdominal obesity				
Yes	9/27	33.3%	Ref	Ref
No	3/619	0.5%	102.7 (25.61–11.60)	<0.0001

*Number of subjects with general obesity/number of subjects in each category. Ref refers to reference point.

respectively. This presents an inverse relationship between coffee consumption and body fat. Findings on the effect of coffee on body fat have been inconsistent. A cross-sectional study among a noninstitutionalized US population showed that coffee consumption was not related to BMI or WC in either gender [36]. However, a study by Lopez-Garcia et al. [37] found that an increase in coffee consumption was associated with less weight gain. Caffeine, the chemical found in coffee, has been shown to have an effect on weight gain and weight loss. Caffeine has been shown to stimulate the utilization of fat in muscle tissue during exercise [38]. In addition, Astrup et al. [39] reported a dose-dependent increase in basal energy expenditure with caffeine intake in healthy subjects who had moderate habitual caffeine consumption attributing the effect to an increase in lactate and triacylglycerol production and increased vascular smooth muscle tone. Acheson et al. [40] suggested that caffeine may stimulate thermogenesis by increasing lipid turnover. All the above mechanisms suggest a beneficial effect of caffeine on energy metabolism thereby resulting in weight loss. A limitation of our study was that information on coffee consumption was self-reported. In addition the quantity, flavor, and frequency of coffee consumed were not also assessed.

Students who were married were 5.7 and 6.1 times at risk of developing general and abdominal obesity. In consonance with our findings a nationwide cross-sectional survey in Iran found that currently and formerly married individuals were more overweight or obese than those never married [41]. Several cross-sectional studies have reported similar relationships [42–45]. However, other studies have also reported inconsistent findings ranging from the lack of association [46, 47] to a protective effect of marriage [48]. The positive relationship between marital status and obesity or abdominal obesity found in this study could be related to the fact that married people engage in less physical activity after marriage, have a more stable dietary pattern, and may place less emphasis on being attractive [41].

Using Chi-square for trend analysis age was not associated with obesity or with abdominal obesity. However, using univariate analysis participants aged 28–37 were 5.7 times at risk of developing obesity. This is in keeping to the fact that general and abdominal obesity increase with increase in age. This is in agreement with several studies conducted among young [49] and older adults [50–52]. The proportion of fat deposited in the abdomen increases as body shape becomes more android with age, due to decreasing height and increasing slackness of abdominal wall muscles. During adulthood, weight gain occurs in the abdominal region, emphasizing the importance of hypertrophic obesity, which is generally android [53]. This change in the adult figure may

Table 4: Risk factors for abdominal obesity using univariate analysis.

Variable	n/N^*	Rate of abdominal obesity	OR (95% CI)	P value
Gender				
Male	0/445	0.0%	123.0 (7.43–2035.00)	<0.0001
Female	24/201	11.9%	Ref	Ref
Physical activity				
Light	6/95	6.3%	Ref	Ref
Moderate	12/315	3.8%	1.7 (0.62–4.67)	0.3888
Vigorous	6/236	2.5%	2.6 (0.81–8.23)	0.1102
Smoking				
Yes	0/7	0.0%	0.6 (0.03–10.76)	1.0000
No	24/639	3.8%	Ref	Ref
Drinks alcohol				
Yes	3/85	3.5%	1.1 (0.310–3.64)	1.0000
No	21/561	3.7%	Ref	
Drinks coffee				
Yes	6/369	1.6%	4.2 (1.65–10.74)	0.0014
No	18/277	6.5%	Ref	Ref
Age				
18–27	21/605	3.5%	2.2 (0.63–7.69)	0.1902
28–37	3/41	7.3%		
Marital status				
Yes	6/38	15.8%	Ref	Ref
No	18/608	3.0%	6.1 (2.28–16.54)	0.0017
Obesity				
Yes	9/12	75.00%	Ref	Ref
No	15/634	2.40%	123.8 (30.41–503.90)	<0.0001

*Number of subjects with distortion/number of subjects in each category. Ref refers to reference point.

influence the positive association between age and excess abdominal adiposity [54].

Students who were abdominally obese were severalfold at risk of developing obesity and those generally obese were also severalfold at risk of developing abdominal obesity. A longitudinal, population-based birth cohort study conducted by Laitinen et al. [55] among 31-year-old men found high BMI as an important predictor of abdominal obesity.

Even though smoking has been shown to be associated with general and abdominal obesity in some studies [56, 57], a significant association was not found in this study. This could be due to the fact that a small proportion of the sample ever smoked. Notwithstanding, several other studies have also found no significant association between smoking and obesity [55].

Alcohol consumption was not a significant risk factor for both obesity and abdominal obesity. Several conflicting findings have been reported on the effect of alcohol on obesity ([58–61]). A study among randomly selected adults aged ≥18 years in Brazil showed that participants who consumed alcohol had a higher probability of being centrally obese among men and women [62]. A similar association has also been reported among Korean adults [63]. Other studies report that light alcohol drinking is known to be associated with lower incidence of obesity [56]. Another study among middle-aged women found that the risk of becoming overweight was almost 30 percent lower for women who consumed one or two alcoholic beverages a day, compared to nondrinkers [64]. The lack of association in our study could be due to the fact that quantity and frequency of alcohol consumed were not measured and students self-reported their consumption status.

Our study is not without limitations. This study was conducted on a sample of only university students without considering young adults from other nonuniversity tertiary students and those out of school. This makes it difficult to generalize the findings to the entire young adult population in Ghana. Even though the findings of this study are comparable to previous studies, its cross-sectional design makes it unable to establish causality.

5. Conclusion

The prevalence of abdominal obesity was higher than general obesity. Associated risk factors of both general and abdominal obesity were being female, engaging in light PA, being married, and nonintake of coffee. Health authorities should design health and nutrition education programs that target young adults in our tertiary institutions.

Conflict of Interests

The right of the authors to examine, analyze, and publish the data of the research is not infringed upon by any contractual agreement or conflict of interests.

Acknowledgments

The authors wish to thank the Metropolitan Director and the Nutrition Officer of the Tamale Metropolitan Health Directorate for making anthropometric instruments for the data collection available to them. They also wish to make special mention of Dr. Nafiu Amidu, Dr. Abass Alhassan, and Mr. Evans Ameade, all of the University for Development Studies, School of Medicine and Health Sciences, for their insightful contributions during the write-up of the paper.

References

[1] W. P. T. James, R. Jackson-Leach, C. Ni Mhurchu et al., "Overweight and obesity (high body mass index)," in *Comparative Quantification of Health Risks: Global and Regional Burden of Disease Attribution to Selected Major Risk Factors*, vol. 1, pp. 497–596, 2004.

[2] WHO, "Reducing Risks, Promoting Healthy Life," The World Health Report", World Health Organization, Geneva, Switzerland, 2002, http://www.who.int/whr/2002/en/whr02_en.pdf?ua=1.

[3] A. H. Mokdad, B. A. Bowman, E. S. Ford, F. Vinicor, J. S. Marks, and J. P. Koplan, "The continuing epidemics of obesity and diabetes in the United States," *The Journal of the American Medical Association*, vol. 286, no. 10, pp. 1195–1200, 2001.

[4] A. H. Mokdad, M. K. Serdula, W. H. Dietz, B. A. Bowman, J. S. Marks, and J. P. Koplan, "The spread of the obesity epidemic in the United States, 1991-1998," *The Journal of the American Medical Association*, vol. 282, no. 16, pp. 1519–1522, 1999.

[5] K. M. Flegal, M. D. Carroll, C. L. Ogden, and C. L. Johnson, "Prevalence and trends in obesity among US adults, 1999-2000," *The Journal of the American Medical Association*, vol. 288, no. 14, pp. 1723–1727, 2002.

[6] A. R. Abubakari, W. Lauder, C. Agyemang, M. Jones, A. Kirk, and R. S. Bhopal, "Prevalence and time trends in obesity among adult West African populations: a meta-analysis," *Obesity Reviews*, vol. 9, no. 4, pp. 297–311, 2008.

[7] V. Mogre, P. P. Mwinlenaa, J. Oladele, and A. Amalba, "Impact of physical activity levels and diet on central obesity among civil servants in Tamale metropolis," *Journal of Medical and Biomedical Sciences*, vol. 1, no. 2, pp. 1–9, 2012.

[8] K. Steyn and A. Damasceno, "Lifestyle and related risk factors for chronic diseases," in *Disease and Mortality in Sub-Saharan Africa*, World Bank, Washington, DC, USA, 2nd edition, 2006.

[9] H. S. Kruger, T. Puoane, M. Senekal, and M.-T. van der Merwe, "Obesity in South Africa: challenges for government and health professionals," *Public Health Nutrition*, vol. 8, no. 5, pp. 491–500, 2005.

[10] R. S. Strauss and H. A. Pollack, "Epidemic increase in childhood overweight, 1986-1998," *The Journal of the American Medical Association*, vol. 286, no. 22, pp. 2845–2848, 2001.

[11] M. K. Serdula, D. Ivery, R. J. Coates, D. S. Freedman, D. F. Williamson, and T. Byers, "Do obese children become obese adults? A review of the literature," *Preventive Medicine*, vol. 22, no. 2, pp. 167–177, 1993.

[12] R. C. Whitaker, J. A. Wright, M. S. Pepe, K. D. Seidel, and W. H. Dietz, "Predicting obesity in young adulthood from childhood and parental obesity," *The New England Journal of Medicine*, vol. 337, no. 13, pp. 869–873, 1997.

[13] V. Mogre, E. Aneyire, and E. Gyamfi, "Physical activity and BMI status of school-age children in Tamale, Northern Ghana," *Pakistan Journal of Nutrition*, vol. 12, no. 5, pp. 484–490, 2013.

[14] H. Ene-Obong, V. Ibeanu, N. Onuoha, and A. Ejekwu, "Prevalence of overweight, obesity, and thinness among urban school-aged children and adolescents in southern Nigeria," *Food and Nutrition Bulletin*, vol. 33, no. 4, pp. 242–250, 2012.

[15] T. C. Mosha and S. Fungo, "Prevalence of overweight and obesity among children aged 6–12 years in Dodoma and Kinondoni municipalities, Tanzania," *Tanzania Journal of Health Research*, vol. 12, no. 1, pp. 6–16, 2010.

[16] WHO, "Waist circumference and waist-hip ratio: report of a WHO expert consultation," WHO, Geneva, Switzerland, 2008.

[17] J. C. Seidell, "Waist circumference and waist/hip ratio in relation to all-cause mortality, cancer and sleep apnea," *European Journal of Clinical Nutrition*, vol. 64, no. 1, pp. 35–41, 2010.

[18] E. Sobngwi, J.-C. N. Mbanya, N. C. Unwin et al., "Physical activity and its relationship with obesity, hypertension and diabetes in urban and rural Cameroon," *International Journal of Obesity*, vol. 26, no. 7, pp. 1009–1016, 2002.

[19] J. Addo, L. Smeeth, and D. A. Leon, "Obesity in urban civil servants in Ghana: association with pre-adult wealth and adult socio-economic status," *Public Health*, vol. 123, no. 5, pp. 365–370, 2009.

[20] N. Yahia, A. Achkar, A. Abdallah, and S. Rizk, "Eating habits and obesity among Lebanese university students," *Nutrition Journal*, vol. 7, article 32, 2008.

[21] WHO, "Obesity: preventing and managing the global epidemic," WHO, Geneva, Switzerland, 2000.

[22] WHO, "Global physical activity surveillance," 2009, http:// www.who.int/chp/steps/GPAQ/en/index.html.

[23] T. Armstrong and F. Bull, "Development of the World Health Organization global physical activity questionnaire (GPAQ)," *Journal of Public Health*, vol. 14, no. 2, pp. 66–70, 2006.

[24] B. E. Ainsworth, W. L. Haskell, M. C. Whitt et al., "Compendium of physical activities: an update of activity codes and MET intensities," *Medicine & Science in Sports & Exercise*, vol. 32, no. 9, pp. S498–S504, 2000.

[25] P. Chhabra, V. Grover, K. Aggarwal, and A. T. Kannan, "Nutritional status and blood pressure of medical students in Delhi," *Indian Journal of Community Medicine*, vol. 31, pp. 248-251, 2006.

[26] A. S. Hazizi, B. M. Hamdi, Y. M. Leong, and T. Izumi, "Assessment of physical activity among undergraduate students in a local university using a pedometer," *Health and Environment Journal*, vol. 3, no. 1, 2012.

[27] U. A. Onyechi and A. C. Okolo, "Prevalence of obesity among undergraduate students, living in halls of residence, University of Nigeria, Nsukka campus, Enugu state," *Animal Research International*, vol. 5, no. 3, pp. 928–931, 2008.

[28] K. E. Oghagbon, V. U. Odili, E. K. Nwangwa, and K. E. Pender, "Body mass index and blood pressure pattern of students in a Nigerian University," *International Journal of Health Research*, vol. 2, no. 2, pp. 177–182, 2009.

[29] S. Gopalakrishnan, P. Ganeshkumar, M. V. Prakash, Christopher, and V. Amalraj, "Prevalence of overweight/obesity among the medical students, Malaysia," *The Medical Journal of Malaysia*, vol. 67, no. 4, pp. 442–444, 2012.

[30] R. Huxley, S. Mendis, E. Zheleznyakov, S. Reddy, and J. Chan, "Body mass index, waist circumference and waist: hip ratio as predictors of cardiovascular risk—a review of the literature," *European Journal of Clinical Nutrition*, vol. 64, no. 1, pp. 16–22, 2010.

[31] V. Mogre, P. P. Mwinlennaa, and J. Oladele, "Distorted self-perceived weight status and its associated factors among civil servants in Tamale, Ghana: a cross-sectional study," *Archives of Public Health*, vol. 71, no. 1, article 30, 2013.

[32] I. Danquah, G. Bedu-Addo, K.-J. Terpe et al., "Diabetes mellitus type 2 in urban Ghana: characteristics and associated factors," *BMC Public Health*, vol. 12, no. 1, article 210, 2012.

[33] T. O. Lawoyin, M. C. Asuzu, J. Kaufman et al., "Prevalence of cardiovascular risk factors in an African, urban inner city community," *West African Journal of Medicine*, vol. 21, no. 3, pp. 208–211, 2002.

[34] H. H. Vorster, "The emergence of cardiovascular disease during urbanisation of Africans," *Public Health Nutrition*, vol. 5, no. 1, pp. 239–243, 2002.

[35] E. O. Ojofeitimi, A. O. Adeyeye, A. O. Fadiora et al., "Awareness of obesity and its health hazard among women in a university community," *Pakistan Journal of Nutrition*, vol. 6, no. 5, pp. 502–505, 2007.

[36] D. R. Bouchard, R. Ross, and I. Janssen, "Coffee, tea and their additives: association with BMI and waist circumference," *Obesity Facts*, vol. 3, no. 6, pp. 345–352, 2010.

[37] E. Lopez-Garcia, R. M. van Dam, S. Rajpathak, W. C. Willett, J. E. Manson, and F. B. Hu, "Changes in caffeine intake and long-term weight change in men and women," *The American Journal of Clinical Nutrition*, vol. 83, no. 3, pp. 674–680, 2006.

[38] L. L. Spriet, D. A. MacLean, D. J. Dyck, E. Hultman, G. Cederblad, and T. E. Graham, "Caffeine ingestion and muscle metabolism during prolonged exercise in humans," *American Journal of Physiology*, vol. 262, no. 6, pp. E891–E898, 1992.

[39] A. Astrup, S. Toubro, S. Cannon, P. Hein, L. Breum, and J. Madsen, "Caffeine: a double-blind, placebo-controlled study of its thermogenic, metabolic, and cardiovascular effects in healthy volunteers," *The American Journal of Clinical Nutrition*, vol. 51, no. 5, pp. 759–767, 1990.

[40] K. J. Acheson, G. Gremaud, I. Meirim et al., "Metabolic effects of caffeine in humans: lipid oxidation or futile cycling?" *The American Journal of Clinical Nutrition*, vol. 79, no. 1, pp. 40–46, 2004.

[41] M. Janghorbani, M. Amini, H. Rezvanian et al., "Association of body mass index and abdominal obesity with marital status in adults," *Archives of Iranian Medicine*, vol. 11, no. 3, pp. 274–281, 2008.

[42] C. E. Ross and J. Mirowsky, "Social epidemiology of overweight: a substantive and methodological investigation," *Journal of Health and Social Behavior*, vol. 24, no. 3, pp. 288–298, 1983.

[43] J. Sobal, B. S. Rauschenbach, and E. A. Frongillo Jr., "Marital status, fatness and obesity," *Social Science & Medicine*, vol. 35, no. 7, pp. 915–923, 1992.

[44] S. Evers, "Economic and social factors associated with obesity in adult Canadians," *Nutrition Research*, vol. 7, no. 1, pp. 3–13, 1987.

[45] T. K. Young and G. Sevenhuysen, "Obesity in northern Canadian Indians: patterns, determinants, and consequences," *The American Journal of Clinical Nutrition*, vol. 49, no. 5, pp. 786–793, 1989.

[46] F. Kittel, R. M. Rustin, and M. Dramaix, "Psycho-socio-biological correlates of moderate overweight in an industrial population," *Journal of Psychosomatic Research*, vol. 22, no. 3, pp. 145–158, 1978.

[47] M. Shah, R. W. Jeffrey, P. J. Hannan, and L. Onstad, "Relationship between socio-demographic and behaviour variables, and body mass index in a population with high-normal blood pressure: hypertension prevention trial," *European Journal of Clinical Nutrition*, vol. 43, no. 9, pp. 583–596, 1989.

[48] F. E. M. Braddon, B. Rodgers, M. E. J. Wadsworth, and J. M. C. Davies, "Onset of obesity in a 36 year birth cohort study," *British Medical Journal*, vol. 293, no. 6542, pp. 299–303, 1986.

[49] A. A. Suleiman, O. K. Alboqai, N. Yasein, J. M. El-Qudah, M. F. Bataineh, and B. A. Obeidat, "Prevalence of and factors associated with overweight and obesity among Jordan University students," *Journal of Biological Sciences*, vol. 9, no. 7, pp. 738–745, 2009.

[50] C. U. Odenigbo, O. C. Oguejiofor, and U. M. Odenigbo, "Prevalence of abdominal obesity in senior civil servants in Asaba, Nigeria," *Tropical Journal of Medical Research*, vol. 12, no. 2, pp. 1–3, 2008.

[51] T. Puoane, K. Steyn, D. Bradshaw et al., "Obesity in South Africa: the South African demographic and health survey," *Obesity Research*, vol. 10, no. 10, pp. 1038–1048, 2002.

[52] M. E. Díaz, S. Jiménez, R. G. García, M. Bonet, and I. Wong, "Overweight, obesity, central adiposity and associated chronic diseases in Cuban adults," *MEDICC Review*, vol. 11, no. 4, pp. 23–28, 2009.

[53] S. A. Kaye, A. R. Folsom, R. J. Prineas, J. D. Potter, and S. M. Gapstur, "The association of body fat distribution with lifestyle and reproductive factors in a population study of postmenopausal women," *International Journal of Obesity*, vol. 14, no. 7, pp. 583–591, 1990.

[54] D. J. Lanska, M. J. Lanska, A. J. Hartz, and A. A. Rimm, "Factors influencing anatomic location of fat tissue in 52,953 women," *International Journal of Obesity*, vol. 9, no. 1, pp. 29–38, 1985.

[55] J. Laitinen, K. Pietiläinen, M. Wadsworth, U. Sovio, and M.-R. Järvelin, "Predictors of abdominal obesity among 31-y-old men and women born in Northern Finland in 1966," *European Journal of Clinical Nutrition*, vol. 58, no. 1, pp. 180–190, 2004.

[56] I. I. Chukwuonye, A. Chuku, U. U. Onyeonoro et al., "Prevalence of abdominal obesity in Abia state, Nigeria: results of a population-based house-to-house survey," *Diabetes, Metabolic Syndrome and Obesity*, vol. 2013, no. 6, pp. 285–291, 2013.

[57] S. E. Saarni, K. Pietiläinen, S. Kantonen, A. Rissanen, and J. Kaprio, "Association of smoking in adolescence with abdominal obesity in adulthood: a follow-up study of 5 birth cohorts of Finnish twins," *American Journal of Public Health*, vol. 99, no. 2, pp. 348–354, 2009.

[58] M. Lahti-Koski, P. Pietinen, M. Heliövaara, and E. Vartiainen, "Associations of body mass index and obesity with physical activity, food choices, alcohol intake, and smoking in the 1982–1997 FINRISK studies," *The American Journal of Clinical Nutrition*, vol. 75, no. 5, pp. 809–817, 2002.

[59] M. Fisher and T. Gordon, "The relation of drinking and smoking habits to diet: the lipid research clinics prevalence study," *The American Journal of Clinical Nutrition*, vol. 41, no. 3, pp. 623–630, 1985.

[60] T. Ruf, G. Nagel, H.-P. Altenburg, A. B. Miller, and B. Thorand, "Food and nutrient intake, anthropometric measurements and smoking according to alcohol consumption in the EPIC Heidelberg study," *Annals of Nutrition & Metabolism*, vol. 49, no. 1, pp. 16–25, 2005.

[61] M. Thomson, M. Fulton, R. A. Elton, S. Brown, D. A. Wood, and M. F. Oliver, "Alcohol consumption and nutrient intake in middle-aged Scottish men," *The American Journal of Clinical Nutrition*, vol. 47, no. 1, pp. 139–145, 1988.

[62] S. Lourenco, A. Oliveira, and C. Lopes, "The effect of current and lifetime alcohol consumption on overall and central obesity," *European Journal of Clinical Nutrition*, vol. 66, no. 7, pp. 813–818, 2012.

[63] M. Ryu, H. Kimm, J. Jo, S. J. Lee, and S. H. Jee, "Association between alcohol intake and abdominal obesity among the Korean population," *Epidemiol Health*, vol. 32, Article ID e2010007, 6 pages, 2010.

[64] L. Wang, I.-M. Lee, J. E. Manson, J. E. Buring, and H. D. Sesso, "Alcohol consumption, weight gain, and risk of becoming overweight in middle-aged and older women," *Archives of Internal Medicine*, vol. 170, no. 5, pp. 453–461, 2010.

7

A Single Institution's Overweight Pediatric Population and Their Associated Comorbid Conditions

Sigrid Bairdain,[1] Chueh Lien,[1] Alexander P. Stoffan,[1] Michael Troy,[1] Donald C. Simonson,[2] and Bradley C. Linden[3]

[1] *Department of Pediatric Surgery, Boston Children's Hospital, Harvard Medical School, Boston, MA 02115, USA*
[2] *Division of Endocrinology, Brigham & Women's Hospital, Harvard Medical School, Boston, MA 02115, USA*
[3] *Pediatric Surgical Associates, Children's Hospitals and Clinics of Minnesota, 2530 Chicago Avenue, South, Suite 550, Minneapolis, MN 55404, USA*

Correspondence should be addressed to Bradley C. Linden; blinden@pediatricsurgical.com

Academic Editors: E. Rodríguez and C. Schmidt

Background. Obesity studies are often performed on population data. We sought to examine the incidence of obesity and its associated comorbidities in a single freestanding children's hospital. *Methods.* We performed a retrospective analysis of all visits to Boston Children's Hospital from 2000 to 2012. This was conducted to determine the incidence of obesity, morbid obesity, and associated comorbidities. Each comorbidity was modeled independently. Incidence rate ratios were calculated, as well as odds ratios. *Results.* A retrospective review of 3,185,658 person-years in nonobese, 26,404 person-years in obese, and 25,819 person-years in the morbidly obese was conducted. Annual rates of all major comorbidities were increased in all patients, as well as in our obese and morbidly obese counterparts. Incidence rate ratios (IRR) and odds ratios (OR) were also significantly increased across all conditions for both our obese and morbidly obese patients. *Conclusions.* These data illustrate the substantial increases in obesity and associated comorbid conditions. Study limitations include (1) single institution data, (2) retrospective design, and (3) administrative undercoding. Future treatment options need to address these threats to longevity and quality of life.

1. Introduction

The increased prevalence of overweight and obese children is not new, yet it has been viewed more recently as a public health epidemic [1–3]. According to the Centers for Disease Control and Prevention (CDC), approximately 12.5 million, or 17%, of American children are obese. More recent studies show that over 10% of 2–5-year-olds would be classified as overweight, whereas this number increases to 15% in the adolescent age group [4].

Interestingly, in 2000 the US Preventive Services Task Force (USPSTF) did not find enough evidence to recommend for or against routine screening for overweight status in either children or adolescents as a means of mitigating further health sequelae, yet now the task force is revisiting this idea as of 2010 [5]. It is known that a higher prevalence of comorbid diseases attributable to obesity is seen in both adults and children, especially modifiable cardiovascular risk factors and sequelae. In the long-standing Bogalusa Heart study, body mass indexes (BMI) performed in childhood and adolescence, as a measurement for obesity, predicted intima-media thickness in adults [6].

Obesity is not only related to modifiable cardiovascular risk factors, but also to several other health-related conditions that may persist or worsen in adulthood [7, 8]. This includes asthma, orthopedic disorders, depression and anxiety, liver abnormalities, and endocrine related issues including type 2 diabetes, hyperlipidemia, and polycystic ovarian syndrome (PCOS) [9]. Further studies may reflect resolution in these conditions with increased awareness of the association between obesity and multiple comorbid conditions. However, these studies are often performed on population-based level. Therefore, we sought to examine the incidence of the diverse sequelae of obesity and morbid obesity, as evidenced by

Table 1: Study design: inclusion criteria and definitions of patient groups in a specific year.

Patient group	Inclusion/exclusion filters and definitions
All patients	patients with encounter start dates within a specific year[a]
All patients *with* condition	Include (condition criteria + date criteria)
Obese patients	Include (obesity criteria + date criteria)
Obese patients *with* condition	Include (obesity criteria + date criteria) Include (condition criteria + date criteria)
Obese patients *without* condition	Include (obesity criteria + date criteria) Exclude (condition criteria + date criteria)
Nonobese patients	(*All* patients) minus (*obese* patients)
Nonobese patients *with* condition	(*All* patients *with* condition) minus (*obese* patients *with* condition)
Nonobese patients *without* condition	(*Nonobese* patients) minus (*nonobese* patients *with* condition)

[a]Data provided by the Clinical Research Informatics group at Boston Children's Hospital.

its associated comorbidities in a single, large, free-standing, children's hospital.

2. Methods

2.1. Data Source. This study was conducted with the approval of the Institutional Review Board at Boston Children's Hospital (IRB-P00001304). No individual patient health information was collected in this study. All inpatient and outpatient visits to Boston Children's Hospital between January 1, 2000, and December 31, 2012, were included in the dataset. These visit were queried through the Informatics for Integrating Biology and the Bedside (i2b2) data warehouse platform (i2b2 v. 1.4; USA) implemented at the institution [10]. The i2b2 system allowed investigators to perform queries on an enterprise data repository through its web-based interface [11]. Selected demographics information in Epic computer system and information on hospital-billed diagnoses in Cerner, in the form of International Classification of Diseases, 9th Revision, Clinical Modification (ICD-9) codes, were available through i2b2.

The data collected was not stratified based on age, gender, nor whether the visit was an inpatient or outpatient visit in nature. Using the i2b2 web client, queries were entered in the form of inclusion or exclusion "filter" groups based on ICD-9 codes and date criteria, with date criteria based on the start date of the encounters. Our queries and calculations are described in Table 1. We obtained counts for different "patient groups" by year based on the respective administrative diagnosis. Temporal constraints were set to treat all groups independently as opposed to have the "filter" groups occur in the same financial encounter. To account for the children and adolescents in our study population, both adult and pediatric ICD-9 criteria were used in determining obesity status, utilizing both the BMI categorization standard as defined by World Health Organization and the percentile standard as defined by American Medical Association [12, 13]. ICD-9 code criteria for obesity status and comorbid conditions are further described in Table 2. A single condition was considered met if one or more of its ICD-9 criteria were coded. To help limit the number of "double-counting," a patient was only counted once in each "patient group" regardless of how many ICD-9 criteria of the same condition the patient has met in that particular year.

Table 2: Study design with ICD-9-CM filter criteria.

Condition	ICD-9-CM codes
Obesity condition	
Obese	V85.4, V85.54, 278.01, V85.3, V85.53, 278.00
Morbidly obese	V85.4, V85.54, 278.01
Major comorbid condition	
Type 2 diabetes	250.00, 250.01, 250.02, 250.03
Hyperlipidemia	272.0, 271.1, 272.2, 272.3, 272.4
Hypertension	401, 405
Sleep apnea	327.23
Asthma	493
Depression	296.2, 296.3, 300.4, 311
Orthopedic	732.2, 732.4, 736.4, 736.42
Other comorbid conditions	
Acanthosis nigricans	701.2
NASH	571.8
PCOS	256.4
Glucose intolerance	790.2
Insulin resistance	277.7
LVH	429.3
Elevated blood pressure	796.2
Pseudotumor cerebri	348.2

ICD-9-CM: International Classification of Diseases, 9th Revision, Clinical Modification; NASH: nonalcoholic steatohepatitis; PCOS: polycystic ovary syndrome; LVH: left ventricular hypertrophy.

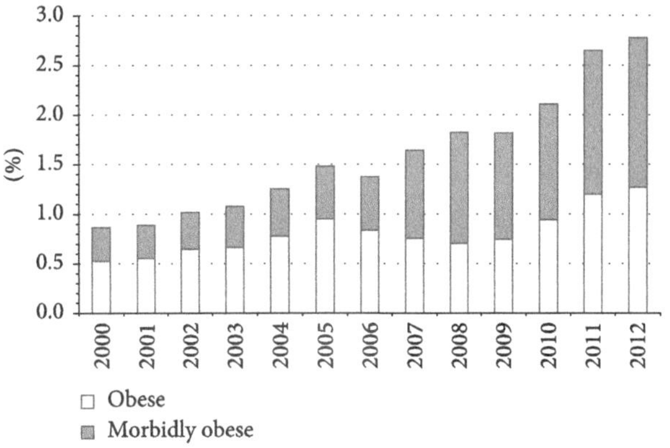

FIGURE 1: This figure illustrates the overall percentage (%) of patients coded as obese and morbidly obese from 2000–2012.

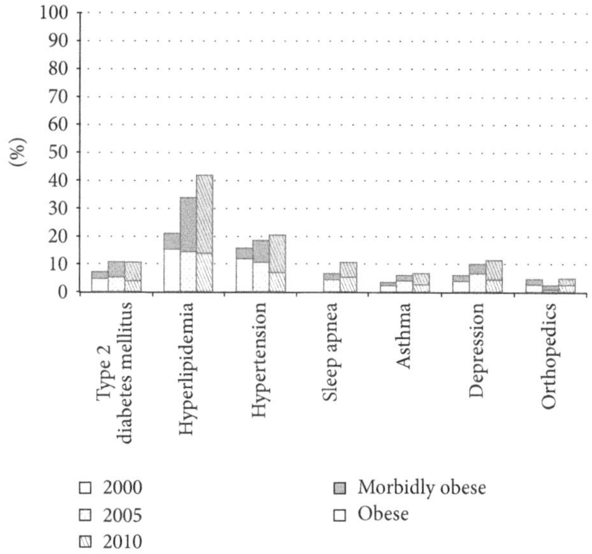

FIGURE 2: This figure illustrates the percentage (%) of patients with major comorbid conditions coded as obese and morbidly obese (not obese) at time points 2000, 2005, and 2010.

2.2. Statistical and Data Analysis. The main comorbid conditions included diabetes mellitus, hypertension, hyperlipidemia, sleep apnea, degenerative joint disease, asthma, and depression. Overall rates of these related comorbid conditions were calculated for obese and morbidly obese versus nonobese patients, as well as the annual increase for all patients over that same time period. Other obesity-related comorbid conditions that we examined included acanthosis nigricans, nonalcoholic steatohepatitis (NASH), PCOS, glucose intolerance, insulin resistance, left ventricular hypertrophy (LVH), elevated blood pressure, and pseudotumor cerebri. The incidence rate ratio (IRR) was then calculated to see if obese and morbidly obese patients were disproportionately affected by these conditions. An odds ratio (OR) was also calculated.

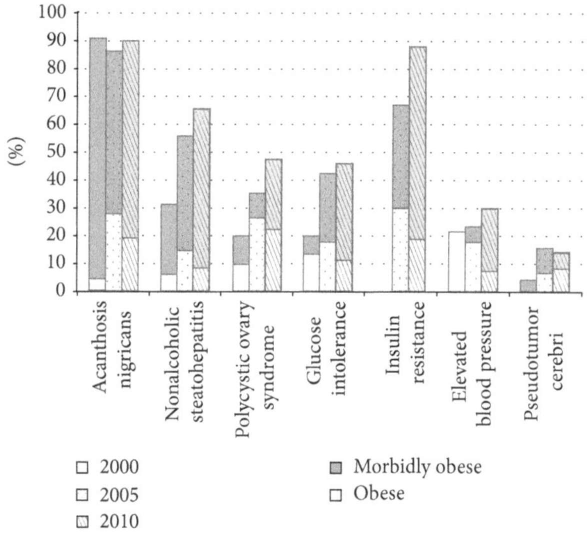

FIGURE 3: This figure illustrates the percentage (%) of patients with "preconditions" coded as obese and morbidly obese (not obese) at time points 2000, 2005, and 2010.

3. Results

In total, a retrospective review of 3,185,658 person-years in nonobese, 26,404 person-years in obese, and 25,819 person-years in the morbidly obese children was conducted. The annual rate of patients coded with obesity increased from 0.86% in 2000 to approximately 2.78% in 2012 at our institution as shown in Figure 1. Figure 1 also illustrates that the annual rate of patients coded with morbid obesity increased from 0.34% in 2000 to 1.51% in 2012. When comparing differing major comorbid conditions, it appeared that the proportions of patients coded as obese or morbidly obese remained constant at the various time points including 2000, 2005, and 2010. On the other hand, when comparing the differing preconditions, it appeared that there was a slight increase in the proportions of patients coded as morbidly obese versus obese. This was especially prominent in the cohort of endocrine conditions including acanthosis nigricans, PCOS, and insulin resistance. A summary of the findings was displayed in Figures 2 and 3.

The annual rate of all major comorbidities (diabetes mellitus, hypertension, hyperlipidemia, sleep apnea, degenerative joint disease, asthma, and depression) increased in all pediatric patients over the study period. Other obesity-related comorbid conditions, or preconditions, including acanthosis nigricans, NASH, PCOS, glucose intolerance, insulin resistance, LVH, elevated blood pressures, hypertension, and pseudotumor cerebri, were also increased among all pediatric patients over the study period. However, when comparing annual rates in obese patients alone, the annual rates for obese patients were higher across all categories as compared to the annual rates calculated in all patients (Table 3).

All of the obesity-related comorbidities were higher among obese versus non-obese patients over the time period from 2000 to 2012. All comorbidities were also higher in the morbidly obese versus non-obese patients over the same time period. All of the "preconditions" were noted to have the

Table 3: Annual increases, odds ratio (OR), and incidence rate ratios (IRR) across 2000–2012.

Comorbidity	Annual increase in all patients 2000 to 2012 (95% CI)	Annual increase in all obese patients 2000 to 2012 (95% CI)	OR in obese versus nonobese patients 2000 to 2012 (95% CI)	OR in morbidly obese versus nonobese patients 2000 to 2012 (95% CI)	IRR in obese versus nonobese patients 2000 to 2012 (95% CI)	IRR in morbidly obese versus nonobese patients 2000 to 2012 (95% CI)
Type 2 diabetes	1.078 (1.050, 1.106)	1.127 (1.003, 1.252)	7.77 (7.47, 8.08)	8.84 (8.39, 9.31)	7.91 (6.61, 9.22)	8.60 (7.15, 10.05)
Hyperlipidemia	1.092 (1.014, 1.171)	1.164 (1.043, 1.285)	38.37 (37.2, 39.5)	52.7 (50.0, 54.6)	33.70 (30.54, 36.87)	43.96 (37.47, 50.44)
Hypertension	1.084 (1.038, 1.130)	1.115 (1.000, 1.230)	14.4 (13.9, 14.9)	15.29 (15.11, 16.49)	13.78 (11.81, 15.76)	12.86 (11.37, 14.36)
Sleep apnea	1.927 (0.569, 3.285)	1.887 (0.854, 2.921)	6.48 (6.12, 6.85)	7.60 (7.07, 8.17)	4.81 (4.51, 5.10)	5.04 (4.79, 5.29)
Asthma	1.049 (1.003, 1.094)	1.130 (1.055, 1.206)	4.23 (4.12, 4.35)	4.00 (3.85, 4.16)	3.78 (3.56, 4.01)	3.23 (2.81, 3.65)
Depression	1.041 (1.003, 1.079)	1.116 (1.026, 1.207)	7.28 (7.02, 7.56)	7.15 (6.78, 7.53)	7.09 (7.75, 6.43)	6.00 (5.07, 6.93)
Orthopedic	1.059 (1.014, 1.103)	1.111 (0.898, 1.323)	2.60 (2.35, 2.88)	2.77 (2.41, 3.81)	2.81 (2.19, 3.43)	3.30 (2.45, 4.14)
Acanthosis nigricans	1.119 (1.028, 1.210)	1.120 (1.036, 1.204)	570.21 (535.49, 607)	1036 (971, 1105)	562.89 (403.52, 722.27)	1104.2 (623.23, 1585.16)
NASH	1.206 (1.057, 1.354)	1.292 (1.081, 1.503)	95 (86.83, 103.97)	160.51 (146, 176)	83.09 (64.27, 101.91)	140.19 (106.73, 173.65)
PCOS	1.079 (1.022, 1.136)	1.171 (1.084, 1.257)	40.1 (38.21, 41.99)	37.52 (35.2, 39.9)	37.73 (34.11, 41.35)	33.43 (28.56, 38.20)
Glucose intolerance	1.392 (1.106, 1.677)	1.592 (1.032, 2.152)	50.68 (47.28, 54.33)	76.63 (70.99, 82.72)	44.17 (36.36, 51.98)	54.11 (40.39, 67.84)
Insulin resistance	2.542 (0.793, 4.291)	3.263 (0.763, 5.7)	528 (472, 590)	955 (853, 969)	334.65 (214.86, 454.43)	558.57 (317.37, 799.76)
LVH	1.199 (1.067, 1.330)	1.384 (0.953, 1.815)	0.97 (0.86, 1.08)	0.65 (0.54, 0.79)	0.81 (0.58, 1.03)	0.69 (0.44, 0.94)
Elevated BP	1.369 (1.007, 1.731)	1.470 (1.077, 1.864)	28.04 (26, 30)	34.54 (31.5, 37.8)	22.68 (18.46, 26.91)	16.89 (9.96, 23.82)
Pseudotumor cerebri	1.164 (1.058, 1.270)	1.662 (0.756, 2.568)	11.28 (9.52, 13.37)	11.34 (8.9, 14.29)	10.83 (7.91, 13.74)	13.27 (5.70, 20.84)

same findings; all the "preconditions" were noted to be higher among obese, as were morbidly obese patients versus non-obese patients from 2000 to 2012. The OR did approximate the IRR with respect to all these conditions. These findings are seen in Table 3.

4. Discussion

This current study illustrates the change in the spectrum of obesity-related comorbid conditions in an overweight, pediatric population at a single institution over the past decade utilizing a hospital database system. As expected, children continue to experience the same comorbidities and preconditions associated with obesity as compared to adults. Among the weaknesses of this study, perhaps the most glaring is that this administrative database may have underestimated the overall incidence of obesity, the overall rate of obesity being only 2-3% at our institution. However, in spite of this, the spectrum of comorbidities seen in our pediatric patients and the knowledge of these have significant clinical implications. Both the medical and surgical treatment of adult obesity has led to associated refinement of treatment modalities; therefore, we hope to do the same with these data that identify the vast host of comorbidities that are most injurious to our children.

On a national level, May et al. have recently published results regarding cardiovascular sequelae in the *National Health and Nutrition Examination Survey (NHANES)* from 1999 to 2008 [14]. Again, the major cardiovascular risk factors including diabetes, hypertension, and hyperlipidemia were elevated across all cohorts but specifically increased in the overweight and obese cohorts. Similar to their study, we also continued to see a dose-response increase in reportable comorbid conditions across both our obese and morbidly obese cohorts. Unlike their study, we did not collect individual data, but rather administrative coding of diagnoses across both inpatient and outpatient visits. Accordingly, there could have been biased introduced with the respective coding, but our hope is that this large sample ameliorated some of the associated, inherent reporting bias.

Comorbid conditions including asymptomatic cardiovascular risk factors (e.g., hypertension, hyperlipidemia) and symptomatic cardiovascular risk factor (e.g., type 2 diabetes) are also prevalent in both the obese and morbidly obese subgroups. In fact, our study shows that hyperlipidemia and hypertension have the broadest effects with both our obese and morbidly-obese populations having the highest weighted OR and IRR. These results are similar to results of a population-based sample of Quebec children and adolescents, where almost one-third of their obese population had unfavorable risk factors; this was evidenced by elevations in apolipoprotein B, high-density lipoprotein cholesterol, triglycerides, insulin, glucose, C-reactive protein, and systolic blood pressure [15]. Thus, despite increased awareness of obesity and intensive medical interventions, obesity and its associated cardiovascular disease risk factors continue to represent an unabated major healthcare burden to this population as a whole.

More importantly, according to Bjørge et al., it is suggested that these comorbidities with cardiovascular implications lend to an increased rate of premature death in early adulthood after adjustment for other confounders [16]. In juxtaposition to this, Park et al. [8] report that the increased risk for morbidity and mortality may be overestimated following adjustment for adult BMI; however, one of the limitations of this study includes that it was a meta-analysis of very small studies. When examining our data more closely, it is very concerning the degree to which certain "preconditions" have arisen, including acanthosis nigricans, nonalcoholic steatohepatitis, glucose intolerance, and insulin resistance. These aforementioned conditions will eventually become lifelong diseases; therefore, it is imperative to continue to reduce those comorbidities with cardiovascular implications, while at the same time providing more longitudinal analysis of obesity's long-term effects.

Obesity and morbid obesity are not only involved in modifiable cardiovascular risk factors, but are also intimately involved in the respiratory system. The evidence correlating the changes in the reactivity and the nature of the pulmonary disease seen with obesity is not new. For example, the NHANES data continues to show that excess weight has stronger association with nonatopic asthma (OR: 2.46, 95% CI: 1.21, 5.21) than atopic asthma (OR: 1.31, 95% CI: 0.70–2.57) [17]. This becomes a vicious cycle for these children as they are often unable to perform activities of daily living and are less likely to perform in exercise programs, which continues to compound weight-related issues. Our data shows that, even beyond an expected increase in asthma, there has also been a substantial increase in those documented with sleep apnea. For example, our data suggests that the odds of having sleep apnea was 6.48 (95% CI: 6.12, 6.85) times more likely if a patient was coded as obese and 7.60 (95% CI: 7.07, 8.17) times more likely if a patient was coded as morbidly obese as compared to normal weight counterparts.

Similar to cardiovascular risk factors, asthma, sleep apnea, and orthopedic problems are also increased in our obese and morbidly obese cohorts. A common theme among these conditions is that they limit the child or adolescent's ability to participate in social activities, which can further alienate this ever-growing proportion of our society. For example, in adults, increasing BMI and subsequent obesity lend itself to knee pain, disability, loss of work productivity, and diminished quality of life [18]. More recent studies in children suggest that obese children report more frequent and severe joint pain with subsequent loss of function [18–21]. Our study did also evaluate the trend between obesity and morbid obesity and depression. It is well known that obesity in children and adolescents results in decreased/reduced health-related quality of life [22]. As referenced by the above orthopedic studies, depression might have been masked as complaints of increased joint pain or inability to perform activities performed by non-obese peers. Further studies are needed to elucidate this connection.

Even though our study did not examine health-related costs specifically, according to one study, the actual cost of obesity is related to the direct costs of its associated medical conditions [23]. Continued attention and US dollars have been driven toward using policy and environmental changes to help combat the obesity epidemic; only in the last decade or so had there been a shift towards medical and operative interventions. Whereas it has been shown in adults that patients with reduced comorbid conditions attained through weight-loss surgery live longer, the same conclusions have yet to be applied to the pediatric population [24]. In fact, Oyetunji et al. remarked that despite this increased prevalence of obesity and morbid obesity among children and adolescents, only approximately 2% of morbidly obese children with a major comorbidity underwent a bariatric procedure [25]. This may be due in part to a myriad of factors including necessity for higher volume centers for pediatric bariatric procedures, as well as concern for permanent procedures to be performed in children and adolescents. However, there is still a need for novel and equitable approaches to pediatric obesity.

This study had important strengths and weaknesses. In the future, we hope to have same functional database as, for example, the National Surgical Quality Improvement Program (NSQIP) database, which relies on specifically trained personnel who use well-defined terms for data collection and dissemination. We encountered visits that had no documentation regarding vital data points including height, weight, or BMI, thus contributing to the underestimation of the prevalence of obesity. Despite these aforementioned weaknesses, this study's strengths included both its size as well as the duration of the data collection. Obese patients, as well as morbidly obese patients, had significant increases in comorbid conditions including hypertension, hyperlipidemia, sleep apnea, orthopedic issues, and type 2 diabetes mellitus as evidenced by the elevated IRR, OR, and tightly controlled confidence intervals.

5. Conclusions

In conclusion, these data show the change in the spectrum of obesity-related comorbid conditions in this pediatric population over the past decade. As expected, the children studied have experienced the same dramatic increases in obesity as seen in the adult population and obesity was independently correlated with major comorbidities. Future research will be needed to implement other treatment options to combat the wide variety of disease sequelae.

Abbreviations

BMI:	Body mass index
IRR:	Incidence rate ratio
NHANES:	National Health and Nutrition Examination Survey
NSQIP:	National Surgical Quality Improvement Program
OR:	Odds Ratio
WLS:	Weight loss surgery.

Disclosure

The authors have no financial relationships to disclose.

Conflict of Interests

The authors have no conflict of interests to disclose.

Acknowledgments

The authors wish to thank Dr. Jonathan Bickel, Nandan Patibandla, and the rest of the Clinical Research Informatics team, all of whom have provided superb assistance in their data collection process.

References

[1] R. E. Andersen, "The spread of the childhood obesity epidemic," *CMAJ*, vol. 163, no. 11, pp. 1461–1462, 2000.

[2] C. B. Ebbeling, D. B. Pawlak, and D. S. Ludwig, "Childhood obesity: public-health crisis, common sense cure," *The Lancet*, vol. 360, no. 9331, pp. 473–482, 2002.

[3] A. P. Rocchini, "Childhood obesity and a diabetes epidemic," *The New England Journal of Medicine*, vol. 346, no. 11, pp. 854–855, 2002.

[4] C. L. Ogden, M. D. Carroll, B. K. Kit, and K. M. Flegal, "Prevalence of obesity and trends in body mass index among US children and adolescents, 1999-2010," *Journal of the American Medical Association*, vol. 307, no. 5, pp. 483–490, 2012.

[5] E. P. Whitlock, E. A. O'Connor, S. B. Williams, T. L. Beil, and K. W. Lutz, "Effectiveness of weight management interventions in children: a targeted systematic review for the USPSTF," *Pediatrics*, vol. 125, no. 2, pp. e396–e418, 2010.

[6] S. Li, W. Chen, S. R. Srinivasan et al., "Childhood cardiovascular risk factors and carotid vascular changes in adulthood: the bogalusa heart study," *Journal of the American Medical Association*, vol. 290, no. 17, pp. 2271–2276, 2003.

[7] E. S. Ford and C. Li, "Defining the metabolic syndrome in children and adolescents: will the real definition please stand up?" *Journal of Pediatrics*, vol. 152, no. 2, pp. 160–164, 2008.

[8] M. H. Park, C. Falconer, R. M. Viner, and S. Kinra, "The impact of childhood obesity on morbidity and mortality in adulthood: a systematic review," *Obesity Reviews*, vol. 13, pp. 985–1000, 2012.

[9] S. E. Messiah, G. Lopez-Mitnik, D. Winegar et al., "Changes in weight and co-morbidities among adolescents undergoing bariatric surgery: 1-year results from the bariatric outcomes longitudinal database," *Surgery for Obesity and Related Diseases*, pp. 1–11, 2012.

[10] S. N. Murphy, M. Mendis, K. Hackett et al., "Architecture of the open-source clinical research chart from informatics for integrating biology and the bedside," *AMIA Annual Symposium Proceedings*, vol. 11, pp. 548–552, 2007.

[11] S. N. Murphy, G. Weber, M. Mendis et al., "Serving the enterprise and beyond with informatics for integrating biology and the bedside (i2b2)," *Journal of the American Medical Informatics Association*, vol. 17, no. 2, pp. 124–130, 2010.

[12] "Obesity: preventing and managing the global epidemic," Report of A WHO consultation, World Health Organ Tech Rep Ser., 2000.

[13] N. F. Krebs, J. H. Himes, D. Jacobson, T. A. Nicklas, P. Guilday, and D. Styne, "Assessment of child and adolescent overweight and obesity," *Pediatrics*, vol. 120, supplement 4, pp. S193–S228, 2007.

[14] A. May, E. V. Kuklina, and P. Yoon, "Prevalence of cardiovascular risk factors among US adolescents, 1999–2008," *Pediatrics*, vol. 129, pp. 1035–1041, 2012.

[15] M. Lambert, E. E. Delvin, E. Levy et al., "Prevalence of cardiometabol-ic risk factors by weight status in a population-based sample of Quebec children and adolescents," *Canadian Journal of Cardiology*, vol. 24, no. 7, pp. 575–583, 2008.

[16] T. Bjørge, A. Engeland, A. Tverdal, and G. D. Smith, "Body mass index in adolescence in relation to cause-specific mortality: a follow-up of 230,000 Norwegian adolescents," *American Journal of Epidemiology*, vol. 168, no. 1, pp. 30–37, 2008.

[17] C. M. Visness, S. J. London, J. L. Daniels et al., "Association of childhood obesity with atopic and nonatopic asthma: results from the National Health and Nutrition Examination Survey 1999–2006," *Journal of Asthma*, vol. 47, no. 7, pp. 822–829, 2010.

[18] S. Bout-Tabaku, M. S. Briggs, and L. C. Schmitt, "Lower extremity pain is associated with reduced function and psychosocial health in obese children," *Clinical Orthopaedics and Related Research*, vol. 471, no. 4, pp. 1236–1244, 2013.

[19] A. L. de Sá Pinto, P. M. de Barros Holanda, A. S. Radu, S. M. F. Villares, and F. R. Lima, "Musculoskeletal findings in obese children," *Journal of Paediatrics and Child Health*, vol. 42, no. 6, pp. 341–344, 2006.

[20] S. D. Stovitz, P. E. Pardee, G. Vazquez, S. Duval, and J. B. Schwimmer, "Musculoskeletal pain in obese children and adolescents," *Acta Paediatrica*, vol. 97, no. 4, pp. 489–493, 2008.

[21] E. D. Taylor, K. R. Theim, M. C. Mirch et al., "Orthopedic complications of overweight in children and adolescents," *Pediatrics*, vol. 117, no. 6, pp. 2167–2174, 2006.

[22] J. B. Schwimmer, T. M. Burwinkle, and J. W. Varni, "Health-related quality of life of severely obese children and adolescents," *Journal of the American Medical Association*, vol. 289, no. 14, pp. 1813–1819, 2003.

[23] A. Wolf and G. A. Colditz, "Current estimates of the economic cost of obesity in the United States," *Obesity Research*, vol. 6, no. 2, pp. 97–106, 1998.

[24] T. D. Adams, R. E. Gress, S. C. Smith et al., "Long-term mortality after gastric bypass surgery," *The New England Journal of Medicine*, vol. 357, no. 8, pp. 753–761, 2007.

[25] T. A. Oyetunji, A. L. Franklin, G. Ortega et al., "Revisiting childhood obesity: persistent underutilization of surgical intervention?" *The American Surgeon*, vol. 78, no. 7, pp. 788–793, 2012.

8

Downregulation of RelA (p65) by Rapamycin Inhibits Murine Adipocyte Differentiation and Reduces Fat Mass of C57BL/6J Mice despite High Fat Diet

Peter D. Ray,[1] Reid A. Maclellan,[2] Jin He,[1] Zhigang Liu,[3] and Jianguo Wu[1]

[1] *Department of Surgery, Division of Plastic Surgery, University of Alabama at Birmingham, 1670 University Boulevard, VHG94, Birmingham, AL 35294, USA*
[2] *Boston Children's Hospital, Department of Plastic and Oral Surgery, Boston, MA 02115, USA*
[3] *Renmin Hospital of Wuhan University, Department of Anesthesiology, Wuhan, Hubei 430060, China*

Correspondence should be addressed to Peter D. Ray; peter.ray@childrensal.org and Jianguo Wu; jgwu@uab.edu

Academic Editors: B. Navia and C. H. Wu

Rapamycin (RAPA) is a clinical immunosuppressive agent first reported in the literature in 1975 after its discovery in a soil sample from the island of Rapa Nui. Aside from the well-documented effects of RAPA on cell division and immunologic response, the literature reveals it to have negative effects on adipocyte and osteocyte differentiation as well. Understanding of the molecular effects of RAPA on cell differentiation is fragmentary in regard to these cell lineages. In this paper, we examined a potential mechanism for RAPA's effects on adipocyte differentiation *in vitro* and *in vivo*. The data point to a unique role of Rel A (p65)—a component of the NF-κB system—in mediating this event. In murine adipose derived stem cell cultures (muADSCs) from C57BL/6J mice, RAPA was found to selectively downregulate RelA/p65, mammalian target of rapamycin (mTOR), and do so in a dose-dependent manner. This implies a novel role for RelA in adipocyte biology. Intracellular lipid accumulation—as subjectively observed—was also decreased in muADSCs treated with RAPA. Mice treated with RAPA had reduced overall body weight and reduced size of both intraabdominal and subcutaneous fat pads. When treated with RAPA, mice fed a high fat diet did not develop obesity and were not different from their regular diet controls in terms of body weight. These results suggested that RAPA inhibits adipogenesis and lipogenesis of muADSCs resulting in a prevention of obesity in C57BL/6J mice. This inhibition is strong enough to negate the effects of a high fat diet and seems to act by downregulating the RelA/p65 mTOR signaling pathway—a key component of the NF-κB family.

1. Introduction

In the 1950s molecular geneticists were trying to determine if proteins built from amino acids were required for the synthesis of nucleic acid chains or vice versa [1]. As a result of this work, the Rel gene was described in *E. coli* in 1969 [2] and so named because when the gene was present it rendered "relaxed" mutants of *E. coli* more stringently dependent on the presence of specific amino acids for successful RNA synthesis. "Rel proteins" share genetic homology and yet initiate different proliferative and/or transformative effects on different cells [3]. The first described "Rel protein" (REV-T) was most intriguing because of its ability to transform cells into malignant populations [4]. A viral form (v-Rel) was then also identified in birds, implying that there existed a related homology across species of these regulator proteins [5]. Due to their ability to drive replication and transformation from bacteria to mammals, the Rel genes were studied extensively in an attempt to understand their relation to malignancy [6, 7].

Further investigation to identify proteins related to c-Rel identified a number of subunits which were found to exist bound to each other as dimers or heterodimers. This led to the concept of a "Rel family of proteins," meaning a set of proteins that regulate transcription and possess the structural ability to form complexes required for DNA binding. Rel family proteins are often described as part of a broader Rel/NF-κB transcription system [8].

Much research has been done on the NF-κB system since its discovery by Sen more than 25 years ago [9]. The NF-κB family members form complexes, combining as dimers from five possible subunits: p50, p52, c-Rel, RelB, and/or RelA (p65). Of these, the first two (p50 and p52) have motifs that contain nuclear localization sequences. The other Rel family members are the transcriptionally active components that exist in the cytoplasm of a cell bound to an inhibitor of Kappa B (IκB) [10].

NF-κB/Rel protein translocation is generally understood to occur by two distinct pathways: canonical (conforming to well-established patterns) and noncanonical (unique pattern). The canonical pathway, which is triggered by inflammatory stimuli, controls innate immunity and protects hepatocytes, lymphocytes, and macrophages from programmed cell death. It involves NF-κB1 (p50). As mentioned previously, an inhibitor, IκB, masks the nuclear localization sequence as a baseline. This masking retains inactive NF-κB dimers, usually p50/p62, in the cytoplasm. Engagement of receptors on the cell surface activates phosphorylation of IκB by its kinases (inhibitor of kappa B kinases or IKKs). IκB degrades as a result and releases the dimer for nuclear translocation.

The alternate (or noncanonical) NF-κB pathway, driven by NF-κB2, operates at the interface of innate and adaptive immunity, meaning that it is intimately involved when fighting off foreign cells [11]. The exclusive partner of NF-κB2 p100 and p52 is RelB. NF-κB2 activation is regulated by NF-κB inducing kinase (NIK), which appears to have an obligatory function in immune cell differentiation based on studies from knockout models [12–14]. In the alternate noncanonical pathway, phosphorylation of NF-κB2 (p100) is mediated by IKKα and NIK to trigger release of p52-RelB dimers for nuclear translocation [15].

What is unknown, however, is the importance of the Rel A component of the NF-κB system as it has not been shown to either induce malignancy or contribute to immune response. Given the clinical finding of poor wound healing in human transplant patients taking the drug RAPA (personal observation), we hypothesized that there may be a mechanism at work on the nonimmunologic level (as a side effect) which impaired subcutaneous tissue regeneration. We hypothesized that an impairment of stem cell differentiation may play a role and found that in the mouse model the RAPA effect involved the Rel A segment of the NF-κB system.

The mammalian target of rapamycin (mTOR) is at the crossroads of a nutrient-hormonal signaling network that is involved in specific pathological responses, including obesity [16]. mTOR forms two distinct signaling complexes known as mTOR complex 1 and mTOR complex 2 (mTORC1 and mTORC2). mTORC1 and mTORC2 contain shared and unique partners, distinct substrates and have differing sensitivities to rapamycin, the molecular functions of which remain poorly understood [17]. mTORC1 is sensitive to rapamycin and promotes anabolism while inhibiting catabolic cellular processes. Growth factors and nutrients promote mTORC1-dependent protein synthesis, cell growth, and metabolism [18]. Conversely, insufficient levels of these factors, or signals of cell stress, rapidly suppress mTORC1 and mTORC1—controlled anabolic processes [19, 20]. Reduced mTORC1 signaling also activates autophagy, a degradative process that may represent the last line of defense against starvation [19–21]. In contrast, mTORC2 contains exclusively rictor (rapamycin-insensitive companion of mTOR), mSin1 (mammalian stress-activated map kinase-interacting protein 1), and PRR5/protor (protein observed with rictor 1 and 2). Rictor and mSin1 promote mTORC2 assembly and signaling; the function of PRR5/protor remains obscure [22].

The clinical immunosuppressive agent RAPA is used extensively to prevent graft rejection in transplant patients [23]. Early studies show an inhibitory effect of RAPA on adipocyte glucose uptake [24] and differentiation associated with mTOR pathway [25]. In view of the remarkable effect of brief RAPA treatment in causing loss of both subcutaneous and intra-abdominal fat as well as protecting against high fat diet-induced obesity in C57BL/6J mice, we strove to identify the subunit responsible for its effects.

Here, we show that RAPA selectively downregulates RelA/p65 and inhibits adipogenic differentiation of murine mesenchymal stem cells derived from adipose tissue. The consequence of muADSC exposure to RAPA is inhibition of NF-κB signaling pathway and downregulated expression of mTOR. In contrast, c-Rel and Rel-B were not changed. These findings suggest a practical avenue for antiobesity therapy and insight into mechanisms of wound healing or disrupted regeneration regulated by RelA/p65 expression in mammals. It may explain why transplant surgeons frequently complain about patients who are on RAPA having wound healing problems.

2. Materials and Methods

2.1. Animals. The normal mice (C57/BL6) used in this study were purchased from The Jackson Laboratory (Bar Harbor, ME). The Institutional Animal Care and Use Committee approved all animal protocols used for these experiments.

2.2. Cell Harvest and Culture. For isolation of murine adipose-derived stem cell cultures (muADSC) cells, omental (OM) and subcutaneous (SUB) adipose tissue was excised separately from ten C57/BL6 mice/group (6 months of age) with/without rapamycin and with/without high fat diet. The samples were finely minced and digested using 0.075% collagenase type XI (Sigma, St. Louis, MO) for 45 min at 37°C. Enzyme activity was neutralized by treatment with Dulbecco's modified Eagle's medium (DMEM) containing 10% fetal bovine serum (FBS). The cell suspension was centrifuged at 1200 g for 10 min to separate the floating adipocytes from the stromal vascular faction (SVF). The SVF was resuspended in ammonium chloride (160 mM), incubated at room temperature for 10 min to lyse contaminating red blood cells, and then centrifuged as described above. After filtration of the cell suspension through a 100 mm nylon strainer to remove cellular debris, cell number and viability were determined using trypan blue exclusion. The SVF cells were plated in T75 flasks overnight in control medium

(DMEM, 10% FBS, and 1% penicillin/streptomycin) at 37°C in 5% carbon dioxide (CO_2). After incubation for 24 h, the flasks were washed extensively using phosphate buffered solution (PBS) to remove residual nonadherent cells. The adherent muADSC cells were expanded using serial passaging.

2.3. In Vitro Adipogenic Differentiation Assay. Cell monolayer from basal cultures was expanded in standard growth medium (DMEM + 10% FBS) to ensure mid-log growth phase confluence (60 to 80%). Medium and floating cells from the culture flask were aspirated and discarded. DPBS was added (using 5 to 10 mL). The cell monolayer was then gently rinsed. After removal of the DPBS, 5 to 7 mL of prewarmed TrypLE Express was added to the flask and until the culture surface was completely coated. The cell monolayer was then incubated for 5 to 8 minutes at 37°C or until cells had fully detached. The detached cells were then pipetted into a single cell solution and verified on an inverted microscope. The cell suspension was removed from the flask, transferred into a centrifuge tube, and spun at 100 ×g for 5 to 10 minutes.

Cell viability and total cell density were confirmed using Trypan Blue Stain. The pellet was resuspended in an appropriate volume of culture medium. The muADSC cells were then replated in 6-well plates (100,000 cells per well) in control medium to allow attachment. Twenty-four hours later, the medium was replaced with new control medium or adipose medium (control medium plus insulin (10 mM), dexamethasone (1 mM), isobutyl-methylxanthine (0.5 mM), and indomethacin (200 mM) (all from Sigma-Aldrich)). Cultures were maintained for 14 days, and refed every 3 to 4 days. The cultures then were assessed using Oil Red O stain, which serves as an indicator of intracellular lipid accumulation. The cells were fixed for 10 min at room temperature in 10% neutral buffered formalin and were washed with distilled water. They then were incubated in Oil Red O (Millipore, Temecula, CA) reagent for 30 min and washed 3 times with distilled water. The cells were counterstained with hematoxylin for 1 min and examined under microscope.

2.4. Characterization of muADASC Cells. Flow cytometry was used to characterize muADSC cells obtained from C57/BL6 mice with/without HFD (high fat diet) or with/without rapamycin and grown for 2 passages and 4 passages under control conditions. Cultured cells were trypsinized, spun, and washed in cold PBS 1X (Mediatech, Herndon, VA) containing 2% FBS. The cells then were divided into aliquots and were spun to form a pellet. Cells were blocked using mouse serum (Sigma) diluted 1:10 in PBS and rat anti-mouse CD14/CD31 (BD PharMingen, San Diego, CA) for 10 min on ice. The primary antibodies (applied in optimal amounts) included a biotin-conjugated rat anti-mouse monoclonal antibody against CD34 and CD29 followed by streptavidin-APC, PE-conjugated mouse anti-Sca-1, and FITC-conjugated mouse anti-CD45 and anti-CD44 (all from BD PharMingen, San Diego, CA). Analysis of surface protein expression was performed using appropriate gating on viable CD45-negative cells to eliminate contaminating hematopoietic cells. The isotype antibody control samples obtained for each individual cell population were used to set the dot-plot intercepts used for the analysis.

Table 1: Phenotypic characterization of muADSC cells. FACS analysis of muADSC demonstrating expression of typical surface proteins. Cultured cells used in the experiments were uniformly positive for CD29, CD44, CD73, and Scal-1 and negative for CD14, CD31, CD34, and CD45.

General surface markers for MuADSC at passage 4	
Positive (+)	Negative (−)
CD29	CD14
CD44	CD31
CD73	CD34
Sca-1	CD45

2.5. Western Blotting. Cells were lysed in 1% NP-40 lysis buffer (1% NP-40, 150 mM NaCl, 50 mM Tris-HCl (pH 8.0), and 1 mM sodium orthovanadate) supplemented with protease inhibitors (0.1 mM PMSF, 2 μg/mL each of leupeptin and aprotinin) for 15 min on ice. Total cell lysates were clarified by centrifuging at 10,000 rpm for 5 min at 4°C. The Pierce Protein Assay was used to estimate protein concentrations, with BSA as the standard. Equivalent amounts of cell lysates (20 μg of total protein) were loaded onto 4 to 20% SDS-PAGE gradient gels, transferred onto nitrocellulose membranes, and probed with the appropriate antibodies. Western blot analysis was carried out according to standard procedures using ECL detection (Amersham, Piscataway, NJ), using antibodies reactive to NF-κB family proteins, and DR4 (Santa Cruz Biotech, Santa Cruz, CA). Changes in protein level was determined through densitometry using Adobe Photoshop and normalized for loading against the actin as appropriate.

2.6. Data Analysis and Statistics. Statistical significance was determined using the InStat computer program (GraphPad Software Inc., San Diego, CA).

3. Results

3.1. Phenotypic Characterization of the muADSC Cells. The visceral adipose tissue from 1 mouse yielded approximately 7.0×10^6 nucleated cells. Within 4 passages after the initial plating of the primary culture, muADSC cells appeared as a monolayer of large, flat cells. As the cells approached confluence, they acquired a spindle-shaped or fibroblast-like appearance. We used flow cytometry to evaluate the expression of CD45, Sca-1, CD34, CD44, and CD29 cell-surface antigens on the muADSC cells obtained from C57/BL6. The muADSC cells were negative for CD45, a hematopoietic cell surface marker. Approximately 50% and 10% of the muADSC cells were Sca-1 and CD34 positive, respectively, at the time of isolation (data not shown). As shown in Table 1, muADSC cells were positive for CD29, CD44, CD73, and Sca-1 and were negative for CD14, CD31, CD45, and CD34 at the time of flow cytometry analysis (after 4 passages).

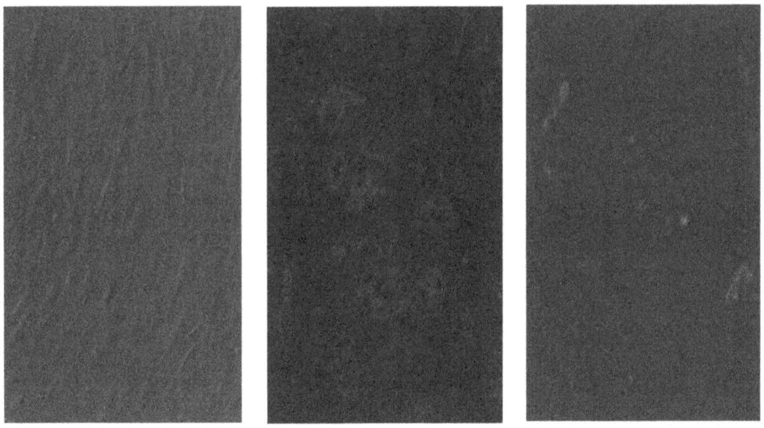

FIGURE 1: Rapamycin (RAPA) inhibited adipogenesis of ADSCs *in vitro*. (a) Resting cells in control media (CM) showed a differentiated contractile phenotype characterized by an irregular shape. (b) Incubation with adipogenic differentiation medium for two weeks induced adipocyte differentiation. Oil Red-O staining of differentiated muADSC without rapamycin treatment show significant numbers of cells and robust phenotype. (c) Differentiating muADSC cells treated with rapamycin and stained with Oil Red-O demonstrated visibly fewer cells and a smaller phenotype.

3.2. muADSC Cells Undergo Adipogenic Differentiation In Vitro. To determine whether muADSC cells undergo adipogenesis, we cultured muADSC cells in adipogenic medium. Oil Red O staining performed 2 weeks later revealed cytoplasmic lipid droplets, which are indicative of the adipogenic phenotype. These results indicate that the muADSC cells cultured in adipogenic medium underwent adipogenic differentiation (Figure 1(b)), whereas muADSC cells maintained in control medium did not (Figure 1(a)).

3.3. Effects of RAPA on Body Weight in LFD- and HFD-Induced Mice. However, surprisingly, RAPA-treated mice had reduced body weight on either the low fat diet (LFD) or high fat diet (HFD) compared to the LFD or HFD control mice. The most marked difference was observed after 1 week of RAPA treatment at 6 months of age when a 8.5 g mean difference (24% weight lost) for LFD-fed mice with/without RAPA and 16 g of mean difference (33% weight lost) for HFD-fed mice with/without RAPA ($N = 10$ each group) in body weight was measured (35.95 ± 0.9293 versus 27.45 ± 0.5843 in LFD-fed mice and 48.73 ± 0.7200 versus 32.66 ± 0.5837 in HFD-fed mice, $P < 0.001$) (Figure 2).

3.4. Effects of RAPA on Fat Pads Mass on the LFD/HFD. The Sub and OM weights of RAPA-treated mice were significantly lower ($P < 0.001$) than those of control mice fed on the LFD or HFD (Table 2). When normalized for body weight, RAPA treatment significantly ($P < 0.001$) reduced Sub by 65% and OM by 72% in RAPA-treated mice with LFD and 47% and 56% in RAPA-treated mice with HFD, respectively. These findings indicated a reduction in fat pad weights and that RAPA prevented the effect of diet on the rate of accretion in fat pad weight.

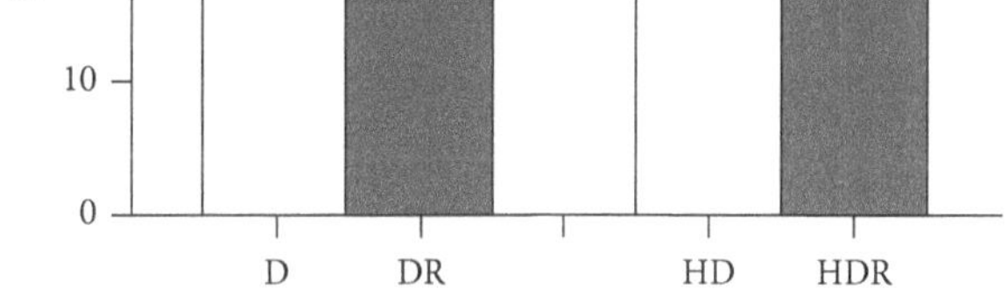

FIGURE 2: Rapamycin (RAPA) reduced body weight of C57BL/6J mice on both high fat and low fat diets. D = 10% fat diet; R = rapamycin; HD = 40% high fat diet; data are expressed as mean ± S.E.M. $n = 10$ mice for each group. $P < 0.001$ (*).

3.5. Effect of RAPA on Adipocyte (ADSCs) Differentiation. When omental or subcutaneous preadipocytes in primary culture were induced to differentiate into adipocytes, the presence of RAPA severely impaired the adipogenesis. Very few cells show the characteristic morphology of rounded, lipid-filled adipocytesunder microscopic visualization as shown in Figure 1. The RAPA-mediated inhibition of adipocyte differentiation was observed to be almost identical in omental or subcutaneous tissue samples.

3.6. Effect of RAPA on the Expression of p65/RelA, mTOR, and the Adipocyte Differentiation Markers in ADSCs Differentiation. RAPA treatment led to a decrease of p65/RelA, mTOR,

Table 2: Effects of rapamycin on fat weights in C57BL/6J mice fed with D (10% fat diet) or HFD (40% fat diet), with or without rapamycin (R). Data are expressed as mean ± SEM. $n = 10$ mice for each group. $P < 0.001$. Sub: subcutaneous; OM: omental.

	D	DR	HD	HDR
Absolute weight (g)				
Sub	1.18 ± 0.054	0.34 ± 0.022**	1.87 ± 0.068	0.66 ± 0.051**
OM	1.45 ± 0.089	0.24 ± 0.029**	1.88 ± 0.109	0.55 ± 0.043**
Percent of body weight (%)				
Sub	3.26 ± 0.102	1.25 ± 0.064**	3.83 ± 0.106	2.02 ± 0.146**
OM	3.69 ± 0.240	0.87 ± 0.091**	3.85 ± 0.177	1.68 ± 0.123**

Data are presented as means ± SEM. The two-tailed P value is <0.0001 (**), extremely significant.

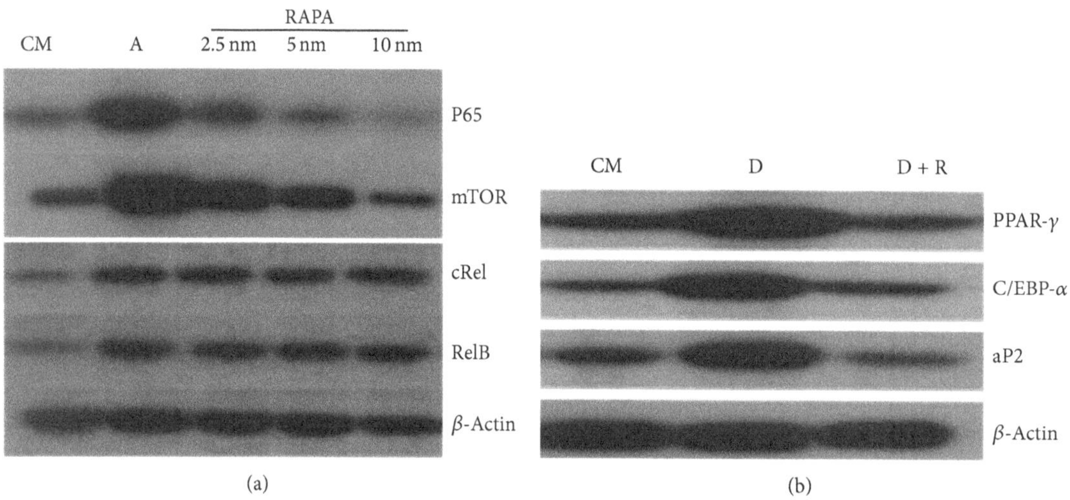

Figure 3: (a) RAPA inhibited the expression of p65/RelA and mTOR during adipocyte differentiation in a dose-dependent manner. Increasing amounts of RAPA were added to muADSC cell culture groups to determine dose dependency. After 6 days posttreatment, total proteins were extracted and Western blot analysis was performed with specific antibodies to RelA, RelB, c-Rel, and mTOR. The antibody to β-actin was used for loading control. (b) RAPA represses the expression of adipogenic marker genes such as PPAR-gamma, C/EBP-α, and aP2 during adipocyte differentiation. 10 nM RAPA was added into muADSC cell cultures. After 6 days posttreatment, total proteins were extracted and Western blot analysis was performed with specific antibodies to PPAR-gamma, C/EBPα, and aP2. Expression of β-actin was used for loading control. The results are representative of three independent experiments.

αP2, C/EPBα, and PPAR-gamma in differentiated ADSCs cells and is dose dependent (Figure 3(b)). ADSCs at baseline were assessed by Western blot analyses. p65/RelA, mTOR, αP2, C/EPBα, and PPAR-gamma were strongly induced in *day 6* differentiated ADSCs compared with undifferentiated ADSCs (Figure 3, lines 2 and 1). Our data suggest that this decrease may contribute to the inhibited adipogenesis in RAPA-treated adipocytes.

4. Discussion

In this study, we examined the effects of rapamycin (RAPA) on obesity of the C57BL/6J mouse strain fed with either low or high fat diets. Results support our prediction that a high fat diet significantly promotes the development of obesity [26] and the treatment of RAPA can reduce body weight gain of mice fed with HDF. The loss of body fat (both omental and subcutaneous) we observed in RAPA-treated mice may be due to a decrease in average adipocyte size or as a result of reduced formation of new adipocytes from precursor cells [27]. The activation of mTORC1 signaling in 3T3-L1 adipocytes by ectopic expression of Rheb inhibits expression of ATGL (adipose triglyceride lipase) and HSL (hormone-sensitive lipase), suppresses lipolysis, increases *de novo* lipogenesis, and promotes intracellular accumulation of triglycerides [28]. Inhibition of mTORC1 signaling by rapamycin or knockdown of raptor stimulates lipolysis primarily *via* activation of ATGL expression [29]. Those findings demonstrate that mTORC1 promotes fat storage in mammalian cells by suppression of lipolysis and stimulation of *de novo* lipogenesis. These result are consistent with RAPA-reduced expression of most adipogenic marker genes including PPAR-gamma, C/EBPα, FAS, αP2, adipsin, and ADD1/SREBP1c, all affecting lipogenesis and adipogenesis [30]. Thus, the ability of RAPA to prevent obesity suggests that RAPA or a molecular derivative without immunologic side effects might be a valuable tool to modulate key energy balance regulators.

Our data also indicate that rapamycin impairs omental and subcutaneous adipocyte differentiation in primary culture. Rapamycin inhibited the characteristic accumulation of intracellular lipid, as well as the expression of αP2, PPAR-gamma, and C/EBPα, the specific markers of adipogenesis. The molecular basis underlying this regulation of RAPA associated mTOR signaling pathway is not fully understood. Rapamycin, upon binding to FKBP12, interacts with mTOR, which then leads to the inhibition of p70 S6 kinase [31]. Recent findings reveal that mTOR itself is a serine kinase. It is capable of autophosphorylation, as well as the phosphorylation (and activation) of p70 S6 kinase. Rapamycin, then, may inhibit p70 S6 kinase as a consequence of blocking the mTOR serine kinase activity. Because insulin is an adipocytedifferentiating hormone and p70 S6 kinase is known to participate in insulin signaling, it was postulated that rapamycin blocked adipogenesis by attenuating insulin signal transduction and blocking critical postconfluent mitoses in the early phase of adipogenesis [32]. We have shown here that rapamycin is effective in attenuating mouse adipocyte differentiation. Both omental and subcutaneous preadipocytes responded similarly to rapamycin, suggesting that preadipocytes derived from either of these anatomic regions use similar insulin signal transduction pathways to trigger adipogenesis.

The precise rapamycin-sensitive pathway regulating adipocyte differentiation remains to be defined. It is possible that the loss of subcutaneous fat that results when humans are given subcutaneous fat injections of glucocorticoids is acting in a similar manner [33]. Insulin is believed to stimulate the mTOR kinase and its phosphorylation of p70 S6 kinase [34], but others have instead reported that p70 S6 kinase phosphorylation is increased indirectly through the inhibition of a mTOR-regulated phosphatase [35]. In addition, mTOR appears to be located upstream of several other signaling proteins in addition to p70 S6 kinase. These include 4EBP-1/PHAS1, a regulator of mRNA translation and cell proliferation, and the cyclin-dependent kinases [36]. Multiple signaling pathways regulated by mTOR may therefore be operative in the preadipocyte.

In summary, we have demonstrated that RAPA dramatically reduced the expression of p65/RelA and inhibited differentiation of ADSCs. At the same time, RAPA revealed no effects on cRel or RelB in our experiments. Our studies provide new insight into the current understanding of the biological function of NF-κB, especially the p65/RelA, in adipocytes differentiation. Targets downstream of mTOR by modulating p65/RelA should be the focus of future studies on the regulation of adipogenesis.

Conflict of Interests

The authors declare that there is no conflict of interests regarding the publication of this paper.

Acknowledgments

This work was supported by (1) John W. Kirklin Research and Education Fellowship Award and (2) The University Children's Surgical Group Research and Education Fellowship Award.

References

[1] A. B. Pardee and L. S. Prestidge, "The dependence of nucleic acid synthesis on the presence of amino acids in *Escherichia coli*," *Journal of Bacteriology*, vol. 71, no. 6, pp. 677–683, 1956.

[2] N. Fiil, "A functional analysis of the rel gene in *Escherichia coli*," *Journal of Molecular Biology*, vol. 45, no. 2, pp. 195–203, 1969.

[3] J. A. Didonato, F. Mercurio, and M. Karin, "NF-κB and the link between inflammation and cancer," *Immunological Reviews*, vol. 246, no. 1, pp. 379–400, 2012.

[4] S. Sarkar and T. D. Gilmore, "Transformation by the vRel oncoprotein requires sequences carboxy-terminal to the Rel Homology domain," *Oncogene*, vol. 8, no. 8, pp. 2245–2252, 1993.

[5] D. Carrasco, C. A. Rizzo, K. Dorfman, and R. Bravo, "The v-rel oncogene promotes malignant T-cell leukemia/lymphoma in transgenic mice," *The EMBO Journal*, vol. 15, no. 14, pp. 3640–3650, 1996.

[6] E. Brownell, C. A. Kozak, and J. R. Fowle III, "Comparative genetic mapping of cellular rel sequences in man, mouse, and the domestic cat," *American Journal of Human Genetics*, vol. 39, no. 2, pp. 194–202, 1986.

[7] J. A. DiDonato, "Nf-κB and the link between inflammation and cancer," *Immunological Reviews*, vol. 246, no. 1, p. 397, 2012.

[8] H. R. Bose Jr., "The Rel family: models for transcriptional regulation and oncogenic transformation," *Biochimica et Biophysica Acta*, vol. 1114, no. 1, pp. 1–17, 1992.

[9] R. Sen, "The origins of NF-κB," *Nature Immunology*, vol. 12, pp. 686–688, 2011.

[10] G. Bonizzi and M. Karin, "The two NF-κB activation pathways and their role in innate and adaptive immunity," *Trends in Immunology*, vol. 25, no. 6, pp. 280–288, 2004.

[11] M. Magnani, R. Crinelli, M. Bianchi, and A. Antonelli, "The ubiquitin-dependent proteolytic system and other potential targets for the modulation of nuclear factor-κB (NF-κB)," *Current Drug Targets*, vol. 1, no. 4, pp. 387–399, 2000.

[12] L. Burkly, C. Hession, L. Ogata et al., "Expression of relB is required for the development of thymic medulla and dendritic cells," *Nature*, vol. 373, no. 6514, pp. 531–536, 1995.

[13] F. Weih, D. Carrasco, S. K. Durham et al., "Multiorgan inflammation and hematopoietic abnormalities in mice with a targeted disruption of RelB, a member of the NF-κB/Rel family," *Cell*, vol. 80, no. 2, pp. 331–340, 1995.

[14] T. Yamada, T. Mitani, K. Yorita et al., "Abnormal immune function of hemopoietic cells from alymphoplasia (aly) mice, a natural strain with mutant NF-κB-inducing kinase," *Journal of Immunology*, vol. 165, no. 2, pp. 804–812, 2000.

[15] U. Senftleben, Y. Cao, G. Xiao et al., "Activation by IKKα of a second, evolutionary conserved, NF-κB signaling pathway," *Science*, vol. 293, no. 5534, pp. 1495–1499, 2001.

[16] S. B. Yang, A. C. Tien, G. Boddupalli, A. W. Xu, Y. N. Jan, and L. Y. Jan, "Rapamycin ameliorates age-dependent obeesity associated with increased mTOR sginaling in hypothalamic POMC neurons," *Neuron*, vol. 75, no. 3, pp. 425–436, 2012.

[17] R. Loewith, E. Jacinto, S. Wullschleger et al., "Two TOR complexes, only one of which is rapamycin sensitive, have distinct roles in cell growth control," *Molecular Cell*, vol. 10, no. 3, pp. 457–468, 2002.

[18] S. Wullschleger, R. Loewith, and M. N. Hall, "TOR signaling in growth and metabolism," *Cell*, vol. 124, no. 3, pp. 471–484, 2006.

[19] C. F. Kurat, K. Natter, J. Petschnigg et al., "Obese yeast: triglyceride lipolysis is functionally conserved from mammals to yeast," *The Journal of Biological Chemistry*, vol. 281, no. 1, pp. 491–500, 2006.

[20] J. Huang and B. D. Manning, "The TSC1-TSC2 complex: a molecular switchboard controlling cell growth," *Biochemical Journal*, vol. 412, no. 2, pp. 179–190, 2008.

[21] S. Grönke, A. Mildner, S. Fellert et al., "Brummer lipase is an evolutionary conserved fat storage regulator in Drosophila," *Cell Metabolism*, vol. 1, pp. 323–330, 2005.

[22] M. Laplante and D. M. Sabatini, "MTOR signaling in growth control and disease," *Cell*, vol. 149, no. 2, pp. 274–293, 2012.

[23] C. Venzina, A. Kudeliski, and S. N. Sehgal, "Rapamycin (AY-22, 989), a new antifungal antibiotic," *The Journal of Antibiotics*, vol. 28, no. 10, p. 721, 1975.

[24] M. J. Pereira, J. Palming, M. Rizell et al., "MTOR inhibition with rapamycin causes impaired insulin signalling and glucose uptake in human subcutaneous and omental adipocytes," *Molecular and Cellular Endocrinology*, vol. 355, no. 1, pp. 96–105, 2012.

[25] X. Xiang, J. Zhao, G. Xu, Y. Li, and W. Zhang, "mTOR and the differentiation of mesenchymal stem cells," *Acta Biochimica et Biophysica Sinica*, vol. 43, no. 7, pp. 501–510, 2011.

[26] S. Lin, T. C. Thomas, L. H. Storlien, and X. F. Huang, "Development of high fat diet-induced obesity and leptin resistance in C57Bl/6J mice," *International Journal of Obesity and Related Metabolic Disorders*, vol. 24, no. 5, pp. 639–646, 2000.

[27] M. Rosenbaum, R. L. Leibel, and J. Hirsch, "Obesity," *The New England Journal of Medicine*, vol. 337, no. 6, pp. 396–407, 1997, Erratum in: *The New England Journal of Medicine*, vol. 338, no. 3, p. 555, 1998.

[28] P. Chakrabarti, T. English, J. Shi, C. M. Smas, and K. V. Kandror, "Mammalian target of rapamycin complex 1 suppresses lipolysis, stimulates lipogenesis, and promotes fat storage," *Diabetes*, vol. 59, no. 4, pp. 775–781, 2010.

[29] P. Polak, N. Cybulski, J. N. Feige, J. Auwerx, M. A. Rüegg, and M. N. Hall, "Adipose-specific knockout of raptor results in lean mice with enhanced mitochondrial respiration," *Cell Metabolism*, vol. 8, no. 5, pp. 399–410, 2008.

[30] I. Bakan and M. Laplante, "Connecting mTORC1 signaling to SREBP-1 activation. Connecting mTORC1 signaling to SREBP-1 activation," *Current Opinion in Lipidology*, vol. 23, no. 3, pp. 226–234, 2012.

[31] K. Jastrzebski, K. M. Hannan, E. B. Tchoubrieva, R. D. Hannan, and R. B. Pearson, "Coordinate regulation of ribosome biogenesis and function by the ribosomal protein S6 kinase, a key mediator of mTOR function," *Growth Factors*, vol. 25, no. 4, pp. 209–226, 2007.

[32] D. Cota, "Mammalian target of rapamycin complex 1 (mTORC1) signaling in energy balance and obesity," *Physiology and Behavior*, vol. 97, no. 5, pp. 520–524, 2009.

[33] R. I. Scheinman, A. Gualberto, C. M. Jewell, J. A. Cidlowski, and A. S. Baldwin Jr., "Characterization of mechanisms involved in transrepression of NF-κB by activated glucocorticoid receptors," *Molecular and Cellular Biology*, vol. 15, no. 2, pp. 943–953, 1995.

[34] F. Tremblay and A. Marette, "Amino acid and insulin signaling via the mTOR/p70 S6 kinase pathway. A negative feedback mechanism leading to insulin resistance in skeletal muscle cells," *The Journal of Biological Chemistry*, vol. 276, no. 41, pp. 38052–38060, 2001.

[35] B. Magnuson, B. Ekim, and D. C. Fingar, "Regulation and function of ribosomal protein S6 kinase (S6K) within mTOR signalling networks," *Biochemical Journal*, vol. 441, no. 1, pp. 1–21, 2012.

[36] T. Ikenoue, S. Hong, and K. Inoki, "Chapter 11 monitoring mammalian target of rapamycin (mTOR) activity," *Methods in Enzymology*, vol. 452, pp. 165–180, 2009.

9

Carotid Intima Media Thickness Is Independently Associated with Male Gender, Middle Age, and IGF-1 in Metabolically Healthy Obese Individuals

Hala Abd El-Hafez,[1] Mohamed M. Elrakhawy,[2] Azza A. El-Baiomy,[3] and Mervat M. El-Eshmawy[1]

[1] *Internal Medicine Department, Mansoura Specialized Medical Hospital, Faculty of Medicine, Mansoura University, Mansoura 35516, Egypt*
[2] *Radiology Department, Mansoura University Hospital, Faculty of Medicine, Mansoura University, Egypt*
[3] *Clinical Pathology Department, Mansoura University Hospital, Faculty of Medicine, Mansoura University, Egypt*

Correspondence should be addressed to Hala Abd El-Hafez; hala_ahmed204@yahoo.com

Academic Editors: K.-C. Huang, N. M. Lalic, and D. Malkova

Background/Aims. The effect of benign obesity on subclinical cardiovascular disease is still questionable. The purpose of this study was to assess carotid intima media thickness (CIMT), as a marker of subclinical atherosclerosis, and to evaluate its relation to age, sex, and IGF-1 in metabolically healthy obese (MHO) subjects. *Methods.* A total of 75 MHO subjects and 80 age, and sex matched healthy nonobese control subjects were included in the study. Body mass index (BMI), waist circumference (WC), blood pressure, fasting plasma glucose, fasting insulin, HOMA-IR, lipid profile, insulin like growth factor-1 (IGF-1), and CIMT were assessed in all subjects. *Results.* MHO subjects had significantly higher CIMT and lower IGF-1 than healthy nonobese controls. Mean CIMT was significantly higher in MHO men age subgroup range from 30 to 50 years than in their age range matched (premenopausal) MHO women subgroup. In MHO subjects, CIMT was positively correlated with age, BMI, WC, SBP, HOMA-IR, TG, and LDL-C, and negatively correlated with IGF-1. Regression analysis revealed that middle age, male sex and IGF-1 remained independently associated with CIMT in MHO subjects. *Conclusion.* CIMT is elevated and IGF-1 is reduced in MHO subjects, and CIMT is independently associated with male gender, middle age, and IGF-1. Definition of healthy obesity may be broadened to include IMT measurement.

1. Introduction

Metabolically healthy obese (MHO) term refers to obese individuals who are relatively insulin sensitive and normotensive and have favourable glucose and lipid profile inspite of high levels of obesity [1, 2]. Evidence suggests that MHO individuals as based on BMI criteria may account for as much as 20–30% of obese population [3, 4]. MHO subset of individuals is relatively protected from obesity related cardiometabolic disturbances that increase cardiovascular disease (CVD) risk in metabolically abnormal obese [5]. However, data concerning the exact risk of CVD in MHO as compared to healthy normal weight individuals is limited, and most data are confined to women at narrow age range.

Carotid artery intima media thickness (CIMT) is a noninvasive surrogate marker of subclinical atherosclerosis and an indicator of CVD risk [6, 7]. In addition, IMT is associated with age, male gender, obesity, and traditional risk factors [8–11].

Beside traditional CVD risk factors, obesity is associated with changes in insulin like growth factor-1 (IGF-1) [12, 13] which may be linked to atherosclerosis. Previous studies concerning the association between IGF-1 and atherosclerosis have led to conflicting results; some authors found positive association between IGF-1 and IMT in men [14] and in both men and women [15], while others found inverse association between IGF-1 and carotid IMT in healthy women [16]. Another study in middle aged subjects showed that IMT and

IGF-1 are positively associated in women and inversely in men [17].

Greater subclinical CVD burden in metabolically benign obese individuals compared to metabolically healthy lean women was recently reported [18]. Further studying of subclinical CVD profile in MHO men and women and investigation of its correlates may help in proper management of MHO individuals. The aim of the present study was to assess carotid intima media thickness (CIMT) as a marker of subclinical atherosclerosis in metabolically healthy obese (MHO) subjects as compared to healthy nonobese subjects. Also we evaluated the relation of CIMT with age, sex, and IGF-1 in MHO subjects.

2. Subjects and Methods

The study comprised 75 MHO subjects (37 men and 38 women, mean age 48.85 ± 11.59 years) and 80 age, and sex, matched healthy nonobese (BMI 20–24.9 kg/m^2) control subjects (Table 1). Obesity was defined as BMI of ≥30 kg/m^2. Healthy obese adults were included in the study, and they were recruited from obesity Clinic of Specialized Medical Hospital, Mansoura University, Egypt. All subjects signed an informed consent to be included in our study. This study was approved by the local ethical committee.

All participants were healthy without known acute or chronic diseases. Exclusion criteria included smoking, alcohol consumption, cardiovascular, inflammatory or metabolic diseases, known or suspected pituitary, thyroid, adrenal or gonadal dysfunction, pregnancy, abnormal liver function tests, and medications (antihypertensive, lipid lowering, hypoglycaemic agents, growth hormone, anabolic steroids, glucocorticoids, hormone replacement, and hormonal contraception).

All participants were subjected to thorough medical history and clinical examination. Anthropometric measurements including height, weight, body mass index (BMI), and waist circumference (WC) were obtained using standardized techniques; height was measured to the nearest 0.5 cm, body weight was measured to the nearest 1.0 kg using mechanical weight scale (in the fasting state in the morning while wearing light clothes and no shoes). BMI was calculated as weight/height^2 (kg/m^2), and WC was measured at the highest point of the iliac crest at the end of normal expiration. Blood pressure (BP) was measured in the sitting position, with a mercury sphygmomanometer after a 10-minute rest. Measures were taken from the upper arm with an appropriately sized cuff. The systolic and diastolic blood pressure were read to the nearest 2 mmHg and recorded at the appearance (phase I) and disappearance (phase V) of Korotkoff's sounds respectively. The lowest of three consecutive readings was recorded.

Metabolically healthy state, defined as having 0 to 1 out of six cardiometabolic abnormalities including (1) BP ≥130/85, (2) fasting triglyceride level ≥150 mg/dL, (3) HDL-C <40 mg/dL in men and <50 mg/dL in women, (4) fasting glucose ≥100 mg/dL (ATP-III cut-off values) [19], (5) HOMA-IR >2.7, (6) high sensitive C-reactive protein (hs-CRP) >3 mg/L (Cutoff values for HOMA-IR and hs-CRP were obtained from Karelis and Rabasa-lhoret) [20].

Table 1: Characteristics of metabolically healthy obese and nonobese control subjects.

Characteristics	Metabolically healthy obese subjects (n = 75)	Nonobese controls (n = 80)	P value
Men/women (n)	37/38	40/40	0.93
Age (years)	48.8 ± 11.6	47.50 ± 12	0.48
BMI (kg/m^2)	34.9 ± 3	22.7 ± 1.8	<0.001*
WC (cm)	104.6 ± 10.5	77.3 ± 6.8	<0.001*
SBP (mmHg)	120.9 ± 9.5	116.9 ± 9.8	0.01*
DBP (mmHg)	75.4 ± 10.5	74.3 ± 7.2	0.44
Fasting glucose (mg/dL)	88 ± 9.2	86.2 ± 8.2	0.18
Fasting insulin (μIU/mlL)	9.3 ± 2.7	7.2 ± 2.5	<0.001*
HOMA-IR	1.9 ± 0.6	1.5 ± 0.6	<0.001*
Total cholesterol (mg/dL)	172 ± 33.1	167.9 ± 24.3	0.37
Triglycerides (mg/dL)	118.6 ± 23.7	111.9 ± 25.9	0.001*
HDL-C (mg/dL)	53.2 ± 7.3	58.6 ± 6.5	<0.001*
LDL-C (mg/dL)	96 ± 25.6	86.6 ± 24	0.02*
hs-CRP (mg/L)	1.6 ± 0.6	0.8 ± 0.3	<0.001*
IGF-1 (ng/mL)	203.7 ± 40.3	229.4 ± 57.5	0.002*
Carotid IMT (mm)	0.78 ± 0.15	0.67 ± 0.1	<0.001*

BMI: body mass index, WC: waist circumference, SBP: systolic blood pressure, DBP: diastolic blood pressure, HOMA-IR: homeostasis model assessment of insulin resistance, HDL-C: high density lipoprotein cholesterol, LDL-C: low density lipoprotein cholesterol, hs-CRP: high sensitivity C-reactive protein, IGF-1: insulin-like growth factor-1, and Carotid IMT: carotid intima media thickness. To converte lipid concentration from mg/dl into mmol/L; for total, HDL, and LDL cholesterol divide mg/dL by 38.6 and for triglycerides divide mg/dL by 88.57. Data are expressed as mean ± standard deviation; *P is significant if <0.05.

2.1. Laboratory Assay. Fasting blood sample (10 mL) was drawn from cubital vein of each participant in the sitting position between 8.00 and 10.00 a.m., after 12 hours of fasting. Each blood sample was divided into two tubes, one of them containing EDTA for preparation of plasma and the other for preparation of serum. Plasma glucose and serum lipids were assayed immediately, and the remaining of the samples were kept in aliquots at −70°C till the time of the rest of assays.

Fasting plasma glucose (FPG) was estimated using commercially available kit supplied by Human (Germany). Fasting serum insulin was assayed by a solid-phase, enzyme-labeled chemiluminescent immunometric assay using immulite analyzer supplied by Siemens (USA). Homeostasis model assessment of insulin resistance (HOMA-IR) index was calculated according to the formula: HOMA-IR = fasting insulin (μU/mL) × fasting glucose (mmol/L)/22.5 [21]. Total cholesterol (TC), triglyceride (TG), and high density lipoprotein cholesterol (HDL-C) were assayed by commercially available kits, Cobas (Integra-400) supplied by Roche Diagnostic, Germany. Low density lipoprotein cholesterol (LDL-C) was calculated according to

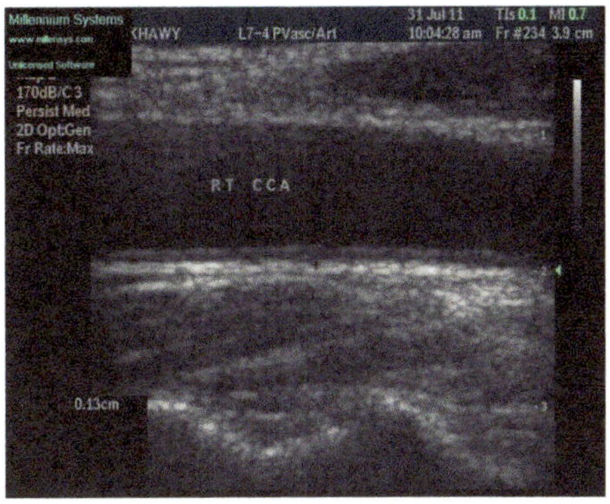

FIGURE 1: B mode longitudinal scan of the right common carotid artery in metabolically healthy obese individual showing clear lumen and carotid intima media thickness measuring 1.3 mm.

Friedewald et al. [22]. High sensitivity CRP (hs-CRP) was estimated using an immunoenzymometric assay supplied by Monobind Inc., Lake Forest, CA 92630, USA. Serum IGF-1 was estimated by immunoenzymometric assay supplied by Roy Bio (USA) with intraassay CV <10%, inter-assay <12%, and no cross-reactivity with other cytokines.

2.2. Measurement of Carotid Intima Media Thickness. Carotid IMT was measured by B mode ultrasound using high frequency transducers 4–7 and 5–12 MHz; all subjects were examined with ATL 5000, USA, and Philips 11xe, The Netherlands. Subjects lie supine with slight head tilt to the contralateral of the examined side, with elevation of the shoulder to stretch the neck in subjects with short neck. Cases were examined by one examiner who was unaware of participant's clinical characteristics. Common carotid artery (CCA) was scanned bilaterally (in the longitudinal and transverse views) 1 cm before carotid bulb over a length of 1 cm at the far wall of both CCAs. IMT thickness was measured at plaque free segments only as the distance between the leading edge of the lumen-intima interface and media-adventitia interface. Two measurements were taken from each side and averaged; then, the mean carotid IMT was calculated as the average of measurements obtained from both CCAs (Figure 1).

2.3. Statistical Analysis. Data entry and analysis were performed using SPSS statistical package version 15. The quantitative data were expressed as mean ± SD. Student's t-test was conducted to compare the mean of continuous variables in two groups. Pearson's correlation coefficient was used to test correlations between variables. Linear regression analysis was done to identify predictors of CIMT. P value <0.05 was considered as significant at a 95% confidence interval.

3. Results

Baseline characteristics of the MHO subjects and nonobese healthy controls are shown in Table 1. MHO subjects had significantly higher SBP, fasting insulin, HOMA-IR, TG, LDL-C, CRP, and CIMT (0.78 ± 0.15 versus 0.67 ± 0.10) and

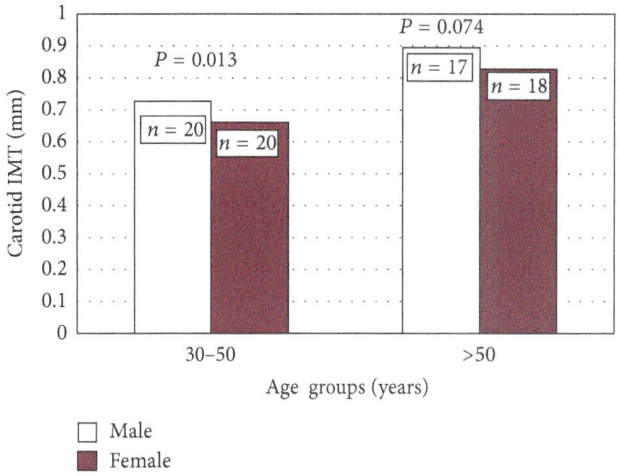

FIGURE 2: Carotid IMT in MHO women subgroups: from 30 to 50 (premenopausal) and above 50 years as compared to their age range matched MHO men subgroups.

significantly lower HDL-C and IGF-1 (203.7 ± 40.3 versus 229.4 ± 57.5) than those of healthy nonobese subjects.

MHO participants were divided into 2 groups according to sex. Compared to MHO women, MHO men showed significantly higher LDL-C and lower HDL-C. No significant difference was observed between MHO men and women regarding fasting insulin, HOMA-IR, TG, hs-CRP, and IGF-1 (Table 2).

CIMT was significantly higher in MHO men than in MHO women (0.82 ± 0.16 versus 0.74 ± 0.14) (Table 2). MHO women were divided into 2 age subgroups with respect to menopausal state: from 30 to 50 year (premenopausal) and above 50 years (after menopause), and they were compared to their age range matched subgroups of MHO men; CIMT was significantly higher in MHO men age subgroup ranged from 30 to 50 years than that in their age ranging matched pre-menopausal MHO women. However, the difference in CIMT between MHO men and women age subgroups above 50 years was insignificant (Figure 2).

The correlation between CIMT and other parameters in MHO subjects is shown in Table 3. CIMT was positively correlated with age, BMI, WC, SBP, HOMA-IR, TG, and LDL-C and negatively correlated with IGF-1.

Regression analysis was done to identify predictors of CIMT in MHO (Table 4). Age, sex, SBP, BMI, WC, HOMA-IR, TG, LDL-C, and IGF-1 were entered in the regression model. Only middle age, male gender, WC, and IGF-1 remained independently and significantly associated with CIMT in MHO subjects.

4. Discussion

The exact effect of metabolic healthy obesity on subclinical cardiovascular disease particularly in relation to age, sex,and different risk factors is not clearly defined. In the current study, we assessed CIMT and its relation to age, sex and IGF-1 in MHO. The main finding was elevated CIMT and reduced IGF-1 in MHO subjects; furthermore, IMT in MHO subjects

TABLE 2: Characteristics of MHO according to gender.

Characteristics	MHO men ($n = 37$)	MHO women ($n = 38$)	P value
Age (years)	49.32 ± 11.78	48.39 ± 11.54	0.73
WC (cm)	109.38 ± 9.35	100.03 ± 9.45	<0.001*
SBP (mmHg)	122.84 ± 9.76	119.08 ± 8.92	0.09
DBP (mmHg)	75.22 ± 13.71	75.66 ± 6.28	0.86
Fasting glucose (mg/dL)	87.62 ± 9.76	88.5 ± 8.78	0.68
Fasting insulin (μIU/mL)	9.58 ± 2.47	9.03 ± 2.92	0.38
HOMA-IR	1.97 ± 0.58	1.93 ± 0.61	0.78
Total cholesterol (mg/dL)	175.05 ± 39.34	169.13 ± 25.88	0.44
Triglycerides (mg/dL)	121.57 ± 22.48	115.84 ± 23.80	0.10
HDL-C (mg/dL)	51.35 ± 8.21	54.97 ± 5.77	0.03*
LDL-C (mg/dL)	100.92 ± 27.44	91.26 ± 23.05	0.03*
hs-CRP (mg/L)	1.50 ± 0.58	1.69 ± 0.58	0.15
IGF-1 (ng/mL)	198.16 ± 40.1	209.08 ± 40.39	0.22
Carotid IMT (mm)	0.82 ± 0.16	0.74 ± 0.14	0.02*

BMI: body mass index, WC: waist circumference, SBP: systolic blood pressure, DBP: diastolic blood pressure, HOMA-IR: homeostasis model assessment of insulin resistance, HDL-C: high density lipoprotein cholesterol, LDL-C: low density lipoprotein cholesterol, hs-CRP: high sensitivity C-reactive protein, IGF-1: insulin-like growth factor-1, and carotid IMT: carotid intima media thickness. To converte lipid concentration from mg/dL into mmol/L, for total, HDL, and LDL cholesterol divide mg/dL by 38.6 and for triglycerides divide mg/dL by 88.57. Data are expressed as mean ± standard deviation; * P is significant if <0.05.

TABLE 3: Correlation between CIMT and different parameters in MHO subjects.

Characteristics	MHO ($n = 75$)	
	r	P
Age (years)	0.57	<0.001*
BMI (kg/m^2)	0.40	<0.001*
WC (cm)	0.54	<0.001*
SBP (mmHg)	0.30	0.01*
DBP (mmHg)	0.07	0.55
Fasting glucose (mg/dL)	0.17	0.14
Fasting insulin (μIU/mL)	0.27	0.02*
HOMA-IR	0.26	0.02*
Total cholesterol (mg/dL)	0.23	0.05
Triglycerides (mg/dL)	0.26	0.02*
HDL-C (mg/dL)	−0.18	0.13
LDL-C (mg/dL)	0.24	0.03*
hs-CRP (mg/L)	0.09	0.46
IGF-1 (ng/mL)	−0.47	<0.001*

CIMT: carotid intima media thickness, MHO: metabolically healthy obese, BMI: body mass index, WC: waist circumference, SBP: systolic blood pressure, DBP: diastolic blood pressure, HOMA-IR: homeostasis model assessment of insulin resistance, HDL-C: high density lipoprotein cholesterol, LDL-C: low density lipoprotein cholesterol, hs-CRP: high sensitivity C-reactive protein, and IGF-1: insulin-like growth factor-1. * P is significant if <0.05.

was independently associated with male gender, middle age, and IGF-1.

Our results are in agreement with previous findings of higher CIMT in metabolically benign overweight/obese

TABLE 4: Regression analysis of clinical and laboratory variables on CIMT among MHO subjects.

Characteristics	MHO ($n = 75$)	
	β	P
Age (years)	0.62	<0.001*
Sex (male)	0.08	0.001*
SBP (mmHg)	0.15	0.21
BMI (kg/m^2)	0.12	0.46
WC (cm)	0.39	<0.001*
HOMA-IR	0.03	0.38
Triglycerides (mg/dL)	0.02	0.79
LDL-C (mg/dL)	0.02	0.63
IGF-1 (ng/mL)	−0.07	0.04*

CIMT: carotid intima media thickness, MHO: metabolically healthy obese, BMI: body mass index, WC: waist circumference, SBP: systolic blood pressure, HOMA-IR: homeostasis model assessment of insulin resistance, LDL-C: low density lipoprotein cholesterol, and IGF-1: insulin-like growth factor-1. * P is significant if <0.05.

women compared to normal weight women [18]. In addition Ärnlöv et al. [23] confirmed that the risk of CVD and mortality is elevated in MHO individuals compared to metabolically healthy and lean individuals. In contrast, Park et al. [24] found similar CIMT in healthy obese and healthy normal weight individuals.

Despite relatively favourable cardiometabolic profile in MHO as compared to metabolically abnormal one [1, 2], MHO individuals appear to have greater subclinical CVD than normal healthy individuals. These data go in line with our findings of less favourable metabolic profile in MHO as indicated by significantly higher fasting insulin, HOMA-IR, TG, and LDL-C, and significantly lower HDL-C. Obesity itself may contribute independently to carotid structure and function abnormalities and early atherosclerotic changes in obese are only partially explained by traditional CV risk factors [25]. Obesity may modulate CCA diameter and may induce adaptive changes in carotid wall thickness independent of metabolic and atherosclerotic factors [26]. In addition to the increase in BP, obesity is associated with an elevation in total blood volume, basic cardiac output, and heart rate, which can induce new intima proliferation through changes in arterial wall stress [27].

In addition, we found significant correlations between CIMT and BMI, WC, SBP, TG, LDL-C, and HOMA-IR in MHO subjects. However, among all previous cardiometabolic variables, only WC was a significant predictor of CIMT. Lakka el al. [28] demonstrated that abdominal obesity can be associated with progressive increase in CIMT independently of general obesity and other risk factors. In healthy individuals, WC as a measure of abdominal obesity correlates better than BMI with subclinical atherosclerosis evaluated by CIMT [29]. De Michele et al. [30] also found a significant association between WHR and carotid wall thickening independent of fasting insulin concentration. We suggest that the presence of visceral obesity is more important than insulin resistance in healthy obese and the effect of insulin resistance may be confounded by WC, and some measured (IGF-1) or unmeasured factors.

Our findings suggest that abdominal obesity in MHO individuals may exert an independent effect on atherosclerosis and it may mediate the effect of obesity on early atherosclerosis so, reduction of WC should be a target not only in metabolically abnormal obese subjects but also in MHO subjects.

Less favourable inflammatory profile indicated by significantly higher hs-CRP levels was detected in MHO subjects. We found insignificant relation between hs-CRP and CIMT. In agreement, Sinning et al. [8] found no independent association between CIMT and CRP. It is suggested that CRP is more predictive for cardiovascular prognosis in subjects of established carotid atherosclerosis [31].

In addition, age was the most significant predictor of CIMT among MHO subjects; this is consistent with previous studies reporting an association between IMT and age in both genders [8, 9]. Aging induces intrinsic changes in the arterial wall including progressive increase in intimal thickness [32], and this constant increase in IMT over age is an effect present in both male and female [33].

In accordance with a previously reported gender difference in IMT [8], we found that MHO men had significantly higher CIMT than MHO women, and the male gender remained independently associated with CIMT; this can be explained in part by a small increase in LDL-C and decrease in HDL-C in our MHO men as compared to MHO women. Furthermore, the difference in CIMT between MHO men and women in the current study seems to be influenced by menopausal status because it was more significant between middle age, than older age, subgroups. Tan et al. [9] reported that traditional risk factors explain only a small amount of gender variance in IMT, supporting the hypothesis that other sex hormone-related, behavioural, or genetic factors may play a role in the gender differences.

IGF-1 is a nontraditional factor which has been linked to atherosclerosis and obesity [12, 34]. We observed that MHO subjects had lower IGF-1 levels than healthy nonobese subjects which goes in line with the negative association between IGF-1 and BMI found by others [12, 13]. The relation between obesity and IGF-1 is complex; it is hypothesized that free IGF-1 increases with body weight until it reaches a level that triggers a negative feedback that would suppress growth hormone secretion (GH) which in turn would result in decreased IGF-1 production in the liver [35].

IGF-1 was a significant negative predictor of CIMT in our MHO subjects. These results are parallel to those of Marini et al., who suggested that low IGF-1 levels could contribute to early atherosclerosis in MHO women compared with non-obese women [16]. On the other hand, increased risk of atherosclerosis among individuals with low IGF-1 was previously reported [34]. In contrast, some found positive association between IGF-1 and IMT in men [14] and in both men and women [15]. Another study in middle aged subjects showed that IMT and IGF-1 are positively associated in women and inversely in men [17]. This seems to be a conflict, however the relation between IGF-1 system and CVD is complex, and there are many positive and negative associations. Both disorders of GH/IGF-1 axis activity including GH deficiency characterized by low serum IGF-1 and acromegaly accompanied by IGF-1 excess are associated with increased intima thickness [36, 37], So, a probably U-shaped association between the GH/IGF-1 axis activity and atherosclerosis was suggested though direct mechanisms of such a relation need to be elucidated [14].

Some speculate that IGF-1 is a proatherogenic by exerting an antiapoptotic effect on vascular smooth muscles and endothelial cells, and by being a promigratory factor [38], however, a detailed atheroprotective effect of IGF-1 has been fully reviewed [39]. Atherosclerosis is a chronic inflammatory disease initiated by oxidative stress, so the association of low IGF-1 with early atherosclerosis in our study is consistent with its potential anti-inflammatory and antioxidant effects [40]; as well as its possible role in endothelial function through its stimulation of endothelial nitric oxide production [41, 42].

Interestingly, physical activity is an important regulator of GH/IGF system [43], also weight loss restored low levels of free IGF-1 to normal [44], this further highlights the beneficial effect of life style based weight reduction in healthy obese.

Our study has some limitations, first, the cross sectional design, second, the sample size being relatively small; however, further prospective evaluation on larger scale study may be recommended. Third, CIMT was assessed by one investigator; however, a reasonable examination protocol was done by an expert radiologist.

In conclusion, CIMT is elevated and IGF-1 is reduced in MHO subjects, and CIMT is independently associated with male gender, middle age, and IGF-1. Definition of healthy obesity may be broadened to include IMT measurement.

List of Abbreviations

MHO:	Metabolically healthy obese
CVD:	Cardiovascular disease
CIMT:	Carotid artery intima media thickness
IGF-1:	Insulin-like growth factor-1
BMI:	Body mass index
WC:	Waist circumference
BP:	Blood pressure
FPG:	Fasting plasma glucose
GH:	Growth hormone
HOMA-IR:	Homeostasis model assessment of insulin resistance index
HDL-C:	High density lipoprotein cholesterol
LDL-C:	Low density lipoprotein cholesterol
hs-CRP:	High sensitive C-reactive protein
CCA:	Common carotid artery.

Conflict of Interests

The authors declare that they have no conflict of interests.

Authors' Contribution

Hala Abd El-Hafez drafted the paper, Mohamed M. Elrakhawy carried out carotid ultrasound, Azza A. El-Baiomy carried out the laboratory studies, and Mervat M.

El-Eshmawy conceived the study, helped to draft the paper and participated in its design and coordination.

References

[1] A. D. Karelis, M. Brochu, and R. Rabasa-Lhoret, "Can we identify metabolically healthy but obese individuals (MHO)?" *Diabetes and Metabolism*, vol. 30, no. 6, pp. 569–572, 2004.

[2] M. Brochu, A. Tchernof, I. J. Dionne et al., "What are the physical characteristics associated with a normal metabolic profile despite a high level of obesity in postmenopausal women?" *Journal of Clinical Endocrinology and Metabolism*, vol. 86, no. 3, pp. 1020–1025, 2001.

[3] R. P. Wildman, P. Muntner, K. Reynolds et al., "The obese without cardiometabolic risk factor clustering and the normal weight with cardiometabolic risk factor clustering: prevalence and correlates of 2 phenotypes among the US population (NHANES 1999-2004)," *Archives of Internal Medicine*, vol. 168, no. 15, pp. 1617–1624, 2008.

[4] A. D. Karelis, D. H. St-Pierre, F. Conus, R. Rabasa-Lhoret, and E. T. Poehlman, "Metabolic and body composition factors in subgroups of obesity: what do we know?" *Journal of Clinical Endocrinology and Metabolism*, vol. 89, no. 6, pp. 2569–2575, 2004.

[5] J. B. Meigs, P. W. F. Wilson, C. S. Fox et al., "Body mass index, metabolic syndrome, and risk of type 2 diabetes or cardiovascular disease," *Journal of Clinical Endocrinology and Metabolism*, vol. 91, no. 8, pp. 2906–2912, 2006.

[6] D. H. O'Learly and J. F. Polak, "Intima media thickness: a tool for atherosclerosis imaging and event prediction," *American Journal of Cardiology*, vol. 90, no. 10, pp. 18–20, 2002.

[7] M. W. Lorenz, H. S. Markus, M. L. Bots, M. Rosvall, and M. Sitzer, "Prediction of clinical cardiovascular events with carotid intima-media thickness: a systematic review and meta-analysis," *Circulation*, vol. 115, no. 4, pp. 459–467, 2007.

[8] C. Sinning, P. S. Wild, F. M. O. Echevarria et al., "Sex differences in early carotid atherosclerosis (from the community-based Gutenberg-Heart study)," *American Journal of Cardiology*, vol. 107, no. 12, pp. 1841–1847, 2011.

[9] T.-Y. Tan, C.-H. Lu, T.-K. Lin, C.-W. Liou, Y.-C. Chuang, and U. Schminke, "Factors associated with gender difference in the intima-media thickness of the common carotid artery," *Clinical Radiology*, vol. 64, no. 11, pp. 1097–1103, 2009.

[10] J. Lo, S. E. Dolan, J. R. Kanter et al., "Effects of obesity, body compositionand adiponectin on carotid intima-media thickness in healthy women," *Journal of Clinical Endocrinology and Metabolism*, vol. 9, no. 5, pp. 11677–11682, 2006.

[11] M. A. Espeland, R. Tang, J. G. Terry, D. H. Davis, M. Mercuri, and J. R. Crouse III, "Associations of risk factors with segment-specific intimal-medial thickness of the extracranial carotid artery," *Stroke*, vol. 30, no. 5, pp. 1047–1055, 1999.

[12] C. S. Lam, M. H. Chen, S. M. Lacey et al., "Circulating insulin-like growth factor-1 and its binding protein-3: metabolic and genetic correlates in the community," *Arteriosclerosis, Thrombosis, and Vascular Biology*, vol. 30, pp. 1479–1484, 2010.

[13] J. M. Faupel-Badger, D. Berrigan, R. Ballard-Barbash, and N. Potischman, "Anthropometric correlates of insulin-like growth factor 1 (IGF-1) and IGF binding protein-3 (IGFBP-3) levels by race/ethnicity and gender," *Annals of Epidemiology*, vol. 19, no. 12, pp. 841–849, 2009.

[14] S. Kawashi, N. Takeda, A. Sasaki et al., "Circulating insulin-like growth factor binding protein-3 is associated with early carotid atherosclerosis.," *Arteriosclerosis, Thrombosis, and Vascular Biology*, vol. 25, pp. 617–621, 2005.

[15] E. Spilcke-Liss, N. Friedrich, M. Dörr et al., "Serum insulin-like growth factor I and its binding protein 3 in their relation to intima-media thickness: results of the Study of Health in Pomerania (SHIP)," *Clinical Endocrinology*, vol. 75, no. 1, pp. 70–75, 2011.

[16] M. A. Marini, E. Succurro, S. Frontoni et al., "Metabolically healthy but obese women have an intermediate cardiovascular risk profile between healthy nonobese women and obese insulin-resistant women," *Diabetes Care*, vol. 30, no. 8, pp. 2145–2147, 2007.

[17] M. Hietaniemi, S. M. Pöykkö, O. Ukkola, M. Päivänsalo, and Y. A. Kesäniemi, "IGF-I concentrations are positively associated with carotid artery atherosclerosis in women," *Annals of Medicine*, vol. 37, no. 5, pp. 373–382, 2005.

[18] U. I. Khan, D. Wang, R. C. Thurston et al., "Burden of subclinical cardiovascular disease in "metabolically benign" and "at-risk" overweight and obese women: the Study of Women's Health Across the Nation (SWAN)," *Atherosclerosis*, vol. 217, no. 1, pp. 179–186, 2011.

[19] S. M. Grundy, J. I. Cleeman, S. R. Daniels et al., "Diagnosis and management of the metabolic syndrome: an American Heart Association/National Heart, Lung, and Blood Institute scientific statement," *Circulation*, vol. 112, no. 17, pp. 2735–2752, 2005.

[20] A. D. Karelis and R. Rabasa-Lhoret, "Inclusion of C-reactive protein in the identification of Metabolically Healthy but Obese (MHO) individuals," *Diabetes and Metabolism*, vol. 34, no. 2, pp. 183–184, 2008.

[21] D. R. Matthews, J. P. Hosker, and A. S. Rudenski, "Homeostasis model assessment: insulin resistance and β-cell function from fasting plasma glucose and insulin concentrations in man," *Diabetologia*, vol. 28, no. 7, pp. 412–419, 1985.

[22] W. T. Friedewald, R. I. Levy, and D. S. Fredrickson, "Estimation of the concentration of low-density lipoprotein cholesterol in plasma, without use of the preparative ultracentrifuge," *Clinical Chemistry*, vol. 18, no. 6, pp. 499–502, 1972.

[23] J. Ärnlöv, E. Ingelsson, J. Sundström, and L. Lind, "Impact of body mass index and the metabolic syndrome on the risk of cardiovascular disease and death in middle-aged men," *Circulation*, vol. 121, no. 2, pp. 230–236, 2010.

[24] J. Park, S. H. Kim, G. Y. Cho et al., "Obesity phenotype and cardiovascular changes," *Journal of Hypertension*, vol. 29, no. 9, pp. 1765–1772, 2011.

[25] E. M. Urbina, T. R. Kimball, C. E. McCoy, P. R. Khoury, S. R. Daniels, and L. M. Dolan, "Youth with obesity and obesity-related type 2 diabetes mellitus demonstrate abnormalities in carotid structure and function," *Circulation*, vol. 119, no. 22, pp. 2913–2919, 2009.

[26] M. Kozakova, C. Palombo, M. Paterni et al., "Body composition and common carotid artery remodeling in a healthy population," *Journal of Clinical Endocrinology and Metabolism*, vol. 93, no. 9, pp. 3325–3332, 2008.

[27] A. Simon, J. Levenson, J. Bouthier, and B. Maarek, "Haemodynamic basis of early modifications of the large arteries in borderline hypertension," *Journal of Hypertension*, vol. 5, no. 2, pp. 179–184, 1987.

[28] T. A. Lakka, H.-M. Lakka, R. Salonen, G. A. Kaplan, and J. T. Salonen, "Abdominal obesity is associated with accelerated progression of carotid atherosclerosis in men," *Atherosclerosis*, vol. 154, no. 2, pp. 497–504, 2001.

[29] J. I. Recio-Rodriguez, M. A. Gomez-Marcos, M. C. Patino-Alonso, C. Agudo-Conde, E. Rodriguez-Sanchez, and L. Garcia-Ortiz, "Abdominal obesity vs general obesity for identifying arterial stiffness, subclinical atherosclerosis and wave reflection in healthy, diabetics and hypertensive," *BMC Cardiovascular Disorders*, vol. 12, article 3, 2012.

[30] M. de Michele, S. Panico, A. Iannuzzi et al., "Association of obesity and central fat distribution with carotid artery wall thickening in middle-aged women," *Stroke*, vol. 33, no. 12, pp. 2923–2928, 2002.

[31] J. J. Cao, A. M. Arnold, T. A. Manolio et al., "Association of carotid artery intima-media thickness, plaques, and C-reactive protein with future cardiovascular disease and all-cause mortality: the Cardiovascular Health study," *Circulation*, vol. 116, no. 1, pp. 32–38, 2007.

[32] L. G. Spagnoli, A. Mauriello, A. Orlandi, G. Sangiorgi, and E. Bonanno, "Age-related changes affecting atherosclerotic risk. Potential for pharmacological intervention," *Drugs and Aging*, vol. 8, no. 4, pp. 275–298, 1996.

[33] A. Tosetto, P. Prati, C. Baracchini, R. Manara, and F. Rodeghiero, "Age-adjusted reference limits for carotid intima-media thickness as better indicator of vascular risk: population-based estimates from the VITA project," *Journal of Thrombosis and Haemostasis*, vol. 3, no. 6, pp. 1224–1230, 2005.

[34] A. Juul, T. Scheike, M. Davidsen, J. Gyllenborg, and T. Jørgensen, "Low serum insulin-like growth factor I is associated with increased risk of ischemic heart disease: a population-based case-control study," *Circulation*, vol. 106, no. 8, pp. 939–944, 2002.

[35] E. E. Calle and R. Kaaks, "Overweight, obesity and cancer: epidemiological evidence and proposed mechanisms," *Nature Reviews Cancer*, vol. 4, no. 8, pp. 579–591, 2004.

[36] D. V. Soares, L. D. Spina, R. R. de Lima Oliveira Brasil et al., "Carotid artery intima-media thickness and lipid profile in adults with growth hormone deficiency after long-term growth hormone replacement," *Metabolism*, vol. 54, no. 3, pp. 321–329, 2005.

[37] A. Colao, P. Marzullo, and G. Lombardi, "Effect of a six-month treatment with lanreotide on cardiovascular risk factors and arterial intima-media thickness in patients with acromegaly," *European Journal of Endocrinology*, vol. 146, no. 3, pp. 303–309, 2002.

[38] H. J. Arnqvist, "The role of IGF-system in vascular insulin resistance," *Hormone and Metabolic Research*, vol. 40, no. 9, pp. 588–592, 2008.

[39] Y. Higashi, S. Sukhanov, A. Anwar, S.-Y. Shai, and P. Delafontaine, "IGF-1, oxidative stress and atheroprotection," *Trends in Endocrinology and Metabolism*, vol. 21, no. 4, pp. 245–254, 2010.

[40] S. Sukhanov, Y. Higashi, S.-Y. Shai et al., "IGF-1 reduces inflammatory responses, suppresses oxidative stress, and decreases atherosclerosis progression in ApoE-deficient mice," *Arteriosclerosis, Thrombosis, and Vascular Biology*, vol. 27, no. 12, pp. 2684–2690, 2007.

[41] F. Perticone, A. Sciacqua, M. Perticone et al., "Low-plasma insulin-like growth factor-I levels are associated with impaired endothelium-dependent vasodilatation in a cohort of untreated, hypertensive caucasian subjects," *Journal of Clinical Endocrinology and Metabolism*, vol. 93, no. 7, pp. 2806–2810, 2008.

[42] M. F. Walsh, M. Barazi, G. Pete, R. Muniyappa, J. C. Dunbar, and J. R. Sowers, "Insulin-like growth factor I diminishes in vivo and in vitro vascular contractility: role of vascular nitric oxide," *Endocrinology*, vol. 137, no. 5, pp. 1798–1803, 1996.

[43] F. Lanfranco, L. Gianotti, R. Giordano, M. Pellegrino, M. Maccario, and E. Arvat, "Ageing, growth hormone and physical performance," *Journal of Endocrinological Investigation*, vol. 26, no. 9, pp. 861–872, 2003.

[44] M. H. Rasmussen, A. Juul, and J. Hilsted, "Effect of weight loss on free insulin-like growth factor-I in obese women with hyposomatotropism," *Obesity*, vol. 15, no. 4, pp. 879–886, 2007.

10

Role of Suppressor Variables in Primary Prevention Obesity Research: Examples from Two Predictive Models

Adam P. Knowlden

Department of Health Science, University of Alabama, Russell Hall 472, P.O. Box 870311, Tuscaloosa, AL 35487-0311, USA

Correspondence should be addressed to Adam P. Knowlden; aknowlden@ches.ua.edu

Academic Editors: A. Krettek and M. C. Wang

Pediatric obesity is a pertinent public health challenge. Child physical activity and screen time behaviors enacted within the context of the family and home environment are important determinants of pediatric obesity. The purpose of this study was to operationalize five, maternal-facilitated, social cognitive theory constructs for predicting physical activity and screen time behaviors in children. A secondary purpose was to elucidate the function of suppressor variables in the design and implementation of family- and home-based interventions seeking to prevent pediatric obesity. Instrumentation included face and content validity of the measurement tool by a panel of experts, test-retest reliability of the theoretical constructs, and predictive validity of the constructs through structural equation modeling. Physical activity and screen time were modeled separately according to the five selected social cognitive theory constructs. Data were collected from 224 mothers with children between four and six years of age. Specification indices indicated satisfactory fit for the final physical activity and screen time models. Through a series of four procedures, the structural models identified emotional coping and expectations as suppressor variables for self-efficacy. Suppressor variables can complement program design recommendations by providing a suggested ordering to construct integration within an intervention.

1. Introduction

Pediatric obesity impacts children worldwide and remains a formidable public health challenge [1]. Elucidating theoretical determinants of pediatric obesity is necessary for the development of primary prevention interventions that can reduce obesity prevalence [2]. Two activity-based behaviors posited to contribute to pediatric obesity include physical activity and screen time [3]. Physical activity is recognized as a modifiable determinant in the prevention of noncommunicable diseases including cardiovascular disease, hypertension, type 2 diabetes mellitus, and obesity [4]. Reduced levels of physical activity increase the likelihood of pediatric obesity. The Framingham Children's Study found that preschool children with lower levels of physical activity gained significantly more subcutaneous fat than did active children [5]. A three-year longitudinal study of preschool children found that increases in leisure physical activity and higher levels of aerobic activity led to decreased body mass index [6]. Recommendations for children include a total of 60 minutes of physical activity each day [3, 7]. Screen time is a primary source of sedentary activity for children and a recognized risk factor for pediatric obesity [8]. Screen time includes leisure time spent in front of a television or computer screen [7]. It is generally recommended that children receive no more than 120 minutes of screen time each day [3, 7].

From a psychosocial perspective, researchers are increasingly recognizing the influence of the family and home environment on factors such as physical activity and screen time that contribute to pediatric obesity [9]. However, there is a dearth of behavioral prediction model research for designing and measuring family- and home-based interventions targeting these behaviors [10]. Social cognitive theory (SCT) is a robust, theoretical framework for eliciting health behavior change [11]. SCT is based on the premise of reciprocal determinism; a casual paradigm that posits that human functioning is the result of environmental, personal, and behavioral factors. SCT is rooted in human potential and emphasizes modeling, symbolizing, forethought, self-regulatory, and self-efficacy capabilities. SCT was selected as the theoretical framework for this study for three primary purposes. First, it was the theory applied most frequently

(n = 2) in a systematic review examining family- and home-based pediatric obesity interventions [10]. Second, although SCT is considered an interpersonal-level behavior change theory, it allows for the reification of the environment, which is beneficial for targeting the home milieu. Finally, SCT is grounded in vicarious learning. Evidence suggests that children develop physical activity attitudes and behaviors primarily through observation of parental role models [9].

The five SCT variables operationalized in this investigation included environment, emotional coping, expectations, self-control, and self-efficacy. The constructs operationalized in this study have been applied throughout various streams of pediatric obesity research and have demonstrated their usefulness in interventions targeting behavior change [12]. In terms of SCT, the environment contains both the social and physical milieu [13]. Environment was selected, as availability and accessibility to physical activity and screen time are important mediators of engagement in these behaviors [14]. These factors are even more pronounced in family- and home-based pediatric interventions, as parents are the foremost role models from whom young children develop activity preferences [9]. Self-efficacy has been identified by Bandura [15] as the most salient determinant of behavior change within SCT. Self-control works in tandem with self-efficacy to promote behavior change and was considered important for actualizing self-efficacy [2]. Sharma et al. [16] identified self-efficacy as a primary predictor for daily physical activity among fifth grade school children. The study [16] also found that self-control was associated with reduction of screen time exposure. Expectations perform an integral role in motivation to modify a behavior and were considered a core construct of SCT [17]. Prior research has identified a dose-response relationship between expectations and physical activity [18]. Emotional coping was deemed important in predicting the targeted behaviors, as young children often initially reject behavior modification [19]. To compensate, parents may use authoritarian parenting techniques, which can produce negative long-term outcomes on a child's perceptions of health behaviors [20]; therefore, it was considered advantageous to provide participants with skills and techniques to reduce stress associated with health behavior change in children. Based on prior family- and home-based pediatric obesity research, mothers were selected as the target population for this investigation [8, 21–24]. Children ages 4 to 6 year were targeted for this study as this age range has been demonstrated to be a strong predictor of future health [8, 25].

Given this backdrop, the purpose of this study was to begin addressing the scarcity of behavioral prediction models required to advance family- and home-based, pediatric obesity, primary prevention intervention research. To accomplish this objective, five SCT maternal-facilitated constructs (environment, expectations, emotional coping, self-control, and self-efficacy) hypothesized to predict physical activity and screen time behaviors in children were operationalized and modeled. The behaviors were modeled separately according to the five SCT constructs. Subsequently, this study reports findings of two models. Model one tests the reliability and validity of the five SCT constructs regressed on physical activity. Model two tests the reliability and validity of the five SCT constructs regressed on screen time. As elucidated in the results section of this report, some theoretical constructs entered into the models were identified as suppressor variables. Suppressor variables control for error variance in one or more independent variables within a regression model. Therefore, a secondary objective of this report was to demonstrate the role of suppressor variables in primary prevention, pediatric obesity research, specifically, to explain how suppressor variables can help to inform intervention design and implementation.

2. Materials and Methods

2.1. Participants. Sample size for model building was established using Westland's [26] structural equation modeling calculator. Respondents included convenience samples of mothers recruited from a large, north American Midwestern University, a large, north American Midwestern Hospital, childcare centers located throughout the Midwest region of north America, as well as a preestablished subject pool.

2.2. Instrumentation. Instrumentation encompassed three stages of data collection and analysis. Stage one evaluated face and content validity of the instrument through a panel of six experts over a two-round review process. Stage two evaluated test-retest reliability of the instrument. Stage three evaluated construct and predictive validity of the instrument through structural equation modeling.

2.3. Stage One Procedures. The initial instrument items were adapted from a previous validated instrument developed by Sharma et al. [16] that examined SCT, physical activity, and screen time predictors of pediatric obesity within a school-based context. The original, self-report instrument was designed to be completed by school children; thus the items were modified for relevancy to mothers with young children. After the initial items were created, a panel of experts was formed. The panel of experts consisted of two pediatric obesity experts, two health behavior experts and two SCT experts. Each panel member was sent a cover letter explaining the purpose of the study, a copy of the draft instrument, and a feedback assessment form to evaluate face and content validity of the instrument. Members were asked to provide a general critique of the instrument and to make suggestions for improvement based upon their individual areas of expertise. Feedback materials were requested to be returned within a two-week time frame. Modifications were made to the instrument based on the jurors' feedback. After incorporating the recommended amendments suggested by the panel, a modified version of the instrument was delivered to the panel for a second round of review. For round two, jurors received a summarized list of all changes made to the instrument, a copy of the revised instrument, and an instrument assessment form. Jurors were requested to submit round two feedback within a two-week period. Once again, panel member recommendations were incorporated. Unanimous agreement concerning the face and content validity of the instrument was reached after round two; thus the panel of experts was disbanded. The final, 40-item instrument was organized into four parts: (1) inclusion/exclusion criteria for participation, (2) 24 hour, maternal-proxy behavioral recall of child physical activity and screen time behaviors, (3) operationalized, maternal-facilitated constructs of SCT, and (4) demographic information.

Part one of the instrument applied inclusion criteria to gauge participant eligibility. For the purposes of this study, eligibility was limited to English-speaking mothers with at least one child in the age range of 4 to 6 years. Exclusion criteria included pregnant mothers, mothers with a child inside the age range of 4 to 6 years with a disability that would interfere with participating in physical activity, a child with a medical condition associated with weight gain, a child prescribed medication associated with weight gain, or a child currently enrolled in an additional weight-management program. Participants were requested to either agree or disagree with each criterion. Those participants unable to satisfy inclusion/exclusion criteria were ineligible to participate. For eligible participants with more than one child in the age range of 4 to 6 years, the respondent was requested to answer the instrument items with their oldest child in mind.

Part two of the instrument assessed the physical activity and screen time behaviors of the participants' children. The physical activity item requested "Yesterday, how many total minutes was your child physically active throughout the day?" Screen time items queried "Yesterday, how many minutes did your child watch TV, DVDs, or movies", "Yesterday how many minutes did your child spend on a computer?", and "How many minutes did your child spend playing video games?" Participants were requested to respond in short answer format by indicating the total quantity of the given behavioral unit in the previous 24 hours. Illustrated examples of each behavior were provided on the instrument to assist comprehension of the requested information.

Part three of the instrument comprised the scales for measuring the maternal-facilitated SCT constructs for child physical activity and screen time behaviors. Both models included three items to assess the home environment of the mother's child to engage in the physical activity and screen time behaviors. For both models, the score range for the environment construct was 3 to 15. Higher scores implied an environment more conducive to increasing physical activity and reducing screen time. For both models, the stem statement "How often do you" was followed by 5-point, Likert-type scales with endpoints ranging from "never" to "always." Sample scale items from model 1 included "participate in physical activity in front of your child in your home, yard, or apartment complex?" and "find fun ways for your child to be physically active in your home, yard, or apartment complex?" Sample scale items from model 2 included "find alternatives to screen time at home for your child?" and "participate in screen time at home with your child?"

Both models included three items to measure the capacity of the mother to assist her child with adjusting emotionally and psychologically to increasing physical activity and reducing screen time. For both models, the score range for the environment construct was 3 to 15. Higher scores indicated stronger emotional coping capabilities of the mother to encourage physical activity and to reduce screen time. For both models, the emotional coping stem statement "How sure are you that you can help your child" was proceeded by 5-point, Likert-type scales with endpoints ranging from "not at all sure" to "completely sure." Sample scale items from model 1 included "adjust to being physically active for 60 minutes each day?" and "manage any negative emotions from them if you encourage them to be physically active?" Sample scale items from model 2 included "manage any negative emotions from them while reducing screen time?" and "adjust to reducing screen time to less than 2 hours per day?"

Expectations were comprised of the multiplicative score of two subconstructs: outcome expectations and outcome expectancies. Both models included four items to measure outcome expectations and four complementary items to measure outcome expectancies of the two behaviors. The summative scores of the outcome expectations and outcome expectancies constructs were multiplied for a potential product score range of 4 to 100. Higher scores indicated stronger maternal expectations regarding engagement in physical activity and refrainment of screen time. For both models, the outcome expectations stem statement "If your child participates in physical activity/screen time every day they will" was proceeded by 5-point, Likert-type scales with endpoints ranging from "not at all likely" to "extremely likely." Sample scale items for both models included "have a better weight?", and "have more energy?" For both models, the outcome expectancies stem statement, "Overall, how important is it to you that your child will" was proceeded by a 5-point, Likert-type scale with endpoints ranging from "not at all important" to "extremely important." Sample scale items for both models included "have more self-confidence?" and "be more relaxed?"

Both models included three items to measure the capacity of the mother to set goals to increase physical activity and decrease screen time. For both models, the score range for the self-control construct was 3 to 15. Higher scores indicated stronger self-regulatory abilities of the mother to promote physical activity and discourage screen time. For both models, the self-control stem statement "How sure are you that you can" was proceeded by 5-point, Likert-type scales with endpoints ranging from "not at all sure" to "completely sure." Sample scale items from model 1 included "reward your child with something they like for being physically active for 60 minutes every day?" and "plan to have your child be physically active for 60 minutes every day?" Sample scale items from model 2 included "set goals to reduce your child's screen time to no more than 2 hours per day?" and "reward your child for reducing screen time?"

Both models included three items to measure the confidence of the mother to increase physical activity and reduce screen time. For both models, the possible score range for the self-efficacy construct was 3 to 15. Higher scores indicated robust self-efficacy capabilities of the mother to increase physical activity and reduce screen time. For both models, self-efficacy stem statement "How confident are you that you can get your child to" was proceeded by 5-point, Likert-type scales with endpoints ranging from "not at all confident" to "completely confident." Sample scale items from model 1 included "physically active for 60 minutes every day?" and "physically active for 60 minutes every day, even if you are tired?" Sample scale items from model 2 included, "spend no more than 2 hours per day with screen time?" and "reduce screen time even if their favorite show is coming on?"

The final section of the instrument was devoted to collecting demographic data. Multiple choice questions were used to obtain race/ethnicity of the mother, marital status of the mother, sex of the child, and race/ethnicity of the child. Self-reported ages of the participant and the child were acquired using short answer format.

2.4. Stage Two and Three Procedures. For stage two, test-retest reliability coefficients were calculated for both exogenous and endogenous variables to assess stability over time. In conducting test-retest analysis, 30 volunteering participants were requested to complete the instrument two times, with two weeks between administrations of the instrument. Acceptable test-retest Pearson's r test-retest coefficient values were set *a priori* at 0.70 [27]. For stage three, Kline's [28] two-step modeling procedure was applied to specify each behavioral model. Confirmatory factor analysis (CFA) was conducted to assess model fit. CFA was evaluated through the model chi-square test (χ^2) with significance testing set *a priori* at P value greater than 0.05 and root mean square error of approximation (RMSEA) less than 1.00 [29]. Additional fit indexes included the goodness-of-fit index (GFI), adjusted goodness-of-fit index (AGFI), normed fit index (NFI), and comparative fit index (CFI), all of which should exceed 0.90 by convention [28]. Convergent validity assessed the extent to which the model indicators of each construct converged adequately. In assessing convergent validity, indicator factor loadings, construct reliability, and average variance extracted were calculated [30]. Factor loading values less than 0.50 were considered for removal. In maintaining conventional standards, average variance extracted was set *a priori* at no less than 0.50 and construct reliability was set at no less than 0.60 [30].

Following development of the measurement models, structural models were built to determine the variance explained in physical activity and screen time behaviors by the maternal-facilitated SCT variables. Significance levels for direct path coefficients were set *a priori* at P-value less than 0.05. Practical significance was gauged by evaluating standardized beta coefficients of each of the statistically significant predictors. Parameters for the two-step modeling processes were estimated using the maximum likelihood method. Metric scales were developed by fixing the first indicator of each latent variable to 1.0. Models were developed with Analysis of Moment Structure (AMOS) software version 18. Construct reliability and average variance extracted were calculated manually by computing formulas developed by Fornell and Larcker [30] with Microsoft Excel 2010. University Institutional Review Board (IRB) approval was sought and obtained prior to collecting participant data.

3. Results

3.1. Descriptive Statistics of Sample and Child Behaviors. Participants (n = 224) were predominantly Caucasian (72%), married (70%) and unemployed/homemakers (49%), with a mean age of 33.2 years (SD = 6.8). Data on two child behaviors were collected from the sample using 24 hour, proxy recall. The possible range for the child physical activity behavior construct was 0 to 500 minutes of physical activity in the previous 24 hours. The desired mean value was a minimum of 60 minutes. The observed range was 0 to 400 minutes with a mean of 101.77 minutes and a standard deviation of 80.52 minutes. The possible range for the child screen time behavior construct was 0 to 1,000 minutes of screen time in the previous 24 hours. The desired mean value was a maximum of 120 minutes. The observed range was 0 to 800 minutes with a mean of 104.65 minutes and a standard deviation of 98.61 minutes.

3.2. Model One: Physical Activity Behavior. Mahalanobis d-squared values identified 18 impactful outliers; therefore, 206 samples were analyzed. Factor loadings, construct reliability values, and average variance extracted percentages satisfied the *a priori* thresholds. With the exception of one construct, child physical activity behavior (r = 0.67), all test-retest reliability coefficient values (n = 31) satisfied the 0.70 *a priori* reliability threshold. The final maternal-facilitated child physical activity behavior measurement model indicated reasonable fit to the data (χ^2 = 189.886, df = 92, P < 0.001; GFI = 0.893, AGFI = 0.842, NFI = 0.901, CFI = 0.946, and RMSEA = 0.072). Analysis of the structural model identified significant direct paths between maternal-facilitated environment (P < 0.001), emotional coping (P = 0.006), self-efficacy (P = 0.010), and child physical activity behavior. Specification indices indicated satisfactory fit for the final model (χ^2 = 51.268, df = 28, P = 0.005; GFI = 0.955, AGFI = 0.911, NFI = 0.940, CFI = 0.971, and RMSEA = 0.064). The model Chi-square test did not satisfy the *a priori* criteria of P-value greater than 0.05; however, the model Chi-square test is highly sensitive to sample sizes that exceed 200 observations [31]. Applying Kline's alternative to the model Chi-square test, model fit was satisfactory (51.268/28 = 1.831). Table 1 summarizes parameter estimates and fit statistics of the structural model. Figure 1 provides an illustration of the final structural model with standardized regression weights.

Collectively, the exogenous variables accounted for 22% of the variance in the child physical activity behavior construct. Emotional coping explained the greatest proportion of variance in the model ($\beta = -0.479$), followed by environment ($\beta = 0.466$) and self-efficacy ($\beta = 0.372$). Of the predictors, only emotional coping had a negative effect on physical activity behavior, which initially suggested that as emotional coping capacity increased physical activity quantity decreased. Further review of the construct's characteristics suggested

Table 1: Parameter estimates for the trimmed maternal-facilitated child physical activity behavior structural model for the sample of mothers ($n = 206$).

Variables	B	SE B	β	P
CPAB ← MF ENV	2.751	0.709	0.466	<0.001
CPAB ← MF SE	2.637	1.028	0.372	0.010
CPAB ← MF EC	−3.115	1.132	−0.479	0.006

Notes: CPAB: child physical activity behavior; MF ENV: maternal-facilitated environment; MF SE: maternal-facilitated self-efficacy; MF EC: maternal-facilitated emotional coping.
$\chi^2 = 51.268$, $df = 28$, $P = 0.005$; GFI = 0.955, AGFI = 0.911, NFI = 0.940, CFI = 0.971, and RMSEA = 0.064.
R^2 value of CPAB for final specified model is 0.22.

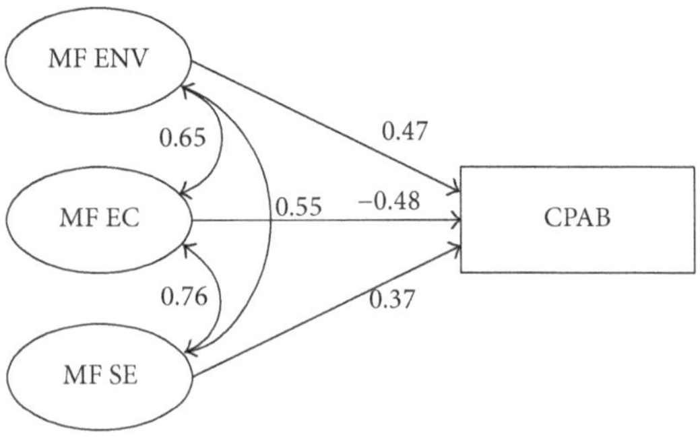

Figure 1: Maternal-facilitated child physical activity behavior structural model illustrating standardized regression weights for the sample of mothers ($n = 206$). Notes: CPAB is child physical activity behavior; MF ENV is maternal-facilitated environment; MF EC is maternal- facilitated emotional coping; MF SE is maternal-facilitated self-efficacy.

that emotional coping acted as a suppressor variable within the model.

3.3. Suppression Variable Procedures. A series of four procedures were applied to determine if emotional coping was functioning as a suppressor variable [32, 33]. The first procedure involved examination of the correlation matrix to determine the relationship between the hypothesized suppressor, the other independent variables in the model, and the outcome variable. Suppressors are characterized by having a minimal direct relationship to the outcome variable, while being significantly correlated to other independent variables in the model [34]. The second procedure involved examining the impact of the hypothesized suppressor on the standardized beta weights of the other independent variables in the model. When included in a regression equation, suppressor variables increase the predictive validity of one or more other independent variables in the model. Concurrently, suppressors only control error variance for those independent variables whose regression weights increase due to its entry into the equation. The third procedure tested the possibility of multicollinearity. Detection of high multicollinearity within a regression model can be determined through examination of the correlational matrix and tolerance and variance inflation factor (VIF) values. Tolerance values less than 0.20 and VIF values greater than 5.0 are generally accepted cutoffs for indicating the presence of multicollinearity [33]. The final procedure included inspection of the suppressor's beta weight. Negative suppression occurs when the beta weight of the suppressor variable in the regression equation is the opposite sign from its correlation with the outcome variable.

Applying the first procedure verified that emotional coping had an insignificant, positive correlation with physical activity behavior ($r = 0.088$); yet, it had a statistically significant correlation with environment ($r = 0.481$) and self-efficacy ($r = 0.601$). The second procedure included examining the effect of the emotional coping variable upon removal from the structural model. Upon removing the hypothesized suppressor, results found that the R value of the physical activity behavior model decreased from 0.22 to 0.14, with the self-efficacy construct becoming statistically insignificant ($P = 0.314$) and the significance level of environment decreasing from a P-value less than 0.001 to P-value equal to 0.001. When the emotional coping variable was reinserted into the model, the total R-value once again increased to its pretest level of 0.22, the self-efficacy construct again became significant ($P = 0.010$), and the environment construct regained its former significance level ($P < 0.001$). Upon reintroduction of the suppressor, regression weights for self-efficacy increased from 0.091 to 0.372, while regression weights for environment increased from 0.318 to 0.466. These findings suggested that emotional coping primarily suppressed self-efficacy but also suppressed the environment construct. Next, multicollinearity was assessed. Of the significant variables in the final model, tolerance values were between 0.577 and 0.739 and VIF levels were between 1.354 and 1.732, indicating an absence of multicollinearity. Finally, the suppressor's beta weight within the regression equation was reviewed. Results found that, despite emotional coping's positive correlation with physical activity behavior, the construct displayed a negative beta weight within the regression equation, implying the status of a negative suppressor.

3.4. Model Two: Screen Time Behavior. Mahalanobis d-squared values identified four impactful outliers; therefore, 220 samples were analyzed. Examination of the initial measurement model found that the first environment indicator had a factor loading value of 0.24. As this fell below the 0.50 threshold, this variable was removed from the measurement model. The remaining factor loadings, construct reliability values, average variance extracted percentages, and test-retest reliability coefficient values satisfied the *a priori* thresholds.

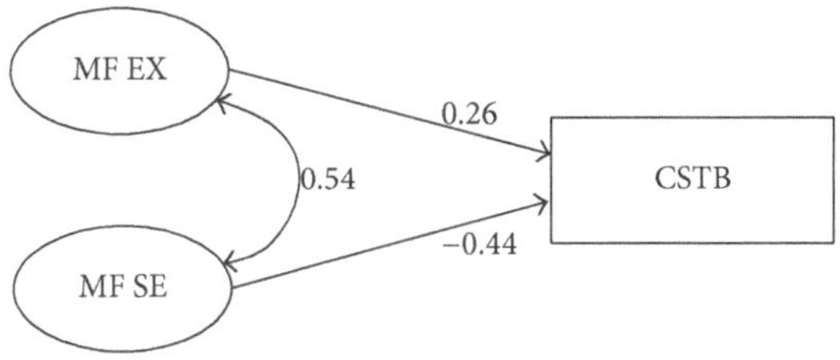

FIGURE 2: Maternal-facilitated child screen time behavior structural model illustrating standardized regression weights for the sample of mothers (n = 220). Notes: CSTB is child screen time behavior; MF EX is maternal-facilitated expectations; MF SE is maternal-facilitated self-efficacy.

The final maternal-facilitated child screen time behavior measurement model indicated reasonable fit to the data (χ^2 = 254.11, df = 94, $P < 0.001$; GFI = 0.873, AGFI = 0.810, NFI = 0.904, CFI = 0.934, and RMSEA = 0.094). Analysis of the structural model identified significant direct paths between maternal-facilitated expectations (P = 0.002), self-efficacy ($P < 0.001$), and child screen time behavior. Specification indices indicated satisfactory fit for the final model (χ^2 = 20.216, df = 16, P = 0.211; GFI = 0.977, AGFI = 0.948, NFI = 0.980, CFI = 0.996, and RMSEA = 0.035). Table 2 summarizes parameter estimates and fit statistics of the structural model. Figure 2 provides an illustration of the final structural model with standardized regression weights.

Combined, emotional coping and environment accounted for 14% of the variance in the child screen time behavior construct. Inspection of the standardized beta weights of the significant variables found self-efficacy explained the greatest proportion of variance in the model (β = −0.479) followed by expectations (β = 0.466). The self-efficacy construct's negative beta weight suggested that as self-efficacy increased screen time behavior decreased. Among the predictors, only expectations had a positive effect on screen time behavior, which initially suggested that as expectations increased screen time quantity increased. Further review of the construct's characteristics suggested that expectations acted as a suppressor variable within the model.

The four procedures for suppressor variable detection were applied. Employing the first procedure verified that expectations had an insignificant, positive correlation with screen time behavior (r = 0.029); yet, it had a statistically significant correlation with self-efficacy (r = 0.491). The second procedure included examining the effect of the expectations variable upon removal from the structural model. Upon removing the hypothesized suppressor, results found that the R-value of the screen time behavior model decreased from 0.14 to 0.08, with the self-efficacy construct retaining its statistical significance in the model ($P < 0.001$). When the expectations variable was re-inserted into the model, the total R-value once again increased to its pretest level of 0.14. Upon reintroduction of the suppressor, standardized regression weights for self-efficacy increased from −0.279 to −0.432. Next, multicollinearity was assessed. Of the significant variables in the final model, tolerance values were between 0.599 and 0.690 and VIF levels were between 1.449 and 1.670, indicating an absence of multicollinearity. Finally, the suppressor's beta weight within the regression equation was reviewed. Results found that expectation's positive correlation with screen time behavior was retained within the regression equation, implying the status of a classical suppressor.

4. Discussion

Suppressor variables are variables that suppress or control for error variance in one or more independent variables in a model [34, 35]. Through this action, suppressor variables unleash the latent predictive power of one or more independent variables in the regression equation, thereby bolstering their beta weight(s) [32]. The term suppressor may initially seem obstructive to a model development; however, researchers have identified three primary advantages of retaining suppressor variables in multiple regressions: (1) increased accuracy of regression coefficients associated with independent variables, (2) improved predictive validity of a model, and (3) enhanced accuracy of a theory building [36].

Researchers have categorized three types of suppression effects in multiple correlations [36, 37]. Classical suppression occurs when the variable in question has a zero or minimal correlation with the dependent variable; yet, it significantly correlates with one or more independent variables in the model [38]. Negative suppression occurs when the beta weight of the suppressor variable in the regression equation is the opposite sign from its correlation with the outcome variable [39]. Reciprocal suppression occurs if both the suppressor and predictor are positively correlated with the outcome variable, yet negatively correlated with one another [40].

An important factor when interpreting suppressor variables is refrainment from the assumption that the negative beta weight of a suppressor implies a negative direct effect on the outcome variable; instead, the suppressor should be viewed as clearing out criterion-irrelevant variance in one or more other predictor variables [41]. To understand how suppressors function from an applied perspective, it is helpful to consider the case published by Horst [42], who was one of the first researchers to publish the suppressor concept. Horst described a study conducted during World War II that sought to predict pilot success in a training program. Measures of mechanical, numerical, spatial, and verbal ability were collected and correlated with training success. Results found that each of the variables, aside from verbal ability, was positively correlated with pilot success. Conversely, verbal ability had a near-zero correlation with pilot success yet was correlated with the other three predictors. Paradoxically, when verbal ability was entered into the regression equation the model's predictive capacity increased, despite verbal ability having insignificant correlation with pilot training. Horst's deduction was that verbal ability was required to read the directions and items included on the tests measuring the other three abilities. As such, verbal ability was acting as a suppressor by removing irrelevant variance from the other predictors, which assisted in clarifying their role in the model.

Table 2: Parameter estimates for the trimmed maternal-facilitated child screen time behavior structural model for the sample of mothers ($n = 220$).

Variables	B	SE B	β	P
CSTB ← MF EX	0.216	0.069	0.262	0.002
CSTB ← MF SE	−2.481	0.510	−0.443	<0.001

Notes: CSTB: child screen time behavior; MF EX: maternal-facilitated expectations; MF SE: maternal-facilitated self-efficacy.
$\chi^2 = 20.216$, $df = 16$, $P = 0.211$; GFI = 0.977, AGFI = 0.948, NFI = 0.980, CFI = 996, and RMSEA = 0.035.
R^2 value of PC STB for final specified model is 0.14.

As Horst [42] concluded, "To include the verbal score with a negative weight served to suppress or subtract irrelevant ability and to discount the scores of those who did well on the test simply because of their verbal ability rather than because of abilities required for success in pilot training (p. 355)."

In the context of the physical activity model, emotional coping was significantly correlated with self-efficacy and environment, which, in turn, were significantly related to physical activity behavior in children. In effect, emotional coping, despite having a minimal direct bivariate relationship with physical activity behavior in children, removed error variance from the self-efficacy and environment constructs. Thus, when included in the model, the emotional coping suppressor purified the role of self-efficacy and environment as predictors of child physical activity behavior. In practical terms, the suppression effect of the emotional coping construct suggests that emotional coping abilities are required to actualize self-efficacy and, to some extent, the home environment for increasing maternal-facilitated physical activity behavior in children. In terms of intervention design, emotional coping should be sufficiently developed in mothers prior to attempting to build self-efficacy or improve the home environment for increasing child physical activity. Results of the screen time model suggested that expectations for screen time behavior suppress criterion-irrelevant variance in the self-efficacy construct. The suppression effect of this variable implies that expectations for the reduction of screen time behavior in children are required to actualize self-efficacy for decreasing this sedentary behavior in children. From an intervention perspective, expectations should be sufficiently developed in mothers prior to attempting to build self-efficacy for decreasing child screen time behavior.

5. Conclusions

The purpose of this study was to model maternal-facilitated, SCT predictors of child physical activity and screen time. The intention of these modeling efforts was to provide design, implementation, and evaluation direction for primary prevention, family- and home-based, pediatric obesity interventions. Unexpectedly, results found that emotional coping and expectations acted as suppressor variables in predicting the maternal-facilitated physical activity and screen time behaviors of children. Other researchers have noted suppressor variables present in SCT models [43–45]; however, this study appears to be the first to identify suppressor variables in SCT models examining pediatric obesity within the context of the family and home environment. From an application orientation, suppressor variables can inform essential groundwork required to fully actualize predictors of a given behavior. From a programmatic perspective, behavioral prediction models are often limited in the fact that they can only provide a recommendation of what constructs to reify in an intervention. Suppressor effects can supplement intervention design recommendations by providing a suggested ordering to theoretical construct integration within an intervention.

Based on the models specified in this study, it is recommended to target the suppressor variables at the outset of intervention implementation. Specifically, to improve child physical activity behavior from a maternally-oriented, family and home-based perspective, the present research suggests, first, to develop emotional coping skills within mothers. Once sufficient levels of emotional coping skills are acquired, self-efficacy and environment for physical activity behavior should be developed. To reduce screen time within a maternally-oriented, family and home-based context, the current research suggests developing expectations for reduction of screen time in mothers prior to reifying self-efficacy for this behavior. Future research should test interventions for developing these constructs in mothers.

Although fit statistics suggested satisfactory reliability and validity of the structural equation models, the results of this research should be considered in light of several limitations. Data for this study were collected from a convenience sample of mothers with children between four and six years of age. As such, the results cannot be generalized to all mothers with children in this age range. The cross-sectional nature of the data restricts the ability to establish causal relationships between the variables. From a measurement perspective, the behavioral data were collected through 24 hour, maternal-proxy self-report. Consequently, the precision of the specified models was limited to the self-reporting accuracy and honesty of the participants. Measurement of the behaviors could be improved with accelerometers and screen time monitors with data collected in a longitudinal fashion. Finally, there are also limitations inherent to the design of this study. Primarily, the data only captured one demographic (mothers) and one environment (home of the child) hypothesized to contribute to the prevention of pediatric obesity. Pediatric obesity is a complex health issue that is impacted by multiple social and environmental variables. Therefore, the current models are inadequate to fully capture all antecedents of pediatric obesity, even if ideal measurement were granted. To the best of the author's knowledge, this is the first study to identify suppressor variables in SCT models examining pediatric obesity within the context of the family and home environment. Subsequently, the findings of this research could be strengthened by reproducing the study with new samples. In particular, it would be beneficial if the identified suppressor effects were confirmed or refuted through similar modeling endeavors.

Disclosure

Portions of this paper were presented at the 2012 American Public Health Association National Convention.

Conflict of Interests

The author declares that there is no conflict of interests regarding the publication of this paper.

Acknowledgment

This study was sponsored by the University of Cincinnati Graduate School Summer Research Fellowship.

References

[1] C. L. Ogden, M. D. Carroll, B. K. Kit, and K. M. Flegal, "Prevalence of obesity and trends in body mass index among US children and adolescents, 1999-2010," *The Journal of the American Medical Association*, vol. 307, no. 5, pp. 483–490, 2012.

[2] T. Baranowski, K. W. Cullen, T. Nicklas, D. Thompson, and J. Baranowski, "Are current health behavioral change models helpful in guiding prevention of weight gain efforts?" *Obesity Research*, vol. 11, supplement 10, pp. 23S–43S, 2003.

[3] G. Rao, "Childhood obesity: highlights of AMA Expert Committee recommendations," *American Family Physician*, vol. 78, no. 1, pp. 56–66, 2008.

[4] U.S. Department of Health and Human Services, *2008 Physical Activity Guidelines for Americans*, U.S. Department of Health and Human Services, Washington, DC, USA, 2008.

[5] L. L. Moore, U.-S. D. T. Nguyen, K. J. Rothman, L. A. Cupples, and R. C. Ellison, "Preschool physical activity level and change in body fatness in young children: the Framingham Children's study," *American Journal of Epidemiology*, vol. 142, no. 9, pp. 982–988, 1995.

[6] R. C. Klesges, L. M. Klesges, L. H. Eck, and M. L. Shelton, "A longitudinal analysis of accelerated weight gain in preschool children," *Pediatrics*, vol. 95, no. 1, pp. 126–130, 1995.

[7] S. E. Barlow, "Expert committee recommendations regarding the prevention, assessment, and treatment of child and adolescent overweight and obesity: summary report," *Pediatrics*, vol. 120, supplement 4, pp. S164–192, 2007.

[8] S. Brophy, R. Cooksey, M. B. Gravenor et al., "Risk factors for childhood obesity at age 5: analysis of the Millennium Cohort study," *BMC Public Health*, vol. 9, article 467, 2009.

[9] E. M. Arredondo, J. P. Elder, G. X. Ayala, N. Campbell, B. Baquero, and S. Duerksen, "Is parenting style related to children's healthy eating and physical activity in Latino families?" *Health Education Research*, vol. 21, no. 6, pp. 862–871, 2006.

[10] A. P. Knowlden and M. Sharma, "Systematic review of family and home-based interventions targeting paediatric overweight and obesity," *Obesity Reviews*, vol. 13, no. 6, pp. 499–508, 2012.

[11] A. Bandura, "Health promotion by social cognitive means," *Health Education and Behavior*, vol. 31, no. 2, pp. 143–164, 2004.

[12] R. K. Dishman, A. L. Dunn, J. F. Sallis, R. J. Vandenberg, and C. A. Pratt, "Social-cognitive correlates of physical activity in a multi-ethnic cohort of middle-school girls: two-year prospective study," *Journal of Pediatric Psychology*, vol. 35, no. 2, pp. 188–198, 2010.

[13] M. D. Hearn, T. Baranowski, J. Baranowski et al., "Environmental influences on dietary behavior among children: availability and accessibility of fruits and vegetables enable consumption," *Journal of Health Education*, vol. 29, no. 1, pp. 26–32, 1998.

[14] K. J. Gruber and L. A. Haldeman, "Using the family to combat childhood and adult obesity," *Preventing Cronic Disease*, vol. 6, no. 3, article A106, 2009.

[15] A. Bandura, "Health promotion from the perspective of social cognitive theory," *Psychology and Health*, vol. 13, no. 4, pp. 623–649, 1998.

[16] M. Sharma, D. I. Wagner, and J. Wilkerson, "Predicting childhood obesity prevention behaviors using social cognitive theory," *International Quarterly of Community Health Education*, vol. 24, no. 3, pp. 191–203, 2005.

[17] A. Bandura, "Social cognitive theory: an agentic perspective," *Annual Review of Psychology*, vol. 52, pp. 1–26, 2001.

[18] M. E. Huhman, L. D. Potter, M. J. Nolin et al., "The influence of the VERB campaign on children's physical activity in 2002 to 2006," *American Journal of Public Health*, vol. 100, no. 4, pp. 638–645, 2010.

[19] L. L. Birch, "Psychological influences on the childhood diet," *The Journal of Nutrition*, vol. 128, no. 2, pp. 407S–410S, 1998.

[20] A. T. Galloway, L. M. Fiorito, L. A. Francis, and L. L. Birch, "'Finish your soup': counterproductive effects of pressuring children to eat on intake and affect," *Appetite*, vol. 46, no. 3, pp. 318–323, 2006.

[21] G. X. Ayala, J. P. Elder, N. R. Campbell et al., "Longitudinal intervention effects on parenting of the aventuras para Niños study," *American Journal of Preventive Medicine*, vol. 38, no. 2, pp. 154–162, 2010.

[22] H. R. Clark, E. Goyder, P. Bissell, L. Blank, and J. Peters, "How do parents' child-feeding behaviours influence child weight? Implications for childhood obesity policy," *Journal of Public Health*, vol. 29, no. 2, pp. 132–141, 2007.

[23] J. Harvey-Berino and J. Rourke, "Obesity prevention in preschool Native-American children: a pilot study using home visiting," *Obesity Research*, vol. 11, no. 5, pp. 606–611, 2003.

[24] A. Jain, S. N. Sherman, L. A. Chamberlin, Y. Carter, S. W. Powers, and R. C. Whitaker, "Why don't low-income mothers worry about their preschoolers being overweight?" *Pediatrics*, vol. 107, no. 5, pp. 1138–1146, 2001.

[25] D. S. L. Gardner, J. Hosking, B. S. Metcalf, A. N. Jeffery, L. D. Voss, and T. J. Wilkin, "Contribution of early weight gain to childhood overweight and metabolic health: a longitudinal study (EarlyBird 36)," *Pediatrics*, vol. 123, no. 1, pp. e67 e73, 2009.

[26] J. C. Westland, "Lower bounds on sample size in structural equation modeling," *Electronic Commerce Research and Applications*, vol. 9, no. 6, pp. 476–487, 2010.

[27] D. F. Polit and C. T. Beck, *Nursing Research: Principles and Methods*, Lippincott Williams & Wilkins, Hagerstown, Md, USA, 7th edition, 2004.

[28] R. B. Kline, *Principles and Practice of Structural Equation Modeling*, The Guilford Press, 2010.

[29] M. W. Browne and R. Cudeck, *Alternative Ways of Assessing Model Fit. Testing Structural Equation Models*, Sage, Newbury Park, Calif, USA, 1993.

[30] C. Fornell and D. F. Larcker, "Evaluating structural equation models with unobservable variables and measurement error," *Journal of Marketing Research*, vol. 18, no. 1, pp. 39–50, 1981.

[31] S. L. Hoe, "Issues and procedures in adopting structural equation modeling technique," *Journal of Applied Quantitative Methods*, vol. 3, no. 1, pp. 76–83, 2008.

[32] D. L. Paulhus, R. W. Robins, K. H. Trzesniewski, and J. L. Tracy, "Two replicable suppressor situations in personality research," *Multivariate Behavioral Research*, vol. 39, no. 2, pp. 303–328, 2004.

[33] D. A. Walker, "Suppressor variable(s) importance within a regression model: an example of salary compression from career services," *Journal of College Student Development*, vol. 44, no. 1, pp. 127–133, 2003.

[34] B. P. Lancaster, *Defining and Interpreting Suppressor Effects: Advantages and Limitations*, Southwest Educational Research Association, San Antonio, Tex, USA, 1999.

[35] K. K. Woolley, *How Variables Uncorrelated with the Dependent Variable Can Actually Make Excellent Predictors: The Important Suppressor Variable Case*, Southwest Educational Research Association, Austin, Tex, USA, 1997.

[36] S. Pandey and W. Elliott, "Suppressor variables in social work research: ways to identify in multiple regression models," *Journal of the Society for Social Work and Research*, vol. 1, no. 1, 2010.

[37] N. K. Gaylord-Harden, J. A. Cunningham, G. N. Holmbeck, and K. E. Grant, "Suppressor effects in coping research with african american adolescents from low-income communities," *Journal of Consulting and Clinical Psychology*, vol. 78, no. 6, pp. 843–855, 2010.

[38] P. Horst, "The role of predictor variables which are independent of the criterion," *Social Science Research Council Bulletin*, vol. 48, pp. 431–436, 1941.

[39] A. Lubin, "Some formulae for use with suppressor variables," *Educational and Psychological Measurement*, vol. 17, no. 2, pp. 286–296, 1957.

[40] A. J. Conger, "A revised definition for suppressor variables: a guide to their identification and interpretation," *Educational and Psychological Measurement*, vol. 34, no. 1, pp. 35–46, 1974.

[41] G. W. Cheung and R. S. Lau, "Testing mediation and suppression effects of latent variables: bootstrapping with structural equation models," *Organizational Research Methods*, vol. 11, no. 2, pp. 296–325, 2008.

[42] P. Horst, *Psychological Measurement and Prediction*, Wadsworth, Belmont, Calif, USA, 1966.

[43] N. E. Betz and K. K. Voyten, "Efficacy and outcome expectations influence career exploration and decidedness," *Career Development Quarterly*, vol. 46, no. 2, pp. 179–189, 1997.

[44] D. R. Lubans, C. Foster, and S. J. H. Biddle, "A review of mediators of behavior in interventions to promote physical activity among children and adolescents," *Preventive Medicine*, vol. 47, no. 5, pp. 463–470, 2008.

[45] P. R. Pintrich and E. V. de Groot, "Motivational and self-regulated learning components of classroom academic performance," *Journal of Educational Psychology*, vol. 82, no. 1, pp. 33–40, 1990.

11

Health Communication Cards as a Tool for Behaviour Change

Carrie L. Matteson,[1] Thomas D. N. Merth,[2] and Diane T. Finegood[1]

[1] *Department of Biomedical Physiology and Kinesiology, Simon Fraser University, WMC 2805, 8888 University Drive, Burnaby, BC, Canada V5A 1S6*
[2] *Faculty of Medicine, University of British Columbia, The Gordon and Leslie Diamond Health Care Centre, 2775 Laurel Street, Vancouver, BC, Canada V5Z 1M9*

Correspondence should be addressed to Carrie L. Matteson; matteson@sfu.ca

Academic Editors: P. J. Geiselman and L. R. Vartanian

Individuals seeking healthcare treatment in the context of obesity often experience difficulty engaging in discussions around their health and face challenges finding consensus with practitioners on care plans that best suit their lives. The complex set of biological, social, and environmental variables that have contributed to the higher prevalence of obesity are well illustrated in the foresight obesity system map. Effectively understanding and addressing key variables for each individual has proven to be difficult, with clinicians facing barriers and limited resources to help address patients' unique needs. However, productive discussions inspired by patient centered care may be particularly effective in promoting behaviour change. Tools based on systems science that facilitate patient centered care and help identify behaviour change priorities have not been developed to help treat adult obesity. This project created and pilot tested a card based clinical communication tool designed to help facilitate conversations with individuals engaged in health behaviour change. The health communication cards were designed to help direct conversation between patients and healthcare providers toward issues relevant to the individual. Use of the cards to facilitate patient driven conversations in clinical care may help to streamline conversations, set realistic care plan goals, and improve long term rates of compliance.

1. Introduction

Obesity is widely recognized as a complex and serious health problem, yet overweight individuals struggle with losing weight and maintaining weight loss. Health professionals often feel ill equipped to offer support that may lead to success for their clients, and attempts to engage patients in conversations about weight reduction have decreased even in patient populations with the most need [1]. Obesity rates are forecasted to increase as much as 33% in the next 20 years [2], potentially adding to an already high annual estimated health care cost of over $140 billion [3]. The current high rates of obesity have emerged from a complex set of biological, social, and environmental variables. The foresight obesity system map illustrates this complexity, demonstrating 109 variables and 304 connections between them [4]. These variables represent the multiple levels of factors associated with obesity, from population to individual level variables. To successfully combat obesity as a society, solutions will likely need to target all of these levels. However, clinical treatment strategies often focus on individual behaviour change, encouraging increased rates of physical activity and decreased caloric intake. Public health initiatives focus on altering environmental stimuli to reach the same end, but barriers such as policy resistance produce lacklustre results in shifting obesity trends.

Individuals commonly seek help for reducing their weight at commercial facilities such as weight loss and physical activity centers, in addition to physicians' offices. For any person seeking help with behaviour change, only a subset of the many individual level variables in the foresight map may be relevant. Effectively understanding and addressing this subset has proven to be difficult, with clinicians often reporting obesity treatment as being "doomed to failure" [5], frustrating, and ineffective [6]. This stance is problematic, as clinicians are able to positively influence patients' health related behaviour by providing patients with some form of behavioural counselling, especially when patients actively participate [7, 8]. Patient centered care may decrease health care costs, as one study found that participants who received patient centered care sought less diagnostic tests and requested less referrals and follow-up medical visits [9].

The Canadian Clinical Practice Guidelines on the Management and Prevention of Obesity provide some guidance to clinicians by addressing pharmaceutical, surgical, cognitive, and behavioural treatment or prevention strategies [10]. The behavioural and cognitive treatment of obesity is important as it is the least invasive, and it may be more successful than pharmacotherapy, especially in maintaining long term weight loss after the treatment has stopped [11]. Behavioural treatment can exist on its own, or as an important component of these other approaches [12]. Discussions inspired by patient centered care may be particularly effective in behaviour change [13]. However, a review of chronic disease care practices in 13 different countries revealed a lack of self-management support, especially in the realm of emotionally based care challenges [14].

Strategies for effective communication between patients and healthcare practitioners are a key element of behavioural treatment. Decision and communication support aids have been utilized in the treatment of other diseases such as cancer and diabetes to help patients understand treatment options and provide personalized care [15–17]. In the United Kingdom, diabetes cards were developed as part of a project to address the difficulty some patients had in articulating specific challenges in managing their diabetes. Cards consisted of statements constructed from written descriptions of the problems and healthcare needs of diabetes patients. In this way, patients were able to develop their own "diabetes care agenda" [16, 18]. No such systems science based tools that facilitate patient centered care and help identify behaviour change priorities have been developed to help treat adult obesity. Based upon the success of previous support aids and patient communication tools, we aim to generate a tool to guide individuals with health behaviour change.

This project created and pilot tested a card based clinical communication tool designed to help facilitate conversations with individuals engaged in health behaviour change. The health communication cards were designed to help individuals understand the broad range of variables implicated in obesity and to provide a simple tool for generating patient focused goals. The tool is designed to help direct the conversation between patients and healthcare providers to issues relevant to the individual, as opposed to a more generic and simplistic "one size fits all" discussion of the need for more exercise and less food intake. Use of the cards to facilitate patient driven conversations in clinical care may help to develop autonomy and self-motivation in behaviour change, which are shown to improve long term rates of compliance [19].

2. Methods

2.1. Statement Development for Health Communication Cards. Card statements were chosen to represent the broad range of factors implicated in obesity at the level of the individual while including cognitive and behavioural variables found to be important in obesity treatment. These issues were drawn from a system map illustrating the complex influences on obesity in addition to the clinically relevant cognitive and behavioural concepts identified in the treatment literature. The foresight obesity system map was used to construct cards describing individual level variables because it serves as a comprehensive overview of many different areas implicated in obesity with a complex systems lens [4]. All seven clusters on the map (food production, food consumption, individual physical activity, individual psychology, social psychology, physical activity environment, and physiology) were utilized to generate statements worded to describe a problem that an individual might face based on the variables illustrated in the map. For example, the variable "food variety" was converted to the statement "I do not try new foods often," while the variable "cost of physical exercise" was converted to "Physical activity is too expensive."

Specific cognitive and behavioural variables implicated in obesity and shown to be effective treatment targets were further explored and used to inform the development of the cards. These variables include eating self-efficacy [20, 21], exercise self-efficacy [22, 23], binge eating behaviour [23, 24], flexible cognitive restraint, disinhibition, and hunger [25–28]. Validated and widely used tools to assess these variables provided background for generating statements in these areas. For example, the weight efficacy lifestyle questionnaire assesses eating self-efficacy and has a series of statements that assess self-efficacy in situations where food is readily available. The card "I do not feel confident in my ability to resist overeating when many kinds of food are available (such as at a buffet)" was created to reflect this. The intention was to capture a full range of issues that may be relevant to individuals as they try to communicate the details surrounding their individual circumstances regarding health behaviour change. A total of 64 card statements were generated for the health communication cards.

2.2. Semistructured Interviews and Focus Group. All subjects were actively trying to make changes in eating and exercise behaviours and were purposively recruited to participate in either semistructured interviews ($n = 10$) or a focus group ($n = 8$). A research design flow chart is shown in Figure 1. Ethical approval was obtained by the Simon Fraser University Office of Research Ethics. For interviews, two trained researchers worked with patients at an internal medicine specialist's office. Adult patients who were overweight or obese, were seeking treatment for a weight related condition, could speak and read English, and had an appointment during that time were eligible. The recruiting physician spoke to all patients seeking treatment for a weight related condition about the project, and interested individuals were directed to the on-site researchers. After obtaining signed, informed consent, participants contributed to individually recorded conversations regarding their challenges and successes with lifestyle change while sorting through the health communication card deck.

Insights gained through interview data analysis were used to modify the interview script in order to further explore targeted lines of inquiry during a focus group located in a different clinical context and geographic location. Participants

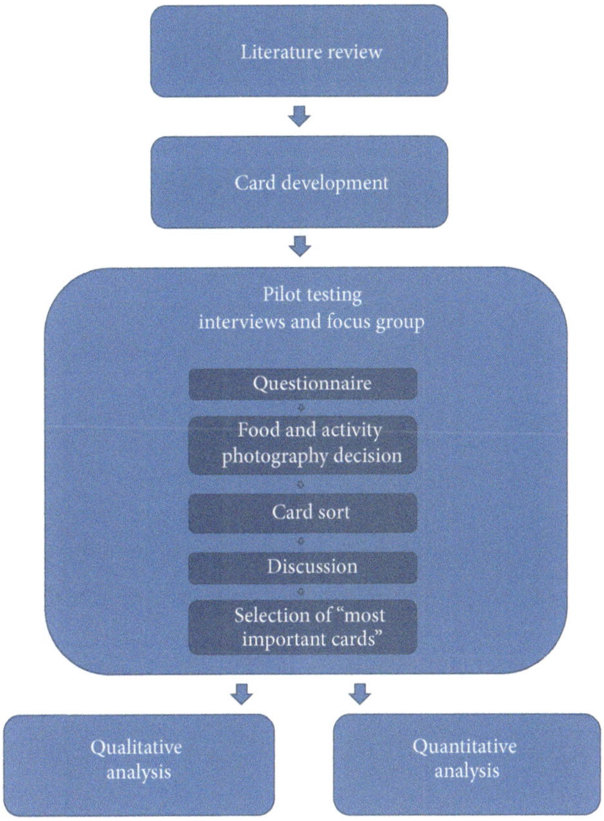

FIGURE 1

were individuals participating in a weight loss surgery support group. The group was self-organized by patients who had undergone bariatric surgery some time in the past and included members who were waiting for surgery. The intent of the group is to provide treatment information, postoperative support, and guidance with health behaviour change to group members at any stage in the surgical continuum (from presurgical treatment to many years post-op). Support group members were comprised of adults who spoke English, were self-seeking support with regard to lifestyle change, and had access to bariatric surgery. The health communication cards project was introduced by the group founder and core facilitator at a meeting in advance of the focus group date. All individuals interested in participating were asked to attend the next regular meeting. After obtaining signed, informed consent, participants engaged in a focus group discussion about behaviour change and provided feedback regarding their experiences with the health communication cards. The discussion was facilitated by the same two researchers who previously conducted the individual interviews.

The protocols for interviews and the focus group were similar. Participants first completed a questionnaire to assess basic demographic and health information. As an opening exercise, participants were shown two sets of contrasting photographs. The first set of photographs displayed similar foods representing a weekly grocery shop, but one image contained more packaged foods while the other had more fresh and organic foods. The next set of images depicted leisure time activities (such as an exercise ball and active games) in contrast to outdoor sports equipment (such as skates and bikes). Participants were asked to choose which photos reflected healthy living and describe the types of families who might be represented by the images.

All participants sorted through their own deck of health communication cards and were instructed to categorize the cards into two piles: "cards that describe me" and "cards that do not describe me." Conversation about the card sort activity followed, which included discussion around the best uses of the cards and exploration of which types of health workers or social supports participants felt would be most likely to engage in such an activity. Participants were prompted to select their three to five most important cards from the "cards that describe me" pile.

2.3. Quantitative Data Analysis. Demographics information in addition to card selection data were entered into Microsoft Excel 2010 and transferred to SPSS (PASW Statistics 18) for statistical analysis. Graphs and figures summarizing results were produced in both Excel and SPSS. Spearman's correlation coefficients were calculated for age and body mass index (BMI) as they relate to the number of cards selected in the first card sort.

A total of 18 participants completed questionnaires and the card sort activity. Both the interview and focus groups were similar in participant demographic profiles (Table 1). A greater portion of the interview sample participants were single (40%) and had at least one chronic disease (90%) compared to the focus group where no participants were identified as being single and fewer identified as having a chronic disease (37.5%).

2.4. Qualitative Data Analysis. Interpretive description is a qualitative methodology developed to investigate clinical phenomena. This methodology guided the research design, data collection, and analysis [29, 30]. Interview and focus group audio files were transcribed verbatim using Transcribe! transcription software (Seventh String software, Version 8.10, 2010). NVivo qualitative data analysis software (QSR International Pty Ltd. Version 8) was used to track coding themes. All data received multiple passes by two researchers for coding based upon themes generated inductively from the data. Interpretive description [31] served as the conceptual framework for analysis, allowing for a rich understanding of how and why participants may have felt and behaved as they revealed during discussions. Grounding for data display and knowledge development was based on a complex systems approach to obesity [32].

3. Results

3.1. Card Selection Trends. The mean number of cards selected as "applies to me" by any one participant during the card sort was 25.4 (the lowest 5, the highest 41) out of the total 64 health communication cards in the deck (Table 2). There was a significant ($P = 0.01$), negative correlation between age and number of cards selected with Spearman's

Table 1: Participant characteristics.

Variable	Sample 1 [n = 10]	Sample 2 [n = 8]
Sex [m/f]	5/5	4/4
Age	51.0 ± 17.6	50.9 ± 13.6
BMI [kg/m^2]	40.8 ± 8.5	33.7 ± 9.7
Marital status		
Married	3	3
Common law	2	3
Widowed	0	0
Separated	1	1
Divorced	0	1
Single	4	0
Education		
Less than HS	0	0
HS or trade school	4	2
University	3	6
Advanced degree	3	0
Living with others [y/n]	8/2	6/2
Income		
\$0–\$25,000	2	2
\$26–\$50,000	2	0
\$51–\$60,000	2	1
\$61–\$80,000	1	1
\$80,000+	3	4
Weight loss or diet [y/n]	8/2	8/0
Medication [y/n]	9/0	4/4
Chronic disease [y/n]	9/1	3/5

Table 2: Correlation matrix.

		Age	BMI
Number of cards selected as "cards that describe me"	r	−0.58*	0.34
	P value	0.01	0.19
	n	17	17

*Significance at $P < 0.05$.

correlation coefficient −0.58, explaining 34% of the variance in the relationship.

Most cards selected were not different between men and women, although there were several exceptions (Figure 2) in these participant groups. The most frequently chosen cards were not necessarily the ones that participants thought were most important to them. For instance, the two most popular cards in the general card sort were only selected by one participant when asked to narrow their general "applies to me" stack down to the most important cards (Table 3).

3.2. Eating Disorders and Body Dissatisfaction. No men and 44% of women selected the card "I do not pay much attention to changes in my figure," while 56% of women and 11% of men selected the card "I regularly feel disgust, shame, or self-hate from overeating." These selections may highlight some gender sensitivities regarding social norms around food and body image. It is striking that only women reported they did not pay attention to changes in their figure. However, two of the women who made that selection also chose "my body size and shape influence how I value myself," reflecting the conflict and confusion experienced in our society while dealing with weight issues. This pattern of card selection may also be an attempt to clarify that, while they are affected by being overweight, they try not to obsess about their size while engaging in behaviour change. The paradoxical card selections claiming no concern about changes in physical shape while simultaneously reporting that body size influences self-value opens a door for productive conversations around body image sensitivities that may be difficult to broach or may not have come to light without use of the cards.

The cards "I eat way too quickly" and "I often eat too much food and feel uncomfortable" represented items from the binge eating scale [24] and were some of the most popular choices when participants selected cards that described them. Each of these statements were selected by 12 participants. Of the cards chosen most for "cards most important to describe me," four listed feelings or behaviours associated with binge eating. All of these cards were chosen four or more times and represented themes involving weight and shape overvaluation, secrecy when eating, and perceived loss of control (Table 3).

The four most commonly selected cards included statements regarding body image and dieting behaviours, such as

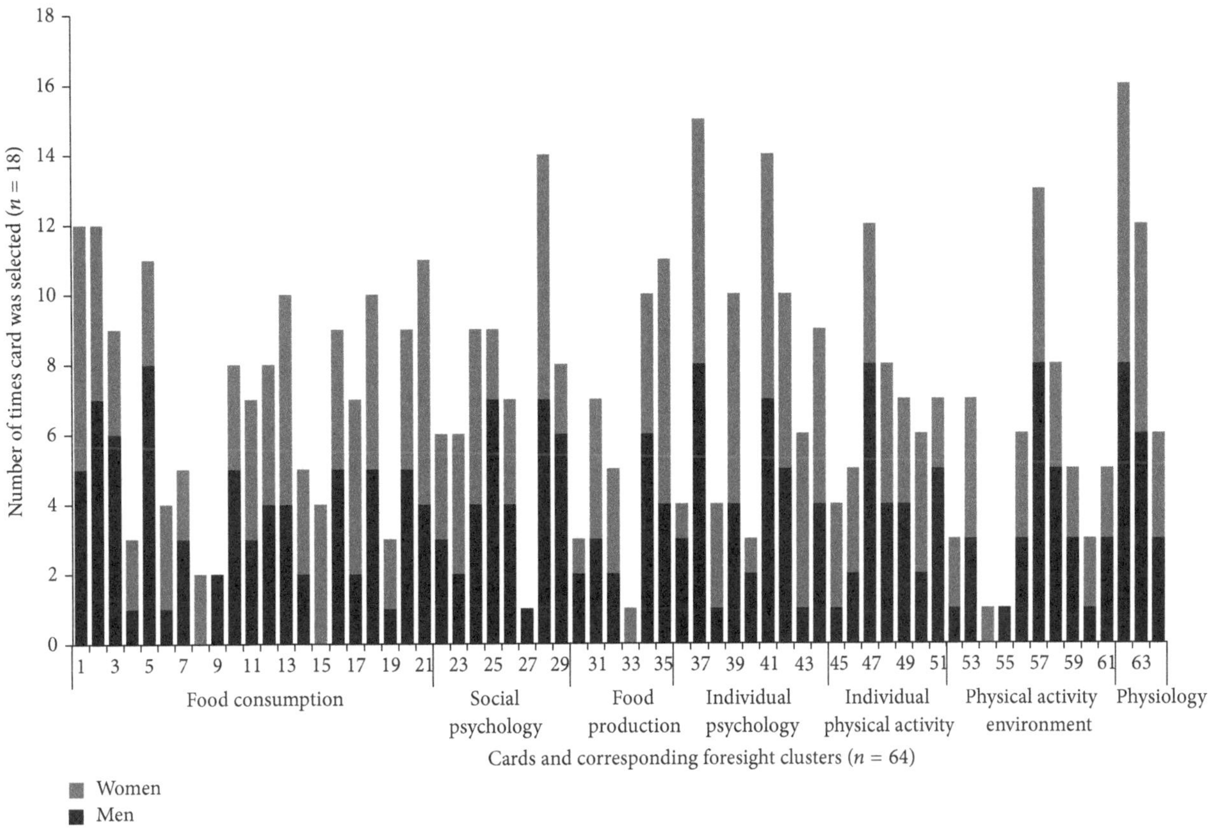

FIGURE 2

TABLE 3: Most frequently selected cards.

"Cards that describe me" [$n = 18$]	"Most important cards" [$n = 18$]	Statement
16	1	I have tried dieting and/or weight loss medication.
15	1	I am a very social person.
14	4	**My body size and shape influence how I value myself.**
12	6	**I eat way too quickly.**
10	5	**Sometimes, even when on a diet or not hungry, I eat sensibly in front of others but splurge while I am alone.**
9	5	I never seem to have free time.
9	4	**I often feel helpless and incapable of controlling my urges to overeat and feel desperate to regain control.**

Note: Bolded statements relate to binge eating disorder behaviours.

"I have tried dieting and/or weight loss medication" (selected by 16 participants), "my body size and shape influence how I value myself" (14 selections), and "I battle between trying to eat healthy and eating foods I like" (14 selections). These statements were selected equally between men and women.

3.3. Individual and Environmental Variables. Some of the card statements described a variable focused on the individual, while some described more environmental or ecological elements (Figure 2). Cards that described individually focused variables were more numerous and were selected more frequently within the psychology based set of statements. Many of the psychological variables were emotional in nature, such as "I do not feel confident in my ability to resist overeating when I am nervous, depressed, or angry."

Individuals recognized both the societal and individual influences on obesity, as overall participants selected equally from both. Nearly all participants chose at least one card from all seven of the clusters represented in the foresight obesity map (Figure 2). However, when participants selected their most important cards, they focused on more proximal issues involving personal behaviours.

3.4. Desire to Connect, Acknowledge Success, and Make Meaning with Health Workers. Although not asked to do so as part of the card sort activity, many participants provided a personal narrative of the reasons behind their overweight or obesity. These reasons included discussions of work, the physical and social environment, childhood, family, and many factors outside their direct control. These stories may have been an attempt to resolve the internal conflicts individuals seemed to have regarding their struggle with weight, validate their experiences and connect with care providers.

One theme that was never specifically asked about but was mentioned by nearly half of the participants was a comparison of cards they would have picked in the past to the cards they currently picked as "applies to me." Participants noted the following:

> *It made me feel good…it made me realize how much I've changed and how much I've realized that there's some of those things that I do not have to worry about.*

> *It made me realize how far I've come.*

Participants spontaneously created a third pile of cards which they said used to describe them but no longer did. There was a sense of pride with this group of individuals who seemed to have turned the corner on their battle with health behaviour change in some way, and the card sorting process was very validating for them. This finding suggests that reflecting on accomplishments around behaviour change when progress has been made can be a positive and motivating experience that may be beneficial for some individuals.

Sorting the cards with or prior to seeing a healthcare worker was generally viewed as something that would make for a better clinical visit. Participants expressed that the cards helped identify concerns and stated that this would be useful in helping stimulate thinking about what they wanted to talk about prior to meeting with the practitioner. Additionally, participants felt that use of the cards may help practitioners provide more thoughtful care instead of listing simplistic diet and exercise advice:

> *…it would be really great having this before, like you know, when I see [my doctor] because I'd know what to tell her, but it just [reminds] me what I really want to talk about.*

> *I think it would be better because I would know specifically what to say…what really affects me…we could just focus on the main thing how I feel.*

> *…it's gotta be better than going in blind and dealing already with those kinds of misconceptions, you know? Like the "oh, you should just eat less and exercise more".*

3.5. Bias in Establishing Appropriate Behaviour Change Targets. A minority of participants initially did not believe that the cards would be helpful in communicating with a healthcare worker. However, once they went through the whole exercise and were asked to choose cards most important to them, they generally found the cards helpful in assisting them to prioritize their efforts in behaviour change:

> *Avoiding generalities that are going to offend us more than help us. You told me I have to lose weight, yeah I did not know it, come on.*

There was total agreement with all participants that physicians were unlikely to spend the time to go through the cards and talk with patients at medical appointments, and specialists or other healthcare workers with the time and experience to engage in meaningful counselling with patients were perceived to be most likely candidates for use of the cards.

Though participants stated that the cards did not introduce any novel variables they had not previously considered, they did report that the cards were helpful in establishing goals and bringing issues top of mind. Both the interview and focus group participants had generally been struggling with obesity for quite some time. Many participants who had completed interviews had previously met with the internal medicine specialist to discuss obesity and related comorbidities, meaning they were integrated into the medical paradigm and likely had multiple interactions and discussions about weight issues. All but one participant in the focus group had undergone bariatric surgery some time in the past 10 years. Therefore, all participants were engaged in the medical model of obesity treatment and could envision how using the cards may impact their experiences with care providers.

Similarly, participants reported that the photograph activity did not provide any opportunity for novel health education. When asked to identify the more healthy photographs of food items and physical activity options, all participants immediately identified the photographs featuring fresh foods and active sports equipment as compared to more packaged foods and sedentary activities. There was not a moment of hesitation or confusion from any participant about the healthy choices, yet some participants reflected personal guilt with "should" statements or remarked about societal beliefs that obese individuals would be more likely to select the less healthy images depicted.

3.6. Using the Cards with Family or Friends. Participants had mixed feelings about using the cards with family and friends with a relatively even split between finding the cards useful in that context or not:

> *I would be able to use it with my partner and I would be able to use it personally, probably we would do it together.*

> *…it's hard, just sometimes they do not know like how I feel. And so maybe like showing them these cards would…show them "ok then, she is struggling."*

> *Well my family, no. Because my husband, 148 lbs and he's been that since grade 12. My daughter wears size 2 and 4 clothes. My son is normal but [lives far away]. For me, no, I do not bring myself*

out to my friends. I do not talk about that kind of thing with my friends really.

Several participants became quite emotional at this stage of the discussion. For example, one participant reported a desire to express more confidence about addressing the issue listed on the card in an effort to appear more accomplished. This finding suggests that the cards helped bring the discussion towards very personal and sensitive issues and is not amenable to online use or some digital applications.

4. Discussion

4.1. Age, Frequency, and Prioritization. There was a negative correlation between age and number of cards selected, which may have been due to the fact that older participants had spent more years engaged in health behaviour change and had already dealt with more of the issues stated on the cards. The fact that younger participants identified with a higher number of card statements may reflect that they experienced, or more fully recognized, increased complexity in their situations. Other studies examining health behaviour change trends have also identified differences related to age, where younger participants were more likely to participate in a treatment program and recognize barriers to change [33, 34]. The most popular card choices were not necessarily the most important issues for everyone (Table 3). This indicates that although some card statements may apply to most patients seeking help with lifestyle change, they are not necessarily the most important when individuals critically consider what they want to change.

4.2. Body Image and Binge Eating Disorder. Research has shown that, in general, women are less satisfied with their bodies compared to men [35] and, unlike men, this lack of satisfaction may not be related to BMI [36]. Our finding that men and women demonstrated variation in card selection related to body image may be reflective of this, or of gender related levels of comfort with discussing body image issues.

Aspects of binge eating behaviour may frequently occur in individuals seeking treatment for obesity. Methods that assess level of binge eating frequently include behavioural, physical, and psychological variables [24, 37]. The two most selected binge eating cards may help identify participants who could benefit from support aimed at the behavioural elements of binge eating (e.g., rate of eating and physical discomfort following overeating). Furthermore, as psychotherapy for treatment of binge eating disorder is costly [38], addressing the behavioural components which may be more prevalent may be a cost-effective way that health practitioners can begin to address some binge eating characteristics in a productive manner.

While card selection patterns featuring body image valuation in parallel with not paying much attention to weight may seem paradoxical, ambivalence is a normal part of any type of attempted behaviour change. Card selection regarding body image may also be related to the well-documented social stigma that overweight and obese individuals experience in their day-to-day lives. Additionally, there is evidence that body weight and shape concerns decrease following bariatric surgery [39]. The women that selected both cards may have lost weight and were satisfied with their body weight and shape and no longer felt the need to monitor these variables as closely. Future use of the cards should explore user rationale for card selection, as this may provide important insight into the interaction between what determines individual differences in self-value and how those variables are dealt with or monitored by each participant.

Discussions around weight can be challenging and subsequently result in patients feeling shame, fear, and ambivalence. These feelings may contribute to apprehension in reporting binge eating behaviours, even when directly asked. Using the cards may not only help with screening for eating disorders, but the process may set the tone for a more gentle and supportive conversation about how patients experience their relationship with food and their own body image concerns. As opposed to a diagnostic tool that definitively categorizes patients, the cards are meant to open conversations about topics that warrant further exploration or follow-up.

4.3. Changing Paradigms and Building Trust in Patient Care. Although no longitudinal data were obtained in this study, many participants noted that they had lost a significant amount of weight and had made important changes to their behaviour. This was also evident from the comparison many participants made about their current card selections and how many more they would have selected in the past. There is evidence that patients who feel more educated on their disease and treatment have better outcomes [40]. In this case, many of the participants may have reached saturation such that any additional information about variables and factors implicated in their obesity was not perceived to be useful. Further research is required to determine whether patients who are just starting to become more educated on their obesity and health related behaviours would benefit from this type of education. Participants brought up the issue of having to "change everything," noting that it is impossible to simply change one thing and that a total "change of attitude has to happen" to attain significant alterations in outcome. Changing one's paradigm may be the most effective but most difficult way to alter one's health related behaviour [41]. Behavioural interventions should focus on making sure patients understand that, although weight changes may be part of the end goal, their target weight may or may not be reached through their process of cumulative attempts to change individual behaviours. Most importantly, they need to understand that, even if weight goals are not attained, the changes made through engaging in more healthy behaviours will positively impact quality of life, health risks, and metabolic variables.

Participants expressed vulnerability when talking about several issues identified on the cards, which revealed various areas of sensitivity that may not necessarily come up during regular clinical visits. Participants seemed to adopt a coping mechanism of focusing on the seemingly more optimistic view of where they wanted to be in terms of their health behaviour change journey, as opposed to where they actually felt they were. Helping individuals self-reflect at this level can be a difficult, emotional, and uncomfortable experience. This process warrants that a high level of trust and comfort with the healthcare provider must exist before patients will open up and discuss the reality of their situation. This is a critical step for developing a relevant and realistic care plan that is truly patient centred. Patients report that increased physician caring, communication, and efforts to partner with them in generating care plans are important elements in building trust [42]. The card sorting process may help to surface latent concerns while building trust into the patient/provider relationship such that more challenging or ambiguous issues may be addressed respectfully over time.

Physicians may also have difficulty sorting through the complexity of the problem. Some participants noted that physicians gave them overly simplistic advice and avoided going into the details of their lifestyle challenges with them. There was frequent frustration that conversations with health providers were didactic and simplistic, suggesting that a conflict exists between overweight patients and the advice they receive from health practitioners. The overly simplistic advice participants often receive leads them to disregard clinical advice and to believe that the health practitioner does not understand their condition. If patients could present their most concerning health issues using cards as a vehicle to direct conversations, this may provide practitioners with a means of addressing obesity that is directly relevant to their patients without ignoring the complex nature of the problem. While no participant in this study hesitated to identify the photographs of the healthier food items and active supports as compared to the less healthy options (suggesting a clear understanding of healthy lifestyle choices), clinical advice often continues to instruct patients what to do (eat less, move more) rather than help them understand how to improve behaviours [43]. The cards help care providers avoid making the error of delivering simplistic information about what healthy behaviours are, and instead direct productive conversations that help patients decide how to best achieve their goals in the context of their lives.

4.4. Establishing Relationships and Goals. Without being explicitly asked, many participants gave detailed accounts of their perceived reasons for being overweight or obese, often in the form of a story. These may have been an attempt to resolve the internal conflict many individuals seemed to struggle with rationalizing between the individual and environmental causes of their health related behaviours. Many of the individually focused cards might have been perceived as putting themselves at fault, while the environmental variables may have alleviated guilt by surfacing contributing factors outside of personal control. This is consistent with other research which found that individuals with obesity frequently provide "blame-absolving narratives to mitigate the negative stereotypes associated with their 'spoiled' body image" [44, 45]. Health practitioners may benefit from emphasizing the broad reasons for obesity with patients who may feel pressure to explain or justify their struggles with weight. Using the cards may also encourage the inclusion of key family members in helpful discussions. A review of studies that assessed behaviour change in couples concluded that involving a patient's partner in diet treatment programs provided better outcomes, especially in the long term, provided that the partner took on a defined active role [46]. This was also true for physical activity related behaviours. Using the cards in clinical settings may be a good start for soliciting improved conversations and support in the context of home and daily life.

Participants who had been engaged in successful behaviour change for some time reported that they would enjoy using the cards as a monitoring device to remind them of how much progress they had made. This unexpected finding suggests that the process of selecting cards may be used to monitor success with behaviour change over time. At present, changes in weight or BMI are the most common outcome measures used to gauge success in obesity treatment [47]. These measures are more likely to miss progress with obtaining healthy habits that do not directly translate into weight loss. For example, increased physical activity lowers cardiometabolic risk even without any associated weight loss [47, 48]. Experiencing success with behaviour change and receiving education about the benefits of lowering key metabolic risk factors with physical activity may help patients to understand that not all individuals will experience the same rate of weight loss even when taking the same actions. Variations in body shape and size are expected, but sometimes difficult to accept for individuals setting size or weight oriented goals. Using the cards to help track behavioural changes may help patients to shift their health goals and build self-efficacy.

Overall, participants found the cards helpful and expressed the desire to use them in a clinical setting, but they doubted physicians would take the time to talk with them long enough to address their concerns. There is evidence that when family doctors do take the time to engage in behavioural counselling around obesity there are positive outcomes, including weight loss [8, 49] and prevention of weight gain [50]. Use of the cards may help patients to connect better with their physicians, while helping physicians feel there are relevant, tangible goals to work toward collectively.

Conflict of Interests

The authors declare no conflict of interests regarding the publication of this paper.

Acknowledgments

The authors gratefully acknowledge all study participants from the interviews and focus group who generously provided their time and insight for this research. They also thank the physicians and medical staff who facilitated the data collection process. This research was funded by CIHR operating Grants 31-711010 and 31-711031.

References

[1] J. L. Kraschnewski, C. N. Sciamanna, H. L. Stuckey et al., "A silent response to the obesity epidemic decline in US physician weight counseling," *Medical Care*, vol. 51, pp. 186–192, 2013.

[2] E. A. Finkelstein, O. A. Khavjou, H. Thompson et al., "Obesity and severe obesity forecasts through 2030," *American Journal of Preventive Medicine*, vol. 42, pp. 563–570, 2012.

[3] E. A. Finkelstein, J. G. Trogdon, J. W. Cohen, and W. Dietz, "Annual medical spending attributable to obesity: payer-and service-specific estimates," *Health Affairs*, vol. 28, no. 5, pp. w822–w831, 2009.

[4] P. Vandenbroeck, J. Goossens, and M. Clemens, *Foresight Tackling Obesities: Future Choices—Obesity System Atlas*, Government Office for Science, 2007.

[5] S. Klein, "Clinical obesity issues from an internist's perspective," *Obesity Research*, vol. 10, supplement 1, pp. 87S–88S, 2002.

[6] J. M. Ferrante, A. K. Piasecki, P. A. Ohman-Strickland, and B. F. Crabtree, "Family physicians' practices and attitudes regarding care of extremely obese patients," *Obesity*, vol. 17, no. 9, pp. 1710–1716, 2009.

[7] C. R. Elley, N. Kerse, B. Arroll, and E. Robinson, "Effectiveness of counselling patients on physical activity in general practice: cluster randomised controlled trial," *British Medical Journal*, vol. 326, no. 7393, pp. 793–796, 2003.

[8] C. Sacerdote, L. Fiorini, R. Rosato, M. Audenino, M. Valpreda, and P. Vineis, "Randomized controlled trial: Effect of nutritional counselling in general practice," *International Journal of Epidemiology*, vol. 35, no. 2, pp. 409–415, 2006.

[9] M. Stewart, J. B. Brown, A. Donner et al., "The impact of patient-centered care on outcomes," *Journal of Family Practice*, vol. 49, no. 9, pp. 796–804, 2000.

[10] D. C. W. Lau, "Synopsis of the 2006 Canadian clinical practice guidelines on the management and prevention of obesity in adults and children," *Canadian Medical Association Journal*, vol. 176, no. 8, pp. 1103–1106, 2007.

[11] K. G. Gotestam, L. Melin, and L. G. Ost, "Behavioral techniques in the treatment of drug abuse: an evaluative review," *Addictive Behaviors*, vol. 1, no. 3, pp. 205–225, 1976.

[12] G. D. Foster, "Clinical implications for the treatment of obesity," *Obesity*, vol. 14, supplement 4, pp. 182S–185S, 2006.

[13] N. Mead and P. Bower, "Patient-centredness: a conceptual framework and review of the empirical literature," *Social Science and Medicine*, vol. 51, no. 7, pp. 1087–1110, 2000.

[14] A. Elissen, E. Notle, C. Knai et al., "Is Europe putting theory into practice? A qualitative study of the level of self-management support in chronic care management approaches," *BMC Health Services Research*, vol. 13, p. 117, 2013.

[15] D. Stacey, R. Samant, and C. Bennett, "Decision making in oncology: a review of patient decision aids to support patient participation," *CA Cancer Journal for Clinicians*, vol. 58, no. 5, pp. 293–304, 2008.

[16] C. Burns and J. Winhall, *Red Health Report: Design Notes 01—the Diabetes Agenda*, Design Council, London, UK, 2006.

[17] J. Neufeind and M. Hannah, "Talking openly: using "6D cards" to facilitate holistic, patient-led communication," *International Journal for Quality in Health Care*, vol. 24, no. 1, Article ID mzr075, pp. 49–54, 2012.

[18] J. Pennington, "Unusual partnerships and new ways of working in Diabetes," *Journal of Diabetes Nursing*, vol. 10, no. 7, pp. 261–264, 2006.

[19] P. J. Teixeira, M. N. Silva, J. Mata, A. L. Palmeira, and D. Markland, "Motivation, self-determination, and long-term weight control," *International Journal of Behavioral Nutrition and Physical Activity*, vol. 9, article 22, 2012.

[20] M. M. Clark, D. B. Abrams, R. S. Niaura, C. A. Eaton, and J. S. Rossi, "Self-efficacy in weight management," *Journal of Consulting and Clinical Psychology*, vol. 59, no. 5, pp. 739–744, 1991.

[21] M. T. Warziski, S. M. Sereika, M. A. Styn, E. Music, and L. E. Burke, "Changes in self-efficacy and dietary adherence: the impact on weight loss in the PREFER study," *Journal of Behavioral Medicine*, vol. 31, no. 1, pp. 81–92, 2008.

[22] A. Bandura, "guide for constructing self-efficacy scales," in *Self-Efficacy Beliefs of Adolescents*, pp. 307–337, Information Age, Greenwich, Conn, USA, 2006.

[23] P. J. Teixeira, S. B. Going, L. B. Sardinha, and T. G. Lohman, "A review of psychosocial pre-treatment predictors of weight control," *Obesity Reviews*, vol. 6, no. 1, pp. 43–65, 2005.

[24] J. Gormally, S. Black, S. Daston, and D. Rardin, "The assessment of binge eating severity among obese persons," *Addictive Behaviors*, vol. 7, no. 1, pp. 47–55, 1982.

[25] A. J. Stunkard and S. Messick, "The three-factor eating questionnaire to measure dietary restraint, disinhibition and hunger," *Journal of Psychosomatic Research*, vol. 29, no. 1, pp. 71–83, 1985.

[26] J. Westenhoefer, A. J. Stunkard, and V. Pudel, "Validation of the flexible and rigid control dimensions of dietary restraint," *International Journal of Eating Disorders*, vol. 26, pp. 53–64, 1999.

[27] G. D. Foster, T. A. Wadden, R. M. Swain, A. J. Stunkard, P. Platte, and R. A. Vogt, "The Eating Inventory in obese women: clinical correlates and relationship to weight loss," *International Journal of Obesity*, vol. 22, no. 8, pp. 778–785, 1998.

[28] F. Bellisle, K. Clément, M. Le Barzic, A. Le Gall, B. Guy-Grand, and A. Basdevant, "The Eating Inventory and body adiposity from leanness to massive obesity: a study of 2509 adults," *Obesity research*, vol. 12, no. 12, pp. 2023–2030, 2004.

[29] S. Thorne, S. R. Kirkham, and K. O'Flynn-Magee, "The Analytic Challenge in Interpretive Description," *International Journal of Qualitative Methods*, vol. 3, article 1, 2004.

[30] S. Thorne, S. R. Kirkham, and J. MacDonald-Emes, "Interpretive description: a noncategorical qualitative alternative for developing nursing knowledge," *Research in Nursing and Health*, vol. 20, no. 2, pp. 169–177, 1997.

[31] S. Thorne, *Interpretive Description*, Left Coast Press, Walnut Creek, Calif, USA, 2008.

[32] D. T. Finegood, T. D. N. Merth, and H. Rutter, "Implications of the foresight obesity system map for solutions to childhood obesity," *Obesity*, vol. 18, no. 1, pp. S13–S16, 2010.

[33] J. Lakerveld, W. IJzelenberg, M. W. Van Tulder et al., "Motives for (not) participating in a lifestyle intervention trial," *BMC Medical Research Methodology*, vol. 8, article 17, 2008.

[34] J. T. Newsom, M. S. Kaplan, N. Huguet, and B. H. McFarland, "Health behaviors in a representative sample of older Canadians: prevalences, reported change, motivation to change, and perceived barriers," *Gerontologist*, vol. 44, no. 2, pp. 193–205, 2004.

[35] I. Esnaola, A. Rodríguez, and A. Goñi, "Body dissatisfaction and perceived sociocultural pressures: gender and age differences," *Salud Mental*, vol. 33, no. 1, pp. 21–29, 2010.

[36] C. Markey and P. Markey, "Romantic partners, weight status, and weight concerns: an examination using the actor-partner interdependence model," *Journal of Health Psychology*, vol. 16, no. 2, pp. 217–225, 2011.

[37] R. L. Spitzer, M. Devlin, B. T. Walsh et al., "Binge eating disorder: a multisite field trial of the diagnostic criteria," *International Journal of Eating Disorders*, vol. 11, no. 3, pp. 191–203, 1992.

[38] M. De Zwaan, "Binge eating disorder and obesity," *International Journal of Obesity*, vol. 25, no. 1, pp. S51–S55, 2001.

[39] J. I. Hrabosky, R. M. Masheb, M. A. White, B. S. Rothschild, C. H. Burke-Martindale, and C. M. Grilo, "A prospective study of body dissatisfaction and concerns in extremely obese gastric bypass patients: 6- and 12-month postoperative outcomes," *Obesity Surgery*, vol. 16, no. 12, pp. 1615–1621, 2006.

[40] A. Robinson and R. Thomson, "Variability in patient preferences for participating in medical decision making: Implication for the use of decision support tools," *Quality in Health Care*, vol. 10, supplement 1, pp. i34–i38, 2001.

[41] L. Malhi, Ö. Karanfil, T. Merth, M. Acheson, A. Palmer, and D. T. Finegood, "Places to intervene to make complex food systems more healthy, green, fair, and affordable," *Journal of Hunger and Environmental Nutrition*, vol. 4, no. 3-4, pp. 466–476, 2009.

[42] D. H. Thom, M. A. Hall, and L. G. Pawlson, "Measuring patients' trust in physicians when assessing quality of care," *Health Affairs*, vol. 23, no. 4, pp. 124–132, 2004.

[43] S. W. Butterworth, "Influencing patient adherence to treatment guidelines," *Journal of Managed Care Pharmacy*, vol. 14, no. 6, pp. S21–S25, 2008.

[44] J. Greener, F. Douglas, and E. van Teijlingen, "More of the same? Conflicting perspectives of obesity causation and intervention amongst overweight people, health professionals and policy makers," *Social Science and Medicine*, vol. 70, no. 7, pp. 1042–1049, 2010.

[45] K. Throsby, ""How could you let yourself get like that?": stories of the origins of obesity in accounts of weight loss surgery," *Social Science and Medicine*, vol. 65, no. 8, pp. 1561–1571, 2007.

[46] T. G. Sher and D. H. Baucom, "Mending a broken heart: a couples approach to cardiac risk reduction," *Applied & Preventive Psychology*, vol. 10, pp. 125–133, 2001.

[47] R. Ross and P. M. Janiszewski, "Is weight loss the optimal target for obesity-related cardiovascular disease risk reduction?" *The Canadian journal of cardiology*, vol. 24, supplement, pp. 25D–31D, 2008.

[48] P. M. Janiszewski and R. Ross, "The utility of physical activity in the management of global cardiometabolic risk," *Obesity*, vol. 17, supplement 3, pp. S3–S14, 2009.

[49] N. Rodondi, J.-P. Humair, W. A. Ghali et al., "Counselling overweight and obese patients in primary care: a prospective cohort study," *European Journal of Cardiovascular Prevention and Rehabilitation*, vol. 13, no. 2, pp. 222–228, 2006.

[50] N. C. W. Ter Bogt, W. J. E. Bemelmans, F. W. Beltman, J. Broer, A. J. Smit, and K. Van Der Meer, "Preventing weight gain by lifestyle intervention in a general practice setting: three-year results of a randomized controlled trial," *Archives of Internal Medicine*, vol. 171, no. 4, pp. 306–313, 2011.

12

Atherosclerosis Burden in Patients with Acute Chest Pain: Obesity Paradox

Kongkiat Chaikriangkrai,[1] Mahwash Kassi,[1] Sayf Khaleel bala,[2] Faisal Nabi,[2] and Su Min Chang[2]

[1] *Department of Medicine, The Methodist Hospital, Houston, TX 77030, USA*
[2] *Methodist DeBakey Heart & Vascular Center, The Methodist Hospital, Houston, TX 77030, USA*

Correspondence should be addressed to Su Min Chang; smchang@houstonmethodist.org

Academic Editors: K.-C. Huang and J. Saleh

Obesity paradox has been described in various populations of coronary artery disease, mainly asymptomatic subjects. However, relationship between obesity and coronary artery calcification detected by cardiac CT in symptomatic patients has rarely been demonstrated. This study seeks to investigate whether the paradoxical relationship between obesity and coronary artery calcification exists in patients with acute chest pain. A final cohort of 1030 chest pain patients presenting at our emergency department who underwent coronary evaluation by multidetector cardiac CT were examined. With absent-to-mild coronary calcification (CAC score < 100) as a referent, multivariable analysis showed that presence of obesity (OR 0.564; 95% CI 0.395, 0.806; P 0.002), body mass index (OR 0.945; 95% CI 0.920, 0.971; $P < 0.001$), body weight (OR 0.987; 95% CI 0.979, 0.995; P 0.001), and body surface area (OR 0.582; 95% CI 0.369, 0.920; P 0.020) were inversely associated with moderate-to-severe coronary calcification (CAC score ≥ 100). This study extends the concept of obesity paradox to symptomatic patients undergoing coronary artery calcium score assessment. However, biological explanation(s) of this paradox remains unanswered.

1. Introduction

Obesity has been believed to be one of the major risk factors and adverse prognosticators, associated with increased mortality risk, for atherosclerotic diseases, especially coronary artery disease (CAD) [1, 2]. Extensive studies have shown that obesity is an independent predictor for CAD and cardiovascular death in multiple populations including a large-scale epidemiological study and a systemic review [3, 4]. Obesity is not only associated with prevalence and death in CAD itself but also related to its major risk factors including hypertension, diabetes mellitus, and dyslipidemia [5]. Body mass index (BMI) which is the index most commonly used in majority of the studies to define obesity has also been shown to be positively associated with increased risk of CAD even in the normal weight range [6]. Pathophysiology of obesity and cardiovascular diseases is complicated and it involves several pathways particularly cardiovascular hemodynamics, systemic inflammation, and leptin metabolism [5]. Given its complexity of interaction and arguable robustness of BMI in defining obesity, it is not surprising that evidences of ability of obesity to be a risk factor and a poor prognosticator are inconsistent among studies. There have been multiple studies describing "obesity paradox," a protective effect of obesity, with various clinical surrogates and outcomes in different populations of CAD including asymptomatic population [5, 7], myocardial infarction [8–10], and patients treated with revascularization [11, 12]. However, in patients with acute chest pain undergoing coronary artery calcification (CAC) evaluation, there have been sparse studies.

This study seeks to primarily examine relationship between obesity and significant CAD in patients with acute chest pain of unknown cardiac significance who were admitted in an observation unit to further support or reject an idea of obesity paradox in this particular population.

2. Materials and Methods

2.1. Study Population. This study is a prospective observational cohort study conducted from September 2005 to

February 2008. Subjects were patients older than 18 years old who were admitted under observational status for further evaluation of acute chest pain suggestive of myocardial ischemia within the previous 24 hours. The evaluation was performed with single-photon emission computed tomography (SPECT) and CAC scoring by multidetector cardiac CT. Exclusion criteria were subjects with noncardiac chest pain based on clinical assessment, elevated troponin on initial blood samples, new or presumably new ST-segment elevation or depression (≥1 mm) on baseline electrocardiogram, hemodynamic or clinical instability defined by systolic blood pressure <90 mmHg or clinical significant atrial/ventricular arrhythmia, history of coronary artery disease based on previous coronary angiography or prior coronary revascularization, and subjects with known or suspected pregnancy. More detailed materials and methods were described elsewhere [13].

2.2. Body Morphology and Obesity. Indices for body morphology used in this study were height in meter, weight in kilogram, body surface area (BSA) in meter^2 calculated by DuBois and DuBois formula [14], and BMI. BMI of each subject was calculated by the following formula: weight in kilogram ÷ (height in meter)^2. Definition of obesity was set at BMI at least 30 kg/m^2.

2.3. CAC Scoring. CAC score was calculated with reconstructed axial images of 2.5 mm thickness as previously described by Agatston et al. [15]. A 16-slice multidetector CT scanner (Philips Precedence, Philips Healthcare, Eindhoven, The Netherlands) was used. Images were acquired during a single breath hold, using prospective ECG gating with imaging triggered at 75% of the R-R interval. Patients were categorized into 2 groups based on their CAC extent: absent-to-mild CAC (CAC score < 100) or moderate-to-severe CAC (CAC score ≥ 100).

2.4. Data Gathering and Processing. During observation period, all clinical information was collected including demographic information, cardiovascular history (i.e., cardiovascular symptoms, history of hypertension, history of diabetes mellitus, history of dyslipidemia, smoking history, history of peripheral arterial disease, history of carotid artery disease, history of abdominal aortic aneurysm, family history of coronary artery disease, and current cardiovascular medication profiles), and blood samples for lipid profiles, cardiac biomarkers, and renal function tests. Clinical information was used to calculate Framingham coronary heart disease 10-year risk score [16], TIMI risk score for acute coronary syndrome [17], and ATP III risk score for coronary artery disease [18].

2.5. Statistical Analysis. Descriptive statistics for studied variables are presented as mean with standard deviation (SD) for normally distributed variables, including age, height, weight, BSA, and BMI, median with range for nonnormally distributed variables, including Framingham coronary heart disease 10-year risk score and TIMI risk score for acute coronary syndrome, and frequency with percentage for categorical variables including binary cardiovascular risk factors and uses of cardiovascular medications. Student's t-test was used to identify differences in mean. Mann-Whitney U test was used to examine differences in medians. χ^2 analysis was used to identify significant heterogeneity in the frequencies. Binary logistic regression was performed to examine relationship between covariables and presence of moderate-to-severe CAC. Odd ratio and 95% confidence interval (CI) were used to describe the relationship. Body morphology indices that had statistical significant difference between CAC groups were included as testing variables. All baseline characteristics that are significant univariable predictors at the level of $P < 0.1$ were entered into multivariable models for each testing variable to identify ability to be an independent predictor. Framingham CAD risk score was entered into multivariable model to represent age, gender, smoking history, dyslipidemia, and hypertension. Other baseline characteristics that were included are history of stroke and history of PAD. All statistical analyses were performed with IBM SPSS/PASW Statistics 20 (SPSS Inc., Chicago, IL). P value < 0.05 was considered statistically significant.

3. Results

3.1. Study Population Characteristics. A total of 5066 patients presented to our ED with acute chest pain between September 2005 and February 2008. The final cohort consisted of 1030 patients. Studied clinical characteristics are shown in Table 1.

The median CAC score in our study population was 0 with 25th and 75th percentile of 0 and 35.75, respectively. Most (624 of 1030; 60.6%) had absent CAC, followed by 21.7% (223 of 1030) with mild CAC (0 < CAC score < 100) and 17.8% (183 of 1030) with moderate-to-severe CAC (CAC score ≥ 100). Patients with moderate-to-severe CAC had expected results for most clinical characteristics. They were older ($P < 0.001$) and tended to be male (P 0.015). They had significantly more history of hypertension ($P < 0.001$), history of dyslipidemia ($P < 0.001$), history of stroke ($P < 0.001$), and history of peripheral arterial disease (PAD) ($P < 0.001$). Other risk factors for CAD were comparable between 2 groups which are history of diabetes (P 0.359), history of cigarette smoking (P 0.099), and family history of CAD (P 0.405). Compared to patients with absent-to-mild coronary calcification, patients with moderate-to-severe coronary calcification had higher median Framingham CAD 10-year risk score ($P < 0.001$), higher median TIMI risk score ($P < 0.001$), higher proportion of high TIMI risk score ($P < 0.001$), and higher proportion of moderately high and high risk in ATP III criteria ($P < 0.001$). There were also significantly higher prevalence of uses of cardiovascular medications including aspirin ($P < 0.001$), angiotensin converting enzyme inhibitors (ACEIs)/angiotensin receptor blockers (ARBs) ($P < 0.001$), beta blockers ($P < 0.001$), calcium channel blockers ($P < 0.001$), and statins ($P < 0.001$) but not diuretics (P 0.101) in moderate-to-severe CAC group compared to absent-to-mild CAC group.

TABLE 1: Baseline characteristics.

Clinical characteristics	All patients (N = 1030)	Absent-to-mild CAC (N = 847)	Moderate-to-severe CAC (N = 183)	P value
Mean age, year (SD)	54.0 (13.5)	51.2 (11.8)	66.8 (13.2)	<0.001
Male, no. (%)	413 (40.1)	522 (61.6)	95 (51.9)	0.015
Risk factors for CAD, no. (%)				
History of hypertension	590 (57.3)	454 (53.6)	136 (74.3)	<0.001
History of diabetes	152 (14.8)	121 (14.3)	31 (16.9)	0.359
History of dyslipidemia	352 (34.2)	261 (30.8)	91 (49.7)	<0.001
History of cigarette smoking	192 (18.6)	150 (17.7)	42 (23.0)	0.099
Family history of CAD	52 (5.0)	45 (5.3)	7 (3.8)	0.405
History of stroke	35 (3.4)	19 (2.2)	16 (8.7)	<0.001
History of PAD	12 (1.2)	5 (0.6)	7 (3.8)	<0.001
Framingham risk score, median (range)	4 (1–30)	2 (1–30)	16 (1–30)	<0.001
TIMI risk score, median (range)	1 (1–4)	1 (1–4)	2 (1–4)	<0.001
1, no. (%)	655 (63.6)	600 (70.8)	55 (30.1)	<0.001
2, no. (%)	258 (25.0)	185 (21.8)	73 (39.9)	
3, no. (%)	106 (10.3)	58 (6.8)	48 (26.2)	
4, no. (%)	11 (1.1)	4 (0.5)	7 (3.8)	
ATP III groups, no. (%)				
Low	366 (35.5)	353 (41.7)	13 (7.1)	<0.001
Moderate	305 (29.6)	258 (30.5)	47 (25.7)	
Moderately high	156 (15.1)	97 (11.5)	59 (32.2)	
High	203 (19.7)	139 (16.4)	64 (35.0)	
Baseline cardiovascular medication use, no. (%)				
Aspirin	190 (18.4)	132 (15.6)	58 (31.7)	<0.001
ACEIs/ARBs	325 (31.6)	249 (29.4)	76 (41.5)	0.001
Beta blockers	164 (15.9)	118 (13.9)	46 (25.1)	<0.001
Diuretics	182 (17.7)	142 (16.8)	40 (21.9)	0.101
Calcium channel blockers	139 (13.5)	97 (11.5)	42 (23.0)	<0.001
Statins	240 (23.3)	167 (19.7)	73 (39.9)	<0.001

3.2. Body Morphology Indices and Obesity. Overall, median BMI was 29.2 kg/m^2 with 25th and 75th percentile of 25.5 kg/m^2 and 34.2 kg/m^2, respectively. There were 223 (21.7%) normal weight patients, 336 (32.6%) overweight patients, and 471 (45.7%) obese patients. Other body morphology indices, differences in median BMI, and differences in mean height, mean weight, and mean BSA are shown in Table 2. Patients with moderate-to-severe CAC had significantly lower median body weight (P 0.005), BSA (P 0.037), and BMI (P 0.001) than those with absent-to-mild CAC. Consistently with BMI, percentage of obesity in the moderate-to-severe CAC group was significantly lower than that in absent-to-mild CAC group (P 0.010).

Binary logistic regression analysis was used to examine these associations. Results are shown in Table 3. Body weight, BSA, BMI values, and presence of obesity are inverse univariable predictors for moderate-to-severe CAC compared to absent-to-mild CAC (body weight: OR 0.989, 95% CI 0.982, 0.997, P 0.005; BSA: OR 0.636, 95% CI 0.415, 0.974, P 0.038; BMI: OR 0.956, 95% CI 0.933, 0.981, P 0.001; presence of obesity: OR 0.651, 95% CI 0.469, 0.905, P 0.011). Multivariable analysis was then evaluated by entering Framingham CAD risk score, history of stroke, and history of PAD into the model to explore confounding effect on each testing univariable predictor. All the testing univariable predictors did not only remain independent predictors for moderate-to-severe CAC compared to absent-to-mild CAC but also showed stronger relationship with greater magnitude in OR and 95% CI (body weight: OR 0.98, 95% CI 0.979,0.995, P 0.001; BSA: OR 0.582, 95% CI 0.369,0.920, P 0.020; BMI: OR 0.945, 95% CI 0.920,0.971, P < 0.001; presence of obesity: OR 0.564, 95% CI 0.395,0.806, P 0.002).

4. Discussion

Our final cohorts of 1030 patients under observation status for acute chest pain evaluation confirmed the concept of obesity paradox in this population. Other body morphology indices including body weight and BSA also showed inverse relationship with moderate-to-severe CAC as well consistently

Table 2: Body morphology indices and obesity categorized by extent of CAC.

Body indices	All patients (N = 1030)	Absent-to-mild CAC (N = 847)	Moderate-to-severe CAC (N = 183)	P value
BMI, median (range)	29.2 (14.8–68.6)	29.4 (17.4–68.6)	27.5 (14.8–57.8)	0.001
Obesity, no. (%)	471 (45.7)	403 (47.6)	68 (37.2)	0.010
Body weight (kg) (SD)	86.4 (23.2)	87.4 (23.5)	82.1 (21.5)	0.005
BSA (m^2) (SD)	2.73 (0.39)	2.74 (0.39)	2.67 (0.38)	0.037
Height (meters) (SD)	1.68 (0.11)	1.68 (0.11)	1.68 (0.11)	0.616

Table 3: Association between body morphology indices and moderate-to-severe CAC.

Body indices	Univariable analysis	P value	Multivariable analysis*	P value
BMI	0.956 (0.933, 0.981)	0.001	0.945 (0.920, 0.971)	<0.001
Obesity	0.651 (0.469, 0.905)	0.011	0.564 (0.395, 0.806)	0.002
Body weight	0.989 (0.982, 0.997)	0.005	0.987 (0.979, 0.995)	0.001
BSA	0.636 (0.415, 0.974)	0.038	0.582 (0.369, 0.920)	0.020

*Adjusted for Framingham CAD risk score, and history of stroke, and history of PAD.

with a recent coronary angiography-based study. Despite the fact that patients with moderate-to-severe CAC were older and had more history of hypertension, dyslipidemia, stroke, and PAD, body morphology indices including BMI were lower in this group. With adjusted logistic regression analysis, presence of obesity, BMI, body weight, and BSA remained independent predictors for moderate-to-severe CAC. In our study, we did not find significant differences in any body composition indices between patients with and without short-term cardiac events.

We chose to use Framingham CAD risk score for an adjustment as a surrogate for age, gender, history of hypertension, and history of dyslipidemia because, with a well-validated risk score as the Framingham CAD risk score, we aimed to minimize confounding effect and interaction between each other in these factors. We also added history of stroke and history of PAD to the adjusted analysis as they are not included in the Framingham risk score and the differences in these baseline characteristics were also significant. We specifically chose moderate-to-severe CAC defined by CAC score of at least 100 as our cutoff for significant CAD as natural history of CAC is over time progressing as suggested by a recent study [19], so robustness of mild CAC in older age group in identifying clinical significant CAD might be arguable. CAC score of at least 100 has also been shown to be associated with significantly higher risk of increased cardiac events including CAD death, nonfatal myocardial infarction, and unstable angina pectoris requiring coronary revascularization [20, 21].

In contrast to several prior CT-based studies which demonstrated positive relationship between BMI and CAC score [22–28], our study found that increased BMI was associated with lower CAC. However, most of the previous studies were conducted on asymptomatic subjects without significant CAD who were at low risk of developing CAD. There is one CT-based study [28], to our knowledge, that investigated this association in patients with significant CAD; however this study contained small number of subjects (N = 115). These discrepancies in findings have been suggested before by Lee et al. that BMI has a U-shaped relationship with CAC [29]. In their report, it was shown that, in young asymptomatic subjects without CAD, initial BMI on enrollment was positively associated with CAC at final follow-up in a linear fashion but BMI at follow-up on years 5, 10, and 15 became progressively U shape. BMI at the final follow-up at year 20 was inversely associated with CAC at final follow-up. Nevertheless, our findings in the present study are consistent with multiple prior coronary angiography-based studies [5, 7, 9–11, 30] which described a paradoxical relationship between CAC and body morphology, mainly BMI as well.

Our study extends the concept of obesity paradox with significant CT-derived CAC to symptomatic patients. The findings in this study support the fact that there is obesity paradox in various CAD populations including stable CAD [7], patients referred for exercise stress testing [11, 31], CAD with acute coronary syndrome requiring coronary angiography [8–10], and CAD requiring revascularization [11, 12]. Whether this concept is an unanswered phenomenon or just an artifact from heterogeneous composition of BMI is still controversial to date. Most studies that described obesity paradox used BMI as a surrogate for obesity. Given that BMI comprises body fat and fat-free mass, "obesity" defined by BMI can theoretically be actually muscle mass which could well explain why subjects with higher BMI in studies had better clinical outcomes or had lower CAC compared to subjects with lower BMI. In evidence, there have been multiple studies focused on cardiorespiratory fitness as it is one of the indices that possibly differentiate higher BMI secondary to body fat from higher BMI secondary to fat-free mass. It has been shown that, in subjects with higher cardiorespiratory fitness, there is no obesity paradox as opposed to subjects with lower cardiorespiratory fitness who demonstrated the paradox [32–34]. Other proposed biological mechanisms to explain inverse relationship between BMI and CAC in significant CAD involve another puzzle called "vascular calcification paradox" proposed by Kovacic et al. [30] which describes the phenomenon that increased bone mineralization is inversely associated with vascular calcification.

The basis of this theory begins with the hypothesis that bigger body size necessitates bigger bony skeletal support. Bigger body size has been shown to be positively associated with higher bone mineralization [35]. In linking all these findings and the theory together, Broussard and Magnus proposed that the obesity paradox might be related to the vascular calcification paradox. This paradox seems to possibly involve Klotho gene which has been shown in mice and human to regulate bone mineralization and vascular calcification [36–38]. The possibility of this theory has also been supported in patients who use bisphosphonate which demonstrated increased bone mass but decreased vascular calcification [39].

In contrast to BMI, BSA has not been studied extensively for associations with CAC or cardiac events. BSA is also a product of weight and height as BMI, although it is a product of multiplication as opposed to division in BMI which might not reflect obesity being as robust as BMI. The results of our study support a recent study by Roy et al. [40] which examined a relationship between BSA and CAC in patients who underwent cardiac CT for coronary artery evaluation. However, the relationship between BSA and CAC score was inverse in our study but positive in their study. They also demonstrated that BSA, but not BMI, is an independent predictor for presence of CAC.

The limitation of this study is the single-center cross-sectional nature of examining association between body morphology and CAC. For all body morphology indices including BMI, we used a single measurement for each patient at the time of presentation to correlate with CAC. All the lack of association between body morphology indices and coronary calcium score in our study cannot reflect changes in these indices in temporal fashion. Also we did not use other body morphology measurements such as waist circumference, hip circumference, or waist-to-hip ratio which might show different results.

Perspectives: in contrast to several previous CT-based studies examining the relationship between BMI and CAC which show positive association in asymptomatic subjects, our study is one of the first large-scale studies which demonstrated that the association is reversed in patients with acute chest pain. However, this reverse relationship between CAC and BMI was described before in symptomatic patients, though with CAC detected by angiography. This raises the possibility of obesity paradox with CAC detected by cardiac CT in this population as well as questions regarding robustness between the two imaging modalities in detecting CAC. Also there could possibly be differences in disease stages or biological mechanisms between asymptomatic subjects and symptomatic patients that could potentially explain this discrepancy. Further investigations are needed to confirm this paradoxical association and to find its biological explanation(s).

5. Conclusion

In patients with acute chest pain who were admitted under observation status for CAC evaluation, we demonstrated an inverse association between body weight, BSA, and BMI and significant CT-derived CAC. These findings extend the concept of obesity paradox to this population. However, biological explanation(s) of this paradox remains unanswered. Further studies are needed to examine the mechanism of this concept.

Novelty and Significance

What Is New?

(i) Our study is a large-scaled study on symptomatic patients that demonstrated paradoxical association between cardiac CT-derived coronary artery calcification and obesity as well as other body morphology indices.

(ii) Most of the previous cardiac CT-based studies were conducted on asymptomatic subjects and showed positive association between obesity and coronary artery calcification.

What Is Relevant?

Obesity paradox in cardiovascular diseases including hypertension has been repeatedly described. Our study extends this concept to a different population with a different imaging modality.

Summary

The present study showed that, in patients with acute chest pain admitted for observation, obesity was an inverse independent predictor for coronary artery calcification detected by cardiac CT.

Conflict of Interests

The authors declare that there is no conflict of interests.

References

[1] H. B. Hubert, M. Feinleib, P. M. McNamara, and W. P. Castelli, "Obesity as an independent risk factor for cardiovascular disease: a 26-year follow-up of participants in the Framingham Heart Study," *Circulation*, vol. 67, no. 5, pp. 968–977, 1983.

[2] G. Whitlock, S. Lewington, P. Sherliker et al., "Body-mass index and cause-specific mortality in 900 000 adults: collaborative analyses of 57 prospective studies," *The Lancet*, vol. 373, no. 9669, pp. 1083–1096, 2009.

[3] P. W. Wilson, R. B. D'Agostino, L. Sullivan, H. Parise, and W. B. Kannel, "Overweight and obesity as determinants of cardiovascular risk: the Framingham experience," *Archives of Internal Medicine*, vol. 162, no. 16, pp. 1867–1872, 2002.

[4] R. P. Bogers, W. J. E. Bemelmans, R. T. Hoogenveen et al., "Association of overweight with increased risk of coronary heart disease partly independent of blood pressure and cholesterol levels: a meta-analysis of 21 cohort studies including more than 300 000 persons," *Archives of Internal Medicine*, vol. 167, no. 16, pp. 1720–1728, 2007.

[5] C. J. Lavie, R. V. Milani, and H. O. Ventura, "Obesity and cardiovascular disease. risk factor, paradox, and impact of

weight loss," *Journal of the American College of Cardiology*, vol. 53, no. 21, pp. 1925–1932, 2009.

[6] W. C. Willett, W. H. Dietz, and G. A. Colditz, "Guidelines for healthy weight," *New England Journal of Medicine*, vol. 341, no. 6, pp. 427–434, 1999.

[7] C. J. Lavie, A. De Schutter, D. Patel, S. M. Artham, and R. V. Milani, "Body composition and coronary heart disease mortality—an obesity or a lean paradox?" *Mayo Clinic Proceedings*, vol. 86, no. 9, pp. 857–864, 2011.

[8] M. Zeller, P. G. Steg, J. Ravisy et al., "Relation between body mass index, waist circumference, and death after acute myocardial infarction," *Circulation*, vol. 118, no. 5, pp. 482–490, 2008.

[9] D. B. Diercks, M. T. Roe, J. Mulgund et al., "The obesity paradox in non-ST-segment elevation acute coronary syndromes: results from the Can Rapid risk stratification of Unstable angina patients Suppress ADverse outcomes with Early implementation of the American College of Cardiology/American Heart Association Guidelines Quality Improvement Initiative," *American Heart Journal*, vol. 152, no. 1, pp. 140–148, 2006.

[10] H. J. Buettner, C. Mueller, M. Gick et al., "The impact of obesity on mortality in UA/non-ST-segment elevation myocardial infarction," *European Heart Journal*, vol. 28, no. 14, pp. 1694–1701, 2007.

[11] A. Romero-Corral, V. M. Montori, V. K. Somers et al., "Association of bodyweight with total mortality and with cardiovascular events in coronary artery disease: a systematic review of cohort studies," *Lancet*, vol. 368, no. 9536, pp. 666–678, 2006.

[12] C. J. Lavie and R. V. Milani, "Obesity and cardiovascular disease: the Hippocrates paradox?" *Journal of the American College of Cardiology*, vol. 42, no. 4, pp. 677–679, 2003.

[13] F. Nabi, S. M. Chang, C. M. Pratt et al., "Coronary artery calcium scoring in the emergency department: identifying which patients with chest pain can be safely discharged home," *Annals of Emergency Medicine*, vol. 56, no. 3, pp. 220–229, 2010.

[14] D. Du Bois and E. F. Du Bois, "A formula to estimate the approximate surface area if height and weight be known,1916," *Nutrition*, vol. 5, no. 5, pp. 303–312, 1989.

[15] A. S. Agatston, W. R. Janowitz, F. J. Hildner, N. R. Zusmer, M. Viamonte Jr., and R. Detrano, "Quantification of coronary artery calcium using ultrafast computed tomography," *Journal of the American College of Cardiology*, vol. 15, no. 4, pp. 827–832, 1990.

[16] P. W. F. Wilson, R. B. D'Agostino, D. Levy, A. M. Belanger, H. Silbershatz, and W. B. Kannel, "Prediction of coronary heart disease using risk factor categories," *Circulation*, vol. 97, no. 18, pp. 1837–1847, 1998.

[17] E. M. Antman, M. Cohen, P. J. L. M. Bernink et al., "The TIMI risk score for unstable angina/non-ST elevation MI: a method for prognostication and therapeutic decision making," *Journal of the American Medical Association*, vol. 284, no. 7, pp. 835–842, 2000.

[18] S. M. Grundy, J. I. Cleeman, C. N. Merz et al., "Implications of recent clinical trials for the National Cholesterol Education Program Adult Treatment Panel III guidelines," *Arteriosclerosis, Thrombosis, and Vascular Biology*, vol. 24, no. 8, pp. e149–e161, 2004.

[19] J. W. McEvoy and M. J. Blaha, "Progression of coronary artery calcification: not down-and-out," *Archives of Internal Medicine*, vol. 170, no. 8, pp. 735–736, 2010.

[20] M. Petretta, S. Daniele, W. Acampa et al., "Prognostic value of coronary artery calcium score and coronary CT angiography in patients with intermediate risk of coronary artery disease," *International Journal of Cardiovascular Imaging*, vol. 28, no. 6, pp. 1547–1556, 2012.

[21] M. J. Pletcher, J. A. Tice, M. Pignone, and W. S. Browner, "Using the coronary artery calcium score to predict coronary heart disease events: a systematic review and meta-analysis," *Archives of Internal Medicine*, vol. 164, no. 12, pp. 1285–1292, 2004.

[22] M. A. Allison and C. M. Wright, "Body morphology differentially predicts coronary calcium," *International Journal of Obesity*, vol. 28, no. 3, pp. 396–401, 2004.

[23] C. H. Hsu, S. G. N. Chang, K. C. Hwang, and P. Chou, "Impact of obesity on coronary artery calcification examined by electron beam computed tomographic scan," *Diabetes, Obesity and Metabolism*, vol. 9, no. 3, pp. 354–359, 2007.

[24] C. K. Kramer, D. Von Mühlen, J. L. Gross, and E. Barrett-Connor, "A prospective study of abdominal obesity and coronary artery calcium progression in older adults," *Journal of Clinical Endocrinology and Metabolism*, vol. 94, no. 12, pp. 5039–5044, 2009.

[25] R. A. Kronmal, R. L. McClelland, R. Detrano et al., "Risk factors for the progression of coronary artery calcification in asymptomatic subjects: results from the Multi-Ethnic Study of Atherosclerosis (MESA)," *Circulation*, vol. 115, no. 21, pp. 2722–2730, 2007.

[26] C. D. Lee, D. R. Jacobs Jr., P. J. Schreiner, C. Iribarren, and A. Hankinson, "Abdominal obesity and coronary artery calcification in young adults: the Coronary Artery Risk Development in Young Adults (CARDIA) Study," *American Journal of Clinical Nutrition*, vol. 86, no. 1, pp. 48–54, 2007.

[27] R. See, S. M. Abdullah, D. K. McGuire et al., "The association of differing measures of overweight and obesity with prevalent atherosclerosis. The dallas heart study," *Journal of the American College of Cardiology*, vol. 50, no. 8, pp. 752–759, 2007.

[28] B. G. Brown, J. Morse, X. Q. Zhao, M. Cheung, E. Marino, and J. J. Albers, "Electron-beam tomography coronary calcium scores are superior to framingham risk variables for predicting the measured proximal stenosis burden," *American Journal of Cardiology*, vol. 88, no. 2A, pp. 23E–26E, 2001.

[29] D. H. Lee, M. W. Steffes, M. Gross et al., "Differential associations of weight dynamics with coronary artery calcium versus common carotid artery intima-media thickness," *American Journal of Epidemiology*, vol. 172, no. 2, pp. 180–189, 2010.

[30] J. C. Kovacic, P. Lee, U. Baber et al., "Inverse relationship between body mass index and coronary artery calcification in patients with clinically significant coronary lesions," *Atherosclerosis*, vol. 221, no. 1, pp. 176–182, 2012.

[31] P. McAuley, J. Myers, J. Abella, and V. Froelicher, "Body mass, fitness and survival in veteran patients: another obesity paradox?" *American Journal of Medicine*, vol. 120, no. 6, pp. 518–524, 2007.

[32] P. A. McAuley, E. G. Artero, X. Sui et al., "The obesity paradox, cardiorespiratory fitness, and coronary heart disease," *Mayo Clinic Proceedings*, vol. 87, no. 5, pp. 443–451, 2012.

[33] P. A. McAuley, P. F. Kokkinos, R. B. Oliveira, B. T. Emerson, and J. N. Myers, "Obesity paradox and cardiorespiratory fitness in 12,417 male veterans aged 40 to 70 years," *Mayo Clinic Proceedings*, vol. 85, no. 2, pp. 115–121, 2010.

[34] K. Goel, R. J. Thomas, R. W. Squires et al., "Combined effect of cardiorespiratory fitness and adiposity on mortality in patients with coronary artery disease," *American Heart Journal*, vol. 161, no. 3, pp. 590–597, 2011.

[35] D. L. Broussard and J. H. Magnus, "Risk assessment and screening for low bone mineral density in a multi-ethnic population of women and men: does one approach fit all?" *Osteoporosis International*, vol. 15, no. 5, pp. 349–360, 2004.

[36] D. E. Arking, D. M. Becker, L. R. Yanek et al., "KLOTHO allele status and the risk of early-onset occult coronary artery disease," *American Journal of Human Genetics*, vol. 72, no. 5, pp. 1154–1161, 2003.

[37] M. Kuro-o, Y. Matsumura, H. Aizawa et al., "Mutation of the mouse klotho gene leads to a syndrome resembling ageing," *Nature*, vol. 390, no. 6655, pp. 45–51, 1997.

[38] N. Bucay, I. Sarosi, C. R. Dunstan et al., "Osteoprotegerin-deficient mice develop early onset osteoporosis and arterial calcification," *Genes and Development*, vol. 12, no. 9, pp. 1260–1268, 1998.

[39] S. Elmariah, J. A. C. Delaney, K. D. O'Brien et al., "Bisphosphonate use and prevalence of valvular and vascular calcification in women: MESA (The Multi-Ethnic Study of Atherosclerosis)," *Journal of the American College of Cardiology*, vol. 56, no. 21, pp. 1752–1759, 2010.

[40] S. K. Roy, I. Zeb, J. Kadakia, D. Li, and M. J. Budoff, "Body surface area is a predictor of coronary artery calcium, whereas body mass index is not," *Coronary Artery Disease*, vol. 23, no. 2, pp. 113–117, 2012.

13

Obesity and Surgical Wound Healing: A Current Review

Yvonne N. Pierpont,[1,2] Trish Phuong Dinh,[2] R. Emerick Salas,[1,2] Erika L. Johnson,[1,2] Terry G. Wright,[1,2] Martin C. Robson,[2] and Wyatt G. Payne[1,2]

[1] *Institute for Tissue Regeneration, Repair & Rehabilitation, Bay Pines VA Health Care System, Bay Pines, FL 33744, USA*
[2] *Division of Plastic Surgery, University of South Florida, Tampa, FL 33620, USA*

Correspondence should be addressed to Wyatt G. Payne; wyatt.payne@va.gov

Academic Editors: K. Abberton, K. C. Huang, and U. J. Magalang

Objective. The correlation between obesity and deficient wound healing has long been established. This review examines the current literature on the mechanisms involved in obesity-related perioperative morbidity. *Methods.* A literature search was performed using Medline, PubMed, Cochrane Library, and Internet searches. Keywords used include obesity, wound healing, adipose healing, and bariatric and surgical complications. *Results.* Substantial evidence exists demonstrating that obesity is associated with a number of postoperative complications. Specifically in relation to wound healing, explanations include inherent anatomic features of adipose tissue, vascular insufficiencies, cellular and composition modifications, oxidative stress, alterations in immune mediators, and nutritional deficiencies. Most recently, advances made in the field of gene array have allowed researchers to determine a few plausible alterations and deficiencies in obese individuals that contribute to their increased risk of morbidity and mortality, especially wound complications. *Conclusion.* While the literature discusses how obesity may negatively affect health on various of medical fronts, there is yet to be a comprehensive study detailing all the mechanisms involved in obesity-related morbidities in their entirety. Improved knowledge and understanding of obesity-induced physiological, cellular, molecular, and chemical changes will facilitate better assessments of surgical risks and outcomes and create efficient treatment protocols for improved patient care of the obese patient population.

1. Introduction

Obesity is a growing and significant healthcare issue [1–4]. In 1910, Dr. Kelly described obesity, stating "to be a storehouse for useless adipose tissue and to carry this handicap around, openly displayed wherever one goes, is one of the most distressing of life's minor ailments [5]." While current viewpoints may be less extreme, obesity continues to carry a social stigma and is increasingly present in our society [2, 4, 6, 7]. According to recent figures, an average prevalence of 35 percent of adult Americans is classified as obese and 5 percent morbidly obese, with this trend continuing [2, 8]. Obesity is responsible for more than 25 percent of the increase in healthcare costs over the past 15 years [2, 4].

Body mass index (BMI) is one of the most objective methods in determining the presence and extent of obesity [9–11]. As BMI increases to obesity levels, morbidity and mortality rates rise dramatically [4, 12–20]. The clinical definition for obesity is a BMI $\geq$ 30 kg/m^2, with severe obesity defined as a BMI $\geq$ 35 kg/m^2 and morbid obesity as a BMI $\geq$ 40 kg/m^2 [2]. Patterns of obesity are affected by internal as well as external and environmental factors, including variables such as age, socioeconomic status, ethnicity, and genetic background [2, 3].

Surgical attempts have been made to correct obesity, such as bariatric surgery and direct surgical excision. Bariatric surgery refers to any of the various surgical procedures performed to treat obesity by modification of the gastrointestinal tract to reduce nutrient intake and/or absorption [12, 14, 21–25]. Direct surgical excision, individualized to each patient's needs, may include circumferential abdominoplasty, panniculectomy, brachioplasty, thighplasty, and/or liposuction [7, 26–28]. Usually performed after massive weight loss following bariatric procedures, surgical excision is an important aspect of treatment for many patients as they often view the redundant tissues as the last barrier to resuming "normalcy", both for cosmetic reasons as well as for physical comfort [29].

From a surgical standpoint, obesity is associated with a multitude of complications including impairments of cutaneous wound healing, total wound failure, and fascial dehiscence [10, 30–39]. Complications can be observed following various surgeries including gastric bypass and panniculectomy [29, 32, 40–42]. While health benefits of bariatric surgery are well recognized, serious complications can result in 2–4% of patients [43]. A 2006 study of postbariatric patients found that over the ensuing six months after surgery, complication rates actually approached 40 percent [2]. These complications included abdominal pain, nutritional deficiencies, endocrine or metabolic disorders, gastrointestinal disorders, and wound compromise. Additionally, patients who have had prior bariatric surgery and subsequently undergo additional surgical procedures may have similar complications as their BMI may persist to be within the obese category [36]. As these postsurgical complications often result in unplanned hospital and emergency room visits, as well as readmissions, there is an imperative need to improve the outcomes of surgery performed on obese patients in order to help decrease health care costs, healing time, and time away from work [2].

Many studies have observed an association between obesity and a myriad of complications [10, 30–39]. Few, however, specifically address the exact mechanisms involved in the deficiencies observed in obese patient wound healing, compared to patients of normal weight. The determination of these mechanisms may allow researchers to pursue a solution, or at least an improvement, to decrease complications and facilitate improved surgical outcomes in the obese patient population.

2. Methods

A literature search was performed using PubMed, Medline, the Cochrane Library, and Internet searches. Keywords used included obesity, wound healing, adipose healing, and bariatric and surgical complications. In addition, a manual search for other articles pertinent to the study was performed. A discussion focusing on the effects of obesity on wound healing, specifically in relation to postoperative complications, is presented. Potential etiologic factors involved and current plausible mechanisms are explained.

3. Discussion

3.1. Complications. Obesity is associated with comorbidities and poor outcomes in a number of medical areas [10, 30–39]. Studies show that even a 10-kilogram weight loss in obese patients can decrease diabetes-related morbidity and mortality by 30% [4, 7, 24]. Improvements are significant in disease processes involving endocrine (diabetes), cardiovascular (hypertension, hyperlipidemia, and coronary artery disease), rheumatic, and hypercoagulation disorders (deep vein thrombosis and pulmonary embolism) [2, 3, 17, 24, 44–46]. Reductions in the severity of symptoms relating to sleep apnea and depression have also been observed [2, 3, 47]. It is important to note that even with the substantial weight loss seen after bariatric procedures, many patients are still considered obese based on their BMI [41, 48].

A higher BMI has repeatedly been correlated with increased mortality resulting from cancers of the uterus, breast, ovary, prostate, colon, and rectum [47, 49]. Baseline values of BMI are an independent predictor of cardiovascular mortality alone [50]. The association of BMI with mortality is further supported by its consistency across different sexes and ethnic groups, with the strength of effect being the main variation [51]. Obese patients suffering a traumatic injury are also at an increased risk of developing multiorgan failure [44]. Since other studies have noted visceral adiposity as having a stronger correlation with increased morbidity and mortality, both BMI and visceral adiposity should be considered as factors that affect the health status of a patient at the time of surgery and during recovery [52–54]. Furthermore, a higher BMI is correlated with increased infection rates in trauma patients [55]. Compared with nonobese surgical patients, obese patients have an increased incidence of surgical complications, including atelectasis, thrombophlebitis, mortality, wound infection, and wound separation [3, 10, 19, 30–32, 34–39, 47, 48, 56–62]. Clearly, there is strong evidence indicating the association between obesity and poorer surgical outcomes, especially in relation to wound healing. However, the mechanisms responsible for these outcomes are not well known nor understood.

Several studies postulate the mechanisms by which obesity increases wound complications. Potential factors include the intrinsic tenuous anatomic properties and poor vascularity of adipose tissue [63–65]. Relative vascular insufficiency, thus decreased oxygen tension, may result in decreased collagen synthesis, decreased capacity to fight infection, and decreased ability to support the necessary mechanisms of the healing cascade [66–73].

3.2. Anatomy. Adipose tissue is a distinct entity often perceived as relatively avascular [6, 74, 75]. From this standpoint, ischemic associations are made and used in an attempt to rationalize responses of adipose tissue to various stressors. A study contradicting this theory of avascularity notes the anatomy of adipose tissue is subdivided into lobules, each made up of thousands of cells which are separated by fibroush septa carring relatively large vessels and neurons [64]. The blood supply to each lobule comes through a vascular pedicle, with fine-meshed capillary retia encompassing every fat cell. The percentage of capillary beds to active cytoplasm in fat cells is in fact similar to that of skeletal muscle, a well-vascularized tissue [5, 64]. As excess adiposity causes an increased demand on the circulation, adipose tissue begins to develop its own vascular system. Vascular insufficiencies arise in obesity because the capillary density does not increase proportionally to the increase in adipose tissue [76]. This may be due to several factors, one of which is a decrease in elastin and an increase in collagen V and VI around the large vessels of adipose tissues, resulting in a profibrotic environment [77, 78]. These changes in the extracellular matrix contribute to fibrosis and increased adipose tissue rigidity, likely hindering the expansion of individual adipocytes. This can also potentially restrict capillary proliferation, leading to impaired angiogenesis. Compounding to this fact is the greater number of large blood vessels in obese individuals. Larger vessels have a greater diffusion barrier so they do not deliver oxygen as efficiently as capillaries. Altogether, decreasing capillary density and increasing number of larger vessels lead to decreased perfusion of adipose tissue and predispose it to a hypoxic environment. This could be a significant detractor for vascular regeneration and oxygen perfusion needed in wound healing. While the strain on circulation created by surplus adipose mass already exists, capillary damage from injury further exacerbates this hypoxic environment.

Structurally, the delicate nature of fat lobules makes it more susceptible to mechanical damage—the *in-situ* resistance ascribed to only the supporting structures [64]. These supportive structures, however, do not develop correspondingly to increasing fat volume [64]. Surgical intervention can render these supportive structures inactive and readily cause adipose weakness. Additionally, fat lobules are units with terminal circulation and severance of the lobule may destroy blood supply, leading to necrosis of the whole unit [64, 65, 73]. Capillary proliferation occurs maximally at the wound surface during normal wound healing. However, necrosed or damaged adipose lobules can complicate this process [31, 64, 79]. With full-thickness skin grafts, complications arise when residual adipose tissue is attached to the graft [64, 65, 80]. Adipose tissue appears to inhibit the flow of wound serum into grafted skin, a process essential to the graft's survival. It is postulated that this interaction is due to the adipocytes' absorption of wound serum with failure to subsequently transfer it to the graft, a theory supported by the substantial edema noted in grafts containing residual adipose tissue, and decreased revascularization of these grafts since fewer capillary links with the dermis exist among the vascular anastomoses between the wound base and the lobules [64, 80]. Decreased angiogenic capacity of adipose tissue in conjunction with decreased oxygenation of graft tissue can lead to hypoxia.

Adipose tissue grafting is notable for variable and often unsatisfactory results due to loss of volume. Fat lobules damaged or severed on removal of the graft are likely to be lost [64]. Rapid revascularization would involve using original vessels, but due to the anatomical features of adipose tissue, this can only occur indirectly. Indirect revascularization possibly results in substantial delay and thus, increased loss of cells incapable of tolerating the ischemic stress as hypoxia may be a risk factor for increased adipocyte death in obese patients [64, 65, 73, 81]. Once becoming necrotic, fat grafts cannot be resorbed but rather need macrophage uptake for elimination [64, 65]. Macrophage recognition of necrotic adipose as a "foreign body" may lead to initiation or perpetuation and extension of the inflammatory phase of an acute or chronic wound. This reaction can be detrimental to ideal healing processes as "foreign bodies" delay the progression of wounds to the fibroproliferative phase, a critical wound healing period where tensile breaking strength quickly increases [61, 82]. Fat necrosis and subsequent foreign body reaction can be substantial if surgical manipulation is not performed along anatomical limits of the fat layer [64].

3.3. Vascularity. Several studies describe the "inherent" decreased vascularity of adipose tissue as leading to its associated wound complications [6, 74, 75]. Increased adiposity sets off a cascade that positively feeds back into impaired angiogenesis and chronic low-grade inflammation. In addition to the overexpression of collagen VI (col6), obesity is associated with increased expression of 11f3-hydroxysteroid dehydrogenase type 1 (11f3HSD1), an intracellular glucocorticoid-amplifying enzyme [83]. Glucocorticoids suppress angiogenesis so the elevated level of 11f3HSD1 amplifies the inhibitory effects of glucocorticoids [84, 85]. As adipose tissue becomes hypoxic from impaired angiogenesis, hypoxia-inducible factor 1 alpha (HIF1α) levels increase [86]. Elevated HIF1α levels initiate local inflammation and fibrosis by activating the collagen I and III cross-linking activity of lysyl oxidase (LOX). Consequently, overexpression of these factors impairs wound healing by suppressing the angiogenic process needed to restore the wound vasculature and contributes to the obesity pathogenesis of hypoxia and fibrosis. Other proposed mechanisms in which excessive adiposity leads to microvascular abnormalities include reduced nitrogen oxide (NO) availability impairing development of microvascular rarefaction and prolonged elevation of free fatty acids in the blood from increased fat mass impairing capillary recruitment [76, 87, 88].

Yet, a few studies debate this viewpoint of inherent decreased vascularity, pointing to the finding that undisturbed adipose is well perfused [58, 64, 65]. Only in particular scenarios is decreased vascularity observed, such as surgical and other traumatic injuries that result in adipose lobule disruption and consequent relative avascularity [64]. In response to ischemic stimulation, obesity in murine models suppresses the ability of adipose-derived endothelial progenitor cells (EPC) to differentiate, reducing the circulating level of EPCs available to function in blood vessel endothelial repair and angiogenesis [89]. Regardless of whether the avascularity is inherent or acquired, the compromise of blood flow and subsequent poor oxygenation can lead to disruption of the normal healing process and/or eventual necrosis of the tissue [64, 90, 91].

Venous insufficiency is another vascular factor associated with the development of chronic wounds and delayed wound healing. The association between obesity and venous insufficiency is well established, but the exact mechanisms for wound disturbances are only beginning to be realized. Understanding of the more advanced clinical stages of venous disease in obese patients has led to a proposal in which raised intra-abdominal pressure may cause the greater reflux, increased vein diameter, increased venous pressure, and ultimately, impaired venous function [92]. Venous insufficiency impairs wound healing by forming a barrier surrounding capillaries and decreasing effective diffusion of oxygen and nutrients from capillaries to surrounding tissue [66–68, 71, 73]. Once venous insufficiency is present, proteinaceous material may accumulate in the interstitium surrounding the capillaries, leading to clotting and eventual fibrosis of these vessels [93, 94]. Additionally, components of intravascular fluid may leak into the surrounding tissues because of increased hydrostatic pressure, inciting an inflammatory response [95]. These factors create a "barrier" through which oxygen and nutrients cannot transverse to supply surrounding tissue. Furthermore, leukocytes may become trapped and accumulate, contributing to poor oxygenation and tissue destruction by releasing lysosomal enzymes and proinflammatory mediators [93, 94]. These mechanisms create a feasible argument for the role of venous insufficiency in contributing to impaired wound healing.

3.4. Cellular and Molecular Alterations. Advances in the field of gene array offer a potential to investigate the changes corresponding with obesity [96]. The discoveries of obesity-induced changes in adipose tissue emphasize that obesity may initiate and perpetuate a chronic low-grade inflammatory process. A study of obese mice demonstrated a progressive increase in proinflammatory cytokine production resulting from the activation of invariant natural killer T (iNKT) cells by the excess lipid. This occurred before or at the time of inflammatory leukocyte recruitment [97]. Furthermore, the iNKT cells influenced other leukocytes to produce proinflammatory cytokines, resulting in an imbalanced proinflammatory cytokine milieu. Other inflammatory mediators that increase concomitantly with adipose tissue mass include angiotensinogen, tumor necrosis factor alpha (TNF-α), leptin, interleukin 6 (IL-6), and transforming growth factor beta (TGF-β). [1] Additionally, pathologic inflammatory changes related to increased macrophages, mononuclear and polymorphonuclear cells, and inflammatory cytokines have been shown in obesity studies to be dependent upon the degree and duration of obesity [1, 96, 98, 99]. [1] As lipopolysaccharide levels increase, the scavenger receptor CD36 enhances adipose tissue inflammation and cell death through its expression on and synergistic modulation of both macrophages and adipocytes [100]. Specifically, the activation state of adipose tissue macrophages shifts from the protective and anti-inflammatory M2-polarized state to an M1 proinflammatory state as a result of diet-induced obesity [101]. M2 macrophages aid in tissue repair and homeostasis and produce anti-inflammatory cytokines [102]. In obese mice, chronic inflammation caused by mediators such as TNF-α can cause skin gamma delta T cells to be unresponsive to damage in the epithelium, preventing the release of cytokines and growth factors that facilitate wound repair and making the wound vulnerable to injury and infection [103]. Thus, the shift in macrophage activation and other immune mediators towards a proinflammatory state likely impairs wound healing in obese patients by compromising immunoregulation and altering the inflammatory stage of wound repair. The view that obesity induces a chronic low-grade inflammatory process is supported by findings of a reduction in macrophage infiltration and chemoattractant gene expression following weight loss [1, 96].

3.5. Oxidative Stress. Obesity, especially abdominal obesity, is positively correlated with oxidative stress [104]. This is partly attributed to a deficiency in adiponectin, an adipose-derived cytokine that protects against oxidative stress and inflammation [105, 106]. Paradoxically, adiponectin concentration decreases with obesity although it is secreted by adipocytes [107]. A deficiency of adiponectin impairs wound healing via two mechanisms. In response to ischemic stimulation, adiponectin stimulates angiogenesis by promoting AMP-activated protein kinase signaling. Secondly, adiponectin activates the ERK signaling pathway to promote keratinocyte proliferation and migration, a critical process in the reepithelialization phase of wound healing [108]. Therefore, decreased adiponectin impairs proper perfusion and reepithelialization of the wound.

Decreased oxygen tension is present in "normal" wounded tissue and is a major factor in the susceptibility of wounds to infection [66, 67, 69, 109, 110]. Baseline oxygen tension was noted to be the lowest in infected wounds, with the most critical range being between 0 and 40 mmHg [71, 73]. The hypovolemia and impaired tissue perfusion of the wound may exacerbate the preexisting relative hypoperfusion of adipose tissue that resulted from the expansion of fat mass without a synchronized increase in blood flow per cell [111]. This can cause a critical reduction in oxygen delivery to adipose tissue, as seen in the impaired tissue perfusion of the morbidly obese during the perioperative period [88].

The hypoperfusion of subcutaneous adipose tissue in obese patients may predispose them to a greater risk of acquiring a surgical site infection [110]. This is likely from a greater risk of ischemia and necrosis and deficiencies in the oxidase system of leukocytes [69, 112, 113]. In the normal, unhindered process, phagocytosis is followed by a burst of oxygen consumption, which coincides with bacterial death [68, 69, 71, 112]. This oxygen consumption is essential to the bactericidal mechanisms of the host's defense system. In an oxygen deficient setting, leukocytes can ingest the bacteria but are unable to kill them [71]. Bacteria cultured from infected wounds of obese patients have been noted to be similar to longstanding wounds of chronic granulomatous disease patients, where the main issue is a defective oxidase system (*i.e., Staphylococcus, E. coli, Klebsiella,* and *Candida)* [68, 70, 71, 112, 114]. The positive feedback interaction between the altered immune responses and local inflammation in adipose tissue contributes to the development of metabolic complications and impaired wound healing in the obese [115].

Infection significantly affects wound healing and preparation of the wound bed. Optimal healing requires eradication of infection [82, 116–119]. Therapies with proven efficacy incorporate minimizing necrosis, bacterial load, and inflammation of the wound bed, all the while maintaining regenerative tissue cells to aid in wound healing [120]. A fine balance exists between the host's defense system and the pathologic effects of bacteria [82, 119, 121]. The faster and more effectively the immune system combats infection, the less disturbed the normal wound healing process and the better the outcome for the patient. Deficiencies in oxygen utilization and increased inflammation associated with adipose tissue partially explain the mechanisms of increased wound infections prominent in obese patients.

Another aspect of wound healing that is potentially affected by hypoxia is fibroblasts' capability to synthesize collagen [73, 93, 94]. Although fibroblasts are able to survive in a hypoxic environment, they cannot proliferate or synthesize collagen properly [73]. Biochemically, the complete absence of oxygen inhibits the hydroxylation of proline and lysine, preventing the final assembly of the collagen molecule [122]. Clinical support of this is evident in the finding of collagen deposition and synthesis being directly proportional to oxygen tension in postsurgical patients [67, 68]. As a result, injured tissues, especially damaged adipose lobules that already have an insufficient vascular supply and experience further oxygen perfusion deficits after an injury, have decreased resources to meet metabolic needs and have a limited ability to effectively produce collagen. Without sufficient collagen IV and V to promote the aggregation of platelets in the subendothelium, hemostasis is delayed and/or impaired [123]. This likely translates into poor wound healing.

Collagen synthesis is an essential part of the wound healing process and subsequent integrity of the wound [124–127]. It is a key element in establishing maximum tensile strength [67, 124–127]. The upregulation of collagen I and III expression has been shown to accelerate cutaneous wound healing in rats [128]. This process is impaired in obesity because excessive adiposity increases the expression of immature type III collagen and disorganized type I collagen fibers [129]. Without the appropriate collagen, the collagen matrix cannot remodel properly, which reduces the mechanical strength and yield required for the recovery of wound strength and healing.

3.6. Micronutrient and Macronutrient Deficiencies. Wound healing involves the well-coordinated processes of hemostasis, inflammation, granulation tissue formation, fibrogenesis, neovascularization, contraction, and reepithelialization [130]. In order for the cellular responses and homeostatic mechanisms to occur properly, there must be sufficient vitamins, minerals, and proteins present, that is, there must be sufficient nutrients available. This requirement necessarily places obese patients at a disadvantage because they suffer from a paradoxical malnutrition resulting from a calorie-dense diet that is high in carbohydrates and fats and low in vitamins and minerals [131]. Eventually, nutritional deficiencies occur. Blood tests and biochemical analysis on bariatric surgery candidates preoperatively revealed an astonishingly high occurrence of micronutrient and macronutrient deficiencies, particularly vitamin B12, 25-OH vitamin D3, zinc, albumin, and iron, with the latter two increasing significantly with BMI [132–136]. Other nutritional deficiencies amongst bariatric surgery candidates include folic acid, ferritin, phosphorus, calcium, magnesium, vitamin A, vitamin B6, vitamin C, and copper [133–135, 137, 138].

Almost immediately after the occurrence of a wound, hemostasis begins to take place. Calcium, predominantly involved as factor IV, is critical in this process as it is required for the activation of many intercellular reactions, serving as a primary catalyst in platelet aggregation and in the production of clotting Factors VIII, IX, and X [123, 139]. Calcium is recruited again later on for the activation of neutrophils, migration of cells, regeneration of epidermal cells, and modulation of keratinocyte proliferation and differentiation. Without sufficient vitamin D, however, calcium cannot be absorbed in the small intestines [140]. Vitamin D deficiency is also associated with obesity [141, 142]. BMI may be a risk factor for vitamin D deficiency, with deficiencies even evident in obese children [143]. Vitamin D has a range of physiological functions, from regulating B cells and bone metabolism to maintaining calcium homeostasis [141, 144]. The role of vitamin D in adipose tissue signaling is being unraveled, with recent findings of vitamin D reducing lipid accumulation in adipocytes and exhibiting an anti-inflammatory effect in adipose tissue [144]. This implies that vitamin D has an immunomodulatory function in adipose tissue and deficiencies may lead to adipocyte dysfunction and impair wound healing.

Proper wound healing also requires the minerals zinc and copper. DNA and RNA polymerases require zinc in the repair processes as it helps the metabolism catalyze more than 200 enzymes, facilitates protein folding, and regulates gene expression [123, 145]. Adipose tissue metabolism requires zinc to regulate the secretion of leptin, an adipocytokine, and promote free fatty acid release and glucose uptake [146]. Obesity is associated with leptin resistance; thus, the abnormal metabolism resulting from zinc deficiency may contribute to impaired wound repair [106]. During the inflammatory and fibrogenesis processes, zinc and zinc metalloenzymes assist in immune and inflammatory responses, collagenesis, matrix degradation, epidermal regeneration, and scar formation [123, 146, 147]. Low zinc intake is associated with low superoxide dismutase activity in obese individuals, likely accounting for why zinc deficiency increases oxidative stress and the inflammatory response [148]. In a clinical study, oral administration of nutritional doses (15 mg elemental zinc) of zinc to burn patients significantly improved outcomes by elevating the level of glutathione (a natural antioxidant), decreasing the incidence of eschar formation, improving the antioxidant status, increasing healing time, and decreasing the mortality rate [149]. In addition, copper is needed by lysyl oxidase in collagenesis and elastic tissue formation and may also have a role in stabilizing epidermal cells [123].

The inflammatory stage may be prolonged if vitamin A is deficient as low vitamin A serum levels correlate with increased oxidative stress and Th1 response, which potentially can heighten the inflammatory processes already involved in the chronic inflammation and fat deposition inherent in obesity [148]. Vitamin A is needed again in collagenesis and epithelialization to increase the rate of collagen synthesis, cross link new collagen, promote epithelialization, and close wounds [23, 150, 151]. Experimental animal studies have shown that vitamin A accelerates the healing of incisions by hastening the formation of granulation tissue [150, 152].

Vitamin A also has the capability of decreasing the severity of bacterial and fungal infections [151]. Due to the increased nutritional requirements for wound healing, it is recommended to give five times the normal supplemental vitamin. A requirement to all patients after an injury, regardless of the patient's nutritional status [150, 151]. Vitamin A can also reverse the negative effects of steroids on wound healing so it may contribute to improved wound healing in various compromised states, for instance, obesity [153–155].

Throughout the process of wound healing, there are also other nutritional factors that are required, such as vitamin B. B complex vitamin deficiencies are concerning as they influence wound healing and other processes [94, 156–160]. B12 injections have been shown to increase the tensile strength of wounds and facilitate superior wound healing [82, 158]. Components of vitamin B complex also serve as cofactors for a number of enzyme systems. Dysfunction of these enzyme systems can affect protein, carbohydrate, and fat metabolism, as well as disturb antibody and white cell functions [70, 157, 158, 160]. Severe deficiencies impair the synthesis of DNA, proteins, and other crucial molecules, leading to megaloblastosis as well as hindering cellular proliferation and repair [161]. Furthermore, megaloblastosis can result in the development of megaloblastic anemia, which may adversely affect circulation. To maintain sufficient vitamin B intake for patients who are severely injured or acutely ill, five to ten times the normal amount of B complex vitamins is usually recommended [64].

Iron is also crucial for proper wound healing. Iron deficiency in the obese may be due to a decrease in dietary iron intake, the effects of obesity-related inflammation on dietary iron absorption, and/or the sequestration of iron as a result of chronic inflammation [148, 162]. Both BMI and inflammation have been shown to predict iron absorption and affect iron fortification response [163]. It is plausible that hepcidin, an inhibitor of intestinal iron absorption and activator of iron sequestration by macrophages, is a mediator as it is directly correlated with the degree of obesity and indirectly correlated with iron absorption [148, 164, 165]. Iron is also required in the hydroxylation of lysine and proline; therefore, insufficiencies of this element can lead to decreased tensile strength in wounds [166, 167]. Additionally, decreased iron absorption may result in iron deficiency anemia. This can diminish oxygen transport and potentiate secondary effects on wound healing due to relative hypoxia in healing tissues [150, 167, 168]. Iron deficiency also results in a dampened leukocyte bactericidal ability, further complicating healing by weakening the wound's defense system [169].

Protein malnutrition also significantly affects wound healing because it is needed for fibroblast proliferation, angiogenesis, and collagen production [150, 161]. An albumin level lower than 2 is associated with a number of wound healing impairments including a prolonged inflammatory phase, decreased fibroplasia, which leads to delayed wound healing, and decreased neovascularization [150]. Additionally, decreased cell synthesis and wound remodeling, diminished wound strength, impaired T-cell function, and phagocyte activity, as well as decreased complement and antibody levels, all contribute to the delayed healing observed in protein deficient states [170–173].

Carbohydrates and fat intake also affect wound metabolism [150, 174]. Together, carbohydrates and fats are the major source of energy in the body and consequently in the wound healing process. The metabolic syndrome commonly associated with obesity may lead to insulin resistance, rendering the body less adept at maximally utilizing glucose, a breakdown product of carbohydrates [175]. Indirectly, insufficient carbohydrates and/or fats will force the body to look for alternate forms of energy, leading to excess oxidation of amino acids to satisfy caloric needs [150]. Following injury, obese patients preferentially oxidize proteins and carbohydrates, possibly from a block in the utilization of free fatty acids [176]. Amino acid use further perpetuates protein malnutrition and their effects on wound healing. Directly, the energy requirement of leukocytes and fibroblasts is increased after injury, and if unfulfilled, can result in impaired wound healing [150]. This altered metabolic function after trauma and injury can reduce the immune response. Cumulatively, all these factors contribute to increasing wound complications and wound failure rates.

3.7. Special Considerations. Gastric bypass (GBP) surgery can be utilized to correct obesity by helping patients achieve and maintain weight loss [2, 36, 47]. An important topic often left unaddressed with patients, however, is the increased risk of possible wound complications following surgery. The nature of GBP surgery leaves patients in a state of "deliberate malnutrition," possibly exacerbating the altered metabolic response and nutritional deficiencies already present in the obese patient. GBP patients, in addition to the normal challenge of maintaining the 25% increase in required protein and caloric intake for wound healing postoperatively, are faced with a new and less effective gastrointestinal anatomy for maintaining the nutrients needed postoperatively [150]. Many post-GBP patients have protein-calorie malnutrition in addition to various vitamin and mineral deficiencies. [177] Post-GBP nutritional deficits in iron, vitamin B12, folate, vitamin A, thiamine, calcium, potassium, and magnesium are relatively common [178, 179]. Following major elective surgery, additional nutritional deficits include reductions in nitrogen, potassium, sulfur, and phosphorus [150]. These deficits are compounded by postsurgical requirements for increased ascorbic acid, thiamin, riboflavin, nicotinamide, and vitamin A, compared to normal daily needs. This further reduction in the quantity of nutrients available for use can lead to an increased risk of medical complications [20, 174]. In a study of postbariatric patients, all of them experienced wound complications following abdominoplasty because they had a reduction of nearly 60% for total tissue protein [177]. These same patients had a reduction of 72% in the amino acid hydroxyproline, a major constituent of collagen, leading to a decrease in tensile strength of the wound. However, a reduction in surgical complications is achievable by giving nutritional supplements to obese patients prior to surgery. Dietary recommendations suggest that unsaturated fatty acids comprise 4–8% of daily caloric intake in injured patients who experience metabolic/physiologic derangements that are prolonged (as in post-GBP patients) [150]. This amount is roughly double the amount recommended for healthy patients [94, 158, 159]. Diet adjustments of post-GBP patients that subsequently undergo panniculectomy or other surgical procedures must be quantified and supplemented in order to maintain sufficient nutritional status. The inability to provide for these requirements can significantly affect patient outcome. Vitamin and protein deficits diminish phagocytic and lymphocytic activity, directly impairing the immune system, after only 4 weeks in this nutritional setting [82, 116, 118]. While nutrition teams closely follow patients postoperatively and advances in supplementation attempt to correct nutritional deficiencies after surgery, the system is by no means perfect as patient noncompliance can negatively impact nutritional and metabolic complications [2, 20, 47, 174].

4. Conclusion

Obesity is a pervasive health issue in today's society. It induces complex negative effects on multiple organ system functions and processes, including issues related to wound healing. Efforts to decipher the origins, physiology, and health consequences of obesity on the human body are an imperative focus in current investigations. Numerous studies have shown the correlation between obesity and abnormal wound healing, with knowledge of the exact mechanisms in the infantile stages. Theories on credible contributing factors are presented in this review.

Healthy adipose tissue is beneficial to the human body as it serves as an insulator and paracrine and endocrine organ, secreting cytokines, growth factors, and immune mediators. Uninjured adipose tissue has a comparable vascular supply to other uninjured tissue types, but its tenuous anatomic configuration leaves it weaker and more susceptible to mechanical damage. Since each lobule is supplied by terminal blood vessels, damage to the area may result in necrosis of the entire lobule.

Problems arise as excessive adiposity modifies the cellular composition and structure of adipose tissue, as well as changing the physiology of the skin and subcutaneous tissues. Obesity induces adipocyte hypertrophy and hyperplasia, eventually impairing the metabolic functions of the adipocytes, such as storing fat. It may be that the metabolic dysfunction is the primary activator in the cascade of obesity-induced problems. Following metabolic dysfunction, inflammatory mediators begin to invade the adipose tissue, leading to a chronic, low-grade inflammatory process that is well associated with obesity. The phenotypic switching of protective M2 macrophages to proinflammatory M1 macrophages exacerbates this problem. As adipocytes grow in size and number, blood vessels develop into the new areas of adipose tissue growth. However, the rate of angiogenesis does not parallel the rate of adipocyte growth. Compounding these properties, obese adipose tissues secrete angiogenic inhibitors and fibrotic mediators. The extracellular matrix remodeling may further impede the process of angiogenesis by creating a stiffer environment and preventing the migration of cells and vessels. Without sufficient supply of blood vessels to oxygenate the area, relative hypoxia ensues. The hypoxia caused by damage to capillaries in wounds and the relative hypoxia in obese individuals likely contribute to higher rates of wound infections in obese patients because of even lower oxygen tension from decreased perfusion and impaired immune system functioning. Additionally, hypoxic wounds impair the synthesis of mature collagen, leading to weaker tissue and deficiencies in the overall healing process. Thus, the microvascular abnormalities as a result of excessive adiposity contribute to obesity-related microangiopathy.

The vascular insufficiencies and altered population of immune mediators present may lengthen the inflammatory stage of wound healing, as well as leaving obese individuals more susceptible to infections. Wound healing is also delayed as a result of macronutrient and micronutrient deficiencies in obese individuals. Without the proper cofactors and enzymes, the process of wound healing is compromised, as well as the integrity of the wound. Nutritional supplements can be given to obese patients preoperatively as a possible solution to decrease wound complications. For bariatric surgery candidates, special considerations need to be made as they are at increased risk of nutrition-related complications.

Although the detrimental effect of obesity on wound healing is established, there is a need for additional studies to determine the comprehensive mechanisms involved in this relationship. Some of the key alterations and deficiencies in obese adipose tissue that already have been determined are presently undergoing investigations that utilize target-specific therapies. Perhaps the breakthrough with obesity and wound healing will be in the realm of growth factors, cytokines, nutritional manipulations, surgical techniques, or in gene array studies. Most likely, interventions will involve a combination of these factors and others. With the prevalence of obesity in today's society and its evidenced effects on health care, the challenge of altering adipose tissue's effect on wound healing remains one which necessitates further exploration.

Conflict of Interests

The authors declare that there is no conflict of interests regarding the publication of this paper.

References

[1] D. R. Cottam, S. G. Mattar, E. Barinas-Mitchell et al., "The chronic inflammatory hypothesis for the morbidity associated with morbid obesity: implications and effect of weight loss," *Obesity Surgery*, vol. 14, no. 5, pp. 589–600, 2004.

[2] W. E. Encinosa, D. M. Bernard, C.-C. Chen, and C. A. Steiner, "Healthcare utilization and outcomes after bariatric surgery," *Medical Care*, vol. 44, no. 8, pp. 706–712, 2006.

[3] S. G. Camden and J. Gates, "Obesity: changing the face of geriatric care," *Ostomy Wound Management*, vol. 52, no. 10, pp. 36–44, 2006.

[4] K. E. Thorpe, C. S. Florence, D. H. Howard, and P. Joski, "The impact of obesity on rising medical spending," *Health Affairs*, Web Exclusives, pp. 480–486, 2004.

[5] H. A. Kelly, "Excision of the fat of the abdominal wall lipectomy," *Surgery, Gynecology & Obstetrics*, vol. 10, article 229, 1910.

[6] J. A. Wilson and J. J. Clark, "Obesity: impediment to postsurgical wound healing," *Advances in Skin & Wound Care*, vol. 17, no. 8, pp. 426–435, 2004.

[7] P. R. Schauer and B. D. Schirmer, "The surgical management of obesity," in *Schwartz's Principles of Surgery*, pp. 997-1016, McGraw Hill Companies, New York, NY, USA, 8th edition, 2005.

[8] K. M. Flegal, D. Carroll, B. K. Kit, and C. L. Ogden, "Prevalence of obesity and trends in the distribution of body mass index among US adults, 1999–2010," *Journal of the American Medical Association*, vol. 307, no. 5, pp. 491–497, 2012.

[9] W. Coutinho, "Latin America consensus on obesity," *Arquivos Brasileiros de Endocrinologia & Metabologia*, vol. 43, pp. 21–67, 1999.

[10] I. Pitanguy, N. F. G. de Amorim, and H. N. Radwanski, "Contour surgery in the patient with great weight loss," *Aesthetic Plastic Surgery*, vol. 24, no. 6, pp. 406–411, 2000.

[11] J. C. Rosen, P. Orosan, and J. Reiter, "Cognitive behavior therapy for negative body image in obese women," *Behavior Therapy*, vol. 26, no. 1, pp. 25–42, 1995.

[12] P. Benotti, G. C. Wood, C. Still, A. Petrick, and W. Strodel, "Obesity disease burden and surgical risk," *Surgery for Obesity and Related Diseases*, vol. 2, no. 6, pp. 600–606, 2006.

[13] M. P. Herman, J. D. Raman, S. Dong, D. Samadi, and D. S. Scherr, "Increasing body mass index negatively impacts outcomes following robotic radical prostatectomy," *Journal of the Society of Laparoendoscopic Surgeons*, vol. 11, no. 4, pp. 438–442, 2007.

[14] K. Jongnarangsin, A. Chugh, E. Good et al., "Body mass index, obstructive sleep apnea, and outcomes of catheter ablation of atrial fibrillation," *Journal of Cardiovascular Electrophysiology*, vol. 19, no. 7, pp. 668–672, 2008.

[15] A. Lübbeke, K. G. M. Moons, G. Garavaglia, and P. Hoffmeyer, "Outcomes of obese and nonobese patients undergoing revision total hip arthroplasty," *Arthritis Care and Research*, vol. 59, no. 5, pp. 738–745, 2008.

[16] J. Parikh, I. Yermilov, M. Mcgory, S. Jain, C. Y. Ko, and M. Maggard, "Is high BMI associated with specific complications after laparoscopic Roux-en-Y gastric bypass?" *American Surgeon*, vol. 73, no. 10, pp. 959–962, 2007.

[17] M. Rogliani, E. Silvi, L. Labardi, F. Maggiulli, and V. Cervelli, "Obese and nonobese patients: complications of abdominoplasty," *Annals of Plastic Surgery*, vol. 57, no. 3, pp. 336–338, 2006.

[18] L. Setälä, A. Papp, S. Joukainen et al., "Obesity and complications in breast reduction surgery: are restrictions justified?" *Journal of Plastic, Reconstructive and Aesthetic Surgery*, vol. 62, no. 2, pp. 195–199, 2009.

[19] F. J. Thomas, L. Goldman, C. M. Mangione et al., "Body mass index as a correlate of postoperative complications and resource utilization," *American Journal of Medicine*, vol. 102, no. 3, pp. 277–283, 1997.

[20] J. L. Mullen, G. P. Buzby, and D. C. Matthews, "Reduction of operative morbidity and mortality by combined preoperative and postoperative nutritional support," *Annals of Surgery*, vol. 192, no. 5, pp. 604–613, 1980.

[21] D. A. Anaya and E. P. Dellinger, "The obese surgical patient: a susceptible host for infection," *Surgical Infections*, vol. 7, no. 5, pp. 473–480, 2006.

[22] R. Bhatheja and D. L. Bhatt, "Clinical outcomes in metabolic syndrome," *Journal of Cardiovascular Nursing*, vol. 21, no. 4, pp. 298–305, 2006.

[23] J. Casey, W. R. Flinn, and J. S. T. Yao, "Correlation of immune and nutritional status with wound complications in patients undergoing vascular operations," *Surgery*, vol. 93, no. 6, pp. 822–826, 1983.

[24] U. Keller, "From obesity to diabetes," *International Journal for Vitamin and Nutrition Research*, vol. 76, no. 4, pp. 172–177, 2006.

[25] Surgery ASfMB, *Bariatric Surgical Society Takes on New Name, New Mission, and New Surgery. Metabolic Surgery Expected to Play Bigger Role in Treating Type 2 Diabetes*, 2013.

[26] A. S. Aly, A. E. Cram, M. Chao, J. Pang, and M. McKeon, "Belt lipectomy for circumferential truncal excess: The University of Iowa experience," *Plastic and Reconstructive Surgery*, vol. 111, no. 1, pp. 398–413, 2003.

[27] D. J. Hurwitz, J. P. Rubin, M. Risin, A. Sajjadian, and S. Sereika, "Correcting the saddlebag deformity in the massive weight loss patient," *Plastic and Reconstructive Surgery*, vol. 114, no. 5, pp. 1313–1325, 2004.

[28] D. J. Hurwitz and T. E. Zewert, "Body contouring surgery in the bariatric surgical patient," *Operative Techniques in Plastic and Reconstructive Surgery*, vol. 8, no. 2, pp. 87–95, 2002.

[29] M. J. Kamper, D. V. Galloway, and F. Ashley, "Abdominal panniculectomy after massive weight loss," *Plastic and Reconstructive Surgery*, vol. 50, no. 5, pp. 441–446, 1972.

[30] R. W. Postlethwait and W. D. Johnson, "Complications following surgery for duodenal ulcer in obese patients," *Archives of Surgery*, vol. 105, no. 3, pp. 438–440, 1972.

[31] K. J. Printen, S. C. Paulk, and E. E. Mason, "Acute postoperative wound complications after gastric surgery for morbid obesity," *American Surgeon*, vol. 41, no. 8, pp. 483–485, 1975.

[32] W. E. Matory Jr., J. O'Sullivan, G. Fudem, and R. Dunn, "Abdominal surgery in patients with severe morbid obesity," *Plastic and Reconstructive Surgery*, vol. 94, no. 7, pp. 976–987, 1994.

[33] J. P. Rubin, "Plastic surgery after massive weight loss," *Contemporary Surgery*, vol. 61, pp. 599–603, 2005.

[34] R. I. Abdel-Moneim, "The hazards of surgery in the obese," *International Surgery*, vol. 70, no. 2, pp. 101–103, 1985.

[35] M. A. Carlson, "Acute wound failure," *Surgical Clinics of North America*, vol. 77, no. 3, pp. 607–636, 1997.

[36] C. E. Yale, "Gastric surgery for morbid obesity. Complications and long-term weight control," *Archives of Surgery*, vol. 124, no. 8, pp. 941–946, 1989.

[37] W. R. Thompson, J. F. Ameral, and M. D. Caldwell, "Complications and weight loss in 150 consecutive gastric exclusion patients. Critical review," *The American Journal of Surgery*, vol. 146, no. 5, pp. 602–612, 1983.

[38] F. M. Grazer and R. M. Goldwyn, "Abdominoplasty assessed by survey, with emphasis on complications," *Plastic and Reconstructive Surgery*, vol. 59, no. 4, pp. 513–517, 1977.

[39] I. Pitanguy, "Abdominal lipectomy," *Clinics in Plastic Surgery*, vol. 2, no. 3, pp. 401–410, 1975.

[40] Z. M. Arthurs, D. Cuadrado, V. Sohn et al., "Post-bariatric panniculectomy: pre-panniculectomy body mass index impacts the complication profile," *The American Journal of Surgery*, vol. 193, no. 5, pp. 567–570, 2007.

[41] M. A. Manahan and M. A. Shermak, "Massive panniculectomy after massive weight loss," *Plastic and Reconstructive Surgery*, vol. 117, no. 7, pp. 2191–2199, 2006.

[42] A. M. Wolf and H. W. Kuhlmann, "Reconstructive procedures after massive weight loss," *Obesity Surgery*, vol. 17, no. 3, pp. 355–360, 2007.

[43] J. F. Finks, K. L. Kole, P. R. Yenumula et al., "Predicting risk for serious complications with bariatric surgery: results from the Michigan bariatric surgery collaborative," *Annals of Surgery*, vol. 254, no. 4, pp. 633–640, 2011.

[44] D. J. Ciesla, E. E. Moore, J. L. Johnson, J. M. Burch, C. C. Cothren, and A. Sauaia, "Obesity increases risk of organ failure after severe trauma," *Journal of the American College of Surgeons*, vol. 203, no. 4, pp. 539–545, 2006.

[45] L. Flancbaum and S. Belsley, "Factors affecting morbidity and mortality of Roux-en-Y gastric bypass for clinically severe obesity: an analysis of 1,000 consecutive open cases by a single surgeon," *Journal of Gastrointestinal Surgery*, vol. 11, no. 4, pp. 500–507, 2007.

[46] P. A. McCullough, M. J. Gallagher, A. T. DeJong et al., "Cardiorespiratory fitness and short-term complications after bariatric surgery," *Chest*, vol. 130, no. 2, pp. 517–525, 2006.

[47] J. Peter Rubin, V. Nguyen, and A. Schwentker, "Perioperative management of the post-gastric-bypass patient presenting for body contour surgery," *Clinics in Plastic Surgery*, vol. 31, no. 4, pp. 601–610, 2004.

[48] J. A. Greco, E. T. Castaldo, L. B. Nanney et al., "The effect of weight loss surgery and body mass index on wound complications after abdominal contouring operations," *Annals of Plastic Surgery*, vol. 61, no. 3, pp. 235–242, 2008.

[49] P. T. Campbell, C. C. Newton, A. N. Dehal, E. J. Jacobs, A. V. Patel, and S. M. Gapstur, "Impact of body mass index on survival after colorectal cancer diagnosis: the cancer prevention study-II nutrition cohort," *Journal of Clinical Oncology*, vol. 30, no. 1, pp. 42–52, 2012.

[50] M. Bombelli, R. Facchetti, D. Fodri et al., "Impact of body mass index and waist circumference on the cardiovascular risk and all-cause death in a general population: data from the PAMELA study," *Nutrition, Metabolism & Cardiovascular Diseases*, vol. 23, no. 7, pp. 650–656, 2013.

[51] S. Y. Park, L. R. Wilkens, S. P. Murphy et al., "Body mass index and mortality in an ethnically diverse population: the Multiethnic Cohort Study," *European Journal of Epidemiology*, vol. 27, no. 7, pp. 489–497, 2012.

[52] J. P. Reis, C. A. MacEra, M. R. Araneta, S. P. Lindsay, S. J. Marshall, and D. L. Wingard, "Comparison of overall obesity and body fat distribution in predicting risk of mortality," *Obesity*, vol. 17, no. 6, pp. 1232–1239, 2009.

[53] M. J. McNeely, J. B. Shofer, D. L. Leonetti, W. Y. Fujimoto, and E. J. Boyko, "Associations among visceral fat, all-cause mortality, and obesity-related mortality in Japanese Americans," *Diabetes Care*, vol. 35, no. 2, pp. 296–298, 2012.

[54] P. E. Serrano, S. A. Khuder, and J. J. Fath, "Obesity as a Risk Factor for Nosocomial Infections in Trauma Patients," *Journal of the American College of Surgeons*, vol. 211, no. 1, pp. 61–67, 2010.

[55] R. M. Pitkin, "Abdominal hysterectomy in obese women," *Surgery Gynecology and Obstetrics*, vol. 142, no. 4, pp. 532–536, 1976.

[56] L. B. Pemberton and W. G. Manax, "Relationship of obesity to postoperative complications after cholecystectomy," *The American Journal of Surgery*, vol. 121, no. 1, pp. 87–90, 1971.

[57] A. J. Derzie, F. Silvestri, E. Liriano, and P. Benotti, "Wound closure technique and acute wound complications in gastric surgery for morbid obesity: a prospective randomized trial," *Journal of the American College of Surgeons*, vol. 191, no. 3, pp. 238–243, 2000.

[58] V. L. Vastine, R. F. Morgan, G. S. Williams et al., "Wound complications of abdominoplasty in obese patients," *Annals of Plastic Surgery*, vol. 42, no. 1, pp. 34–39, 1999.

[59] M. A. Shermak, D. Chang, T. H. Magnuson, and M. A. Schweitzer, "An outcomes analysis of patients undergoing body contouring surgery after massive weight loss," *Plastic and Reconstructive Surgery*, vol. 118, no. 4, pp. 1026–1031, 2006.

[60] D. A. Dubay and M. G. Franz, "Acute wound healing: the biology of acute wound failure," *Surgical Clinics of North America*, vol. 83, no. 3, pp. 463–481, 2003.

[61] H. J. Sugerman, J. M. Kellum Jr., H. D. Reines, E. J. DeMaria, H. H. Newsome, and J. W. Lowry, "Greater risk of incisional hernia with morbidly obese than steroid-dependent patients and low recurrence with prefascial polypropylene mesh," *The American Journal of Surgery*, vol. 171, no. 1, pp. 80–84, 1996.

[62] L. B. Salans, S. W. Cushman, and R. E. Weismann, "Studies of human adipose tissue. Adipose cell size and number in nonobese and obese patients," *Journal of Clinical Investigation*, vol. 52, no. 4, pp. 929–941, 1973.

[63] J. Smahel, "Adipose issue in plastic surgery," *Annals of Plastic Surgery*, vol. 16, no. 5, pp. 444–453, 1986.

[64] B. Markman, "Anatomy and physiology of adipose tissue," *Clinics in Plastic Surgery*, vol. 16, no. 2, pp. 235–244, 1989.

[65] F. Gottrup, R. Firmin, J. Rabkin, B. J. Halliday, and T. K. Hunt, "Directly measured tissue oxygen tension and arterial oxygen tension assess tissue perfusion," *Critical Care Medicine*, vol. 15, no. 11, pp. 1030–1036, 1987.

[66] K. Jonsson, J. A. Jensen, W. H. Goodson III et al., "Tissue oxygenation, anemia, and perfusion in relation to wound healing in surgical patients," *Annals of Surgery*, vol. 214, no. 5, pp. 605–613, 1991.

[67] K. Jonsson, T. K. Hunt, and S. J. Mathes, "Oxygen as an isolated variable influences resistance to infection," *Annals of Surgery*, vol. 208, no. 6, pp. 783–787, 1988.

[68] H. W. Hopf, T. K. Hunt, J. M. West et al., "Wound tissue oxygen tension predicts the risk of wound infection in surgical patients," *Archives of Surgery*, vol. 132, no. 9, pp. 997–1005, 1997.

[69] D. B. Allen, J. J. Maguire, M. Mahdavian et al., "Wound hypoxia and acidosis limit neutrophil bacterial killing mechanisms," *Archives of Surgery*, vol. 132, no. 9, pp. 991–996, 1997.

[70] T. K. Hunt, M. Linsey, M. Sonne, and E. Jawetz, "Oxygen tension and wound infection," *Surgical Forum*, vol. 23, pp. 47–49, 1972.

[71] J. Niinikoski, G. Grislis, and T. K. Hunt, "Respiratory gas tensions and collagen in infected wounds," *Annals of Surgery*, vol. 175, no. 4, pp. 588–593, 1972.

[72] T. K. Hunt and M. P. Pai, "The effect of varying ambient oxygen tensions on wound metabolism and collagen synthesis," *Surgery Gynecology and Obstetrics*, vol. 135, no. 4, pp. 561–567, 1972.

[73] F. X. Hausberger and M. M. Widelitz, "Distribution of labeled erythrocytes in adipose tissue and muscle in the rat," *The American Journal of Physiology*, vol. 204, pp. 649–652, 1963.

[74] D. M. Groszek, "Promoting wound healing in the obese patient," *AORN Journal*, vol. 35, no. 6, pp. 1132–1138, 1982.

[75] O. Gealekman, N. Guseva, C. Hartigan et al., "Depot-specific differences and insufficient subcutaneous adipose tissue angiogenesis in human obesity," *Circulation*, vol. 123, no. 2, pp. 186–194, 2011.

[76] T. Khan, E. S. Muise, P. Iyengar et al., "Metabolic dysregulation and adipose tissue fibrosis: Role of collagen VI," *Molecular and Cellular Biology*, vol. 29, no. 6, pp. 1575–1591, 2009.

[77] M. Spencer, R. Unal, B. Zhu et al., "Adipose tissue extracellular matrix and vascular abnormalities in obesity and insulin resistance," *Journal of Clinical Endocrinology and Metabolism*, vol. 96, no. 12, pp. E1990–E1998, 2011.

[78] J. Hirsch and J. L. Knittle, "Cellularity of obese and nonobese human adipose tissue," *Federation Proceedings*, vol. 29, no. 4, pp. 1516–1521, 1970.

[79] E. Billings Jr. and J. W. May Jr., "Historical review and present status of free fat graft autotransplantation in plastic and reconstructive surgery," *Plastic and Reconstructive Surgery*, vol. 83, no. 2, pp. 368–381, 1989.

[80] J. Ye, "Emerging role of adipose tissue hypoxia in obesity and insulin resistance," *International Journal of Obesity*, vol. 33, no. 1, pp. 54–66, 2009.

[81] M. C. Robson, D. P. Hill, M. E. Woodske, and D. L. Steed, "Wound healing trajectories as predictors of effectiveness of therapeutic agents," *Archives of Surgery*, vol. 135, no. 7, pp. 773–777, 2000.

[82] Z. Michailidou, M. D. Jensen, D. A. Dumesic et al., "Omental 11β-hydroxysteroid dehydrogenase 1 correlates with fat cell size independently of obesity," *Obesity*, vol. 15, no. 5, pp. 1155–1163, 2007.

[83] Z. Michailidou, S. Turban, E. Miller et al., "Increased angiogenesis protects against adipose hypoxia and fibrosis in metabolic disease-resistant 11β-hydroxysteroid dehydrogenase type 1 (HSD1)-deficient mice," *The Journal of Biological Chemistry*, vol. 287, no. 6, pp. 4188–4197, 2012.

[84] G. R. Small, P. W. F. Hadoke, I. Sharif et al., "Preventing local regeneration of qlucocorticoids by 11β-hydroxysteroid dehydrogenase type 1 enhances angiogenesis," *Proceedings of the National Academy of Sciences of the United States of America*, vol. 102, no. 34, pp. 12165–12170, 2005.

[85] N. Halberg, T. Khan, M. E. Trujillo et al., "Hypoxia-inducible factor 1α induces fibrosis and insulin resistance in white adipose tissue," *Molecular and Cellular Biology*, vol. 29, no. 16, pp. 4467–4483, 2009.

[86] R. T. De Jongh, E. H. Serné, R. G. Ijzerman, G. De Vries, and C. D. A. Stehouwer, "Impaired microvascular function in obesity: implications for obesity-associated microangiopathy, hypertension, and insulin resistance," *Circulation*, vol. 109, no. 21, pp. 2529–2535, 2004.

[87] B. I. Levy, E. L. Schiffrin, J.-J. Mourad et al., "Impaired tissue perfusion a pathology common to hypertension, obesity, and diabetes mellitus," *Circulation*, vol. 118, no. 9, pp. 968–976, 2008.

[88] Y. L. Chen, C. L. Chang, C. K. Sun et al., "Impact of obesity control on circulating level of endothelial progenitor cells and angiogenesis in response to ischemic stimulation," *Journal of Translational Medicine*, vol. 10, article 86, 2012.

[89] H. Kiryu, W. Rikihisa, and M. Furue, "Encapsulated fat necrosis: a clinicopathological study of 8 cases and a literature review," *Journal of Cutaneous Pathology*, vol. 27, no. 1, pp. 19–23, 2000.

[90] S. S. Kroll, G. Gherardini, J. E. Martin et al., "Fat necrosis in free and pedicled TRAM flaps," *Plastic and Reconstructive Surgery*, vol. 102, no. 5, pp. 1502–1507, 1998.

[91] A. M. van Rij, C. S. De Alwis, P. Jiang et al., "Obesity and impaired venous function," *European Journal of Vascular and Endovascular Surgery*, vol. 35, no. 6, pp. 739–744, 2008.

[92] W. K. Stadelmann, A. G. Digenis, and G. R. Tobin, "Impediments to wound healing," *The American Journal of Surgery*, vol. 176, no. 2, supplement 1, pp. 39S–47S, 1998.

[93] J. L. Burns, J. S. Mancoll, and L. G. Phillips, "Impairments to wound healing," *Clinics in Plastic Surgery*, vol. 30, no. 1, pp. 47–56, 2003.

[94] G. Yosipovitch, A. DeVore, and A. Dawn, "Obesity and the skin: skin physiology and skin manifestations of obesity," *Journal of the American Academy of Dermatology*, vol. 56, no. 6, pp. 901–916, 2007.

[95] R. Cancello, C. Henegar, N. Viguerie et al., "Reduction of macrophage infiltration and chemoattractant gene expression changes in white adipose tissue of morbidly obese subjects after surgery-induced weight loss," *Diabetes*, vol. 54, no. 8, pp. 2277–2286, 2005.

[96] L. Wu, V. V. Parekh, C. L. Gabriel et al., "Activation of invariant natural killer T cells by lipid excess promotes tissue inflammation, insulin resistance, and hepatic steatosis in obese mice," *Proceedings of the National Academy of Sciences of the United States of America*, vol. 109, no. 19, pp. E1143–E1152, 2012.

[97] F. X. Hausberger, "Pathological changes in adipose tissue of obese mice," *Anatomical Record*, vol. 154, no. 3, pp. 651–660, 1966.

[98] L. Cai, Z. Wang, A. Ji et al., "Scavenger receptor CD36 expression contributes to adipose tissue inflammation and cell death in diet-induced obesity," *PLoS ONE*, vol. 7, no. 5, Article ID e36785, 2012.

[99] C. N. Lumeng, J. L. Bodzin, and A. R. Saltiel, "Obesity induces a phenotypic switch in adipose tissue macrophage polarization," *Journal of Clinical Investigation*, vol. 117, no. 1, pp. 175–184, 2007.

[100] A. Viardot, L. K. Heilbronn, D. Samocha-Bonet et al., "Obesity is associated with activated and insulin resistant immune cells," *Diabetes/Metabolism Research and Reviews*, vol. 28, no. 5, pp. 447–454, 2012.

[101] K. A. Harford, C. M. Reynolds, F. C. McGillicuddy, and H. M. Roche, "Fats, inflammation and insulin resistance: Insights to the role of macrophage and T-cell accumulation in adipose tissue," *Proceedings of the Nutrition Society*, vol. 70, no. 4, pp. 408–417, 2011.

[102] K. R. Taylor, R. E. Mills, A. E. Costanzo, and J. M. Jameson, "$\gamma\delta$ T cells are reduced and rendered unresponsive by hyperglycemia and chronic TNFα in mouse models of obesity and metabolic disease," *PLoS ONE*, vol. 5, no. 7, Article ID e11422, 2010.

[103] M. Sankhla, T. K. Sharma, K. Mathur et al., "Relationship of oxidative stress with obesity and its role in obesity induced metabolic syndrome," *Clinical Laboratory*, vol. 58, no. 5-6, pp. 385–392, 2012.

[104] K. Kawai, A. Kageyama, T. Tsumano et al., "Effects of adiponectin on growth and differentiation of human keratinocytes—implicaiton of impaired wound healing in diabetes," *Biochemical and Biophysical Research Communications*, vol. 374, no. 2, pp. 269–273, 2008.

[105] A. R. Shipman and G. W. M. Millington, "Obesity and the skin," *British Journal of Dermatology*, vol. 165, no. 4, pp. 743–750, 2011.

[106] R. Shibata, N. Ouchi, S. Kihara, K. Sato, T. Funahashi, and K. Walsh, "Adiponectin stimulates angiogenesis in response to tissue ischemia through stimulation of AMP-activated protein kinase signaling," *The Journal of Biological Chemistry*, vol. 279, no. 27, pp. 28670–28674, 2004.

[107] S. Shibata, Y. Tada, Y. Asano et al., "Adiponectin regulates cutaneous wound healing by promoting keratinocyte proliferation and migration via the ERK signaling pathway," *The Journal of Immunology*, vol. 189, no. 6, pp. 3231–3241, 2012.

[108] W. B. Conolly, T. K. Hunt, M. Sonne, and J. E. Dunphy, “Influence of distant trauma on local wound infection,” *Surgery Gynecology and Obstetrics*, vol. 128, no. 4, pp. 713–718, 1969.

[109] T. Hunt, “A new method of determining tissue oxygen tension,” *The Lancet*, vol. 2, no. 7374, pp. 1370–1371, 1964.

[110] M. Di Girolamo, N. S. Skinner Jr., H. G. Hanley, and R. G. Sachs, “Relationship of adipose tissue blood flow to fat cell size and number,” *The American Journal of Physiology*, vol. 220, no. 4, pp. 932–937, 1971.

[111] D. C. Hohn and T. K. Hunt, “Oxidative metabolism and microbicidal activity of rabbit phagocytes: cells from wounds and from peripheral blood,” *Surgical Forum*, vol. 26, pp. 85–87, 1975.

[112] D. A. Anaya and E. P. Dellinger, “The obese surgical patient: a susceptible host for infection,” *Surgical Infections*, vol. 7, no. 5, pp. 473–480, 2006.

[113] D. C. Hohn, R. D. MacKay, B. Halliday, and T. K. Hunt, “Effect of O_2 tension on microbicidal function of leukocytes in wounds and in vitro,” *Surgical Forum*, vol. 27, no. 62, pp. 18–20, 1976.

[114] F. P. de Heredia, S. Gomez-Martinez, and A. Marcos, “Obesity, inflammation and the immune system,” *Proceedings of the Nutrition Society*, vol. 71, no. 2, pp. 332–338, 2012.

[115] T. J. Krizek, M. C. Robson, and E. Kho, “Bacterial growth and skin graft survival,” *Surgical Forum*, vol. 18, article 518, 1967.

[116] M. C. Robson, “Wound infection: a failure of wound healing caused by an imbalance of bacteria,” *Surgical Clinics of North America*, vol. 77, no. 3, pp. 637–650, 1997.

[117] M. C. Robson, T. J. Krizek, and J. P. Heggers, “Biology of surgical infection,” *Current Problems in Surgery*, vol. 10, no. 3, pp. 1–62, 1973.

[118] M. C. Robson, B. D. Stenberg, and J. P. Heggers, “Wound healing alterations caused by infection,” *Clinics in Plastic Surgery*, vol. 17, no. 3, pp. 485–492, 1990.

[119] J. Panuncialman and V. Falanga, “The science of wound bed preparation,” *Surgical Clinics of North America*, vol. 89, no. 3, pp. 611–626, 2009.

[120] S. Udenfriend, “Formation of hydroxyproline in collagen,” *Science*, vol. 152, no. 3727, pp. 1335–1340, 1966.

[121] M. C. Robson, “Infection in the surgical patient: an imbalance in the normal equilibrium,” *Clinics in Plastic Surgery*, vol. 6, no. 4, pp. 493–503, 1979.

[122] A. B. G. Lansdown, B. Sampson, and A. Rowe, “Sequential changes in trace metal, metallothionein and calmodulin concentrations in healing skin wounds,” *Journal of Anatomy*, vol. 195, no. 3, pp. 375–386, 1999.

[123] A. Barbul, S. A. Lazarou, D. T. Efron, H. L. Wasserkrug, and G. Efron, “Arginine enhances wound healing and lymphocyte immune responses in humans,” *Surgery*, vol. 108, no. 2, pp. 331–337, 1990.

[124] W. H. Goodson III and T. K. Hunt, “Development of a new miniature method for the study of wound healing in human subjects,” *Journal of Surgical Research*, vol. 33, no. 5, pp. 394–401, 1982.

[125] J. W. Madden and E. E. Peacock Jr., “Studies on the biology of collagen during wound healing. I. Rate of collagen synthesis and deposition in cutaneous wounds of the rat,” *Surgery*, vol. 64, no. 1, pp. 288–294, 1968.

[126] J. Viljanto, *Biochemical Basis of Tensile Strength in Wound Healing: An Experimental Study with Viscose Cellulose Sponges on Rats*, tr.: Kirjapaino Polytypos, Turku, Finland, 1964.

[127] M. Ganeshkumar, T. Ponrasu, R. Krithika, K. Iyappan, V. S. Gayathri, and L. Suguna, “Topical application of Acalypha indica accelerates rat cutaneous wound healing by up-regulating the expression of Type I and III collagen,” *Journal of Ethnopharmacology*, vol. 142, no. 1, pp. 14–22, 2012.

[128] L. Xing, E. J. Culbertson, Y. Wen, M. C. Robson, and M. G. Franz, “Impaired laparotomy wound healing in obese rats,” *Obesity Surgery*, vol. 21, no. 12, pp. 1937–1946, 2011.

[129] J. P. Cai, B. Harris, V. Falanga, W. H. Eaglstein, P. M. Mertz, and Y. H. Chin, “Recruitment of mononuclear cells into wounded skin: mechanism and modulation,” *Progress in Clinical and Biological Research*, vol. 365, pp. 243–256, 1991.

[130] S. A. Xanthakos, “Nutritional deficiencies in obesity and after bariatric surgery,” *Pediatric Clinics of North America*, vol. 56, no. 5, pp. 1105–1121, 2009.

[131] B. Ernst, M. Thurnheer, S. M. Schmid, and B. Schultes, “Evidence for the necessity to systematically assess micronutrient status prior to bariatric surgery,” *Obesity Surgery*, vol. 19, no. 1, pp. 66–73, 2009.

[132] C. Schweiger, R. Weiss, E. Berry, and A. Keidar, “Nutritional deficiencies in bariatric surgery candidates,” *Obesity Surgery*, vol. 20, no. 2, pp. 193–197, 2010.

[133] V. Moizé, R. Deulofeu, F. Torres, J. M. De Osaba, and J. Vidal, “Nutritional intake and prevalence of nutritional deficiencies prior to surgery in a spanish morbidly obese population,” *Obesity Surgery*, vol. 21, no. 9, pp. 1382–1388, 2011.

[134] C. F. Nicoletti, T. P. Lima, S. P. Donadelli et al., “New look at nutritional care for obese patient candidates for bariatric surgery,” *Surgery for Obesity and Related Diseases*, vol. 9, no. 4, pp. 520–525, 2013.

[135] C. A. Blume, C. C. Boni, D. S. Casagrande et al., “Nutritional profile of patients before and after Roux-en-Y gastric bypass: 3-year follow-up,” *Obesity Surgery*, vol. 22, no. 11, pp. 1676–1685, 2012.

[136] D. A. de Luis, D. Pacheco, O. Izaola, M. C. Terroba, L. Cuellar, and T. Martin, “Zinc and copper serum levels of morbidly obese patients before and after biliopancreatic diversion: 4 years of follow-up,” *Journal of Gastrointestinal Surgery*, vol. 15, no. 12, pp. 2178–2181, 2011.

[137] A. Damms-Machado, A. Friedrich, K. M. Kramer et al., “Pre- and postoperative nutritional deficiencies in obese patients undergoing laparoscopic sleeve gastrectomy,” *Obesity Surgery*, vol. 22, no. 6, pp. 881–889, 2012.

[138] A. B. G. Lansdown, “Calcium: a potential central regulator in wound healing in the skin,” *Wound Repair and Regeneration*, vol. 10, no. 5, pp. 271–285, 2002.

[139] S. Balesaria, S. Sangha, and J. R. F. Walters, “Human duodenum responses to vitamin D metabolites of TRPV6 and other genes involved in calcium absorption,” *The American Journal of Physiology: Gastrointestinal and Liver Physiology*, vol. 297, no. 6, pp. G1193–G1197, 2009.

[140] G. Tamer, B. Mesci, I. Tamer, D. Kilic, and S. Arik, “Is vitamin D deficiency an independent risk factor for obesity and abdominal obesity in women?” *Endokrynologia Polska*, vol. 63, no. 3, pp. 196–201, 2012.

[141] R. Ghergherechi, N. Hazhir, and A. Tabrizi, “Comparison of vitamin D deficiency and secondary hyperparathyroidism in obese and non-obese children and adolescents,” *Pakistan Journal of Biological Sciences*, vol. 15, no. 3, pp. 147–151, 2012.

[142] C. Ding, D. Gao, J. Wilding, P. Trayhurn, and C. Bing, “Vitamin D signaling in adipose tissue,” *British Journal of Nutrition*, vol. 108, no. 11, pp. 1915–1923, 2012.

[143] R. B. Saper and R. Rash, "Zinc: an essential micronutrient," *American Family Physician*, vol. 79, no. 9, pp. 768–772, 2009.

[144] O. Kaidar-Person, B. Person, S. Szomstein, and R. J. Rosenthal, "Nutritional deficiencies in morbidly obese patients: a new form of malnutrition? Part A: vitamins," *Obesity Surgery*, vol. 18, no. 7, pp. 870–876, 2008.

[145] M. Iwata, T. Takebayashi, H. Ohta, R. E. Alcalde, Y. Itano, and T. Matsumura, "Zinc accumulation and metallothionein gene expression in the proliferating epidermis during wound healing in mouse skin," *Histochemistry and Cell Biology*, vol. 112, no. 4, pp. 283–290, 1999.

[146] L. Costarelli, E. Muti, M. Malavolta et al., "Distinctive modulation of inflammatory and metabolic parameters in relation to zinc nutritional status in adult overweight/obese subjects," *Journal of Nutritional Biochemistry*, vol. 21, no. 5, pp. 432–437, 2010.

[147] A. A. Al-Kaisy, S. A. Salih, and H. A. Al-Biati, "Effect of zinc supplement in the prognosis of burn patients in Iraq," *Annals of Burns and Fire Disasters*, vol. 19, no. 3, pp. 115–122, 2006.

[148] S. M. Levenson and E. Seifter, "Dysnutrition, wound healing, and resistance to infection," *Clinics in Plastic Surgery*, vol. 4, no. 3, pp. 375–388, 1977.

[149] M. Freiman, E. Seifter, C. Connerton, and S. M. Levenson, "Vitamin A deficiency and surgical stress," *Surgical Forum*, vol. 21, pp. 81–82, 1970.

[150] D. U. Talas, A. Nayci, S. Atis et al., "The effects of corticosteroids and vitamin A on the healing of tracheal anastomoses," *International Journal of Pediatric Otorhinolaryngology*, vol. 67, no. 2, pp. 109–116, 2003.

[151] S. V. Pollack, "Wound healing: a review. III. Nutritional factors affecting wound healing," *Journal of Enterostomal Therapy*, vol. 9, no. 2, pp. 28–33, 1982.

[152] M. Haws, R. E. Brown, H. Suchy, and A. Roth, "Vitamin A-soaked gelfoam sponges and wound healing in steroid-treated animals," *Annals of Plastic Surgery*, vol. 32, no. 4, pp. 418–422, 1994.

[153] M. F. Trevisani, M. A. Ricci, J. T. Tolland, and W. C. Beck, "Effect of vitamin A and zinc on wound healing in steroid-treated mice," *Current Surgery*, vol. 44, no. 5, pp. 390–393, 1987.

[154] T. K. Hunt, H. P. Ehrlich, J. A. Garcia, and J. E. Dunphy, "Effect of vitamin A on reversing the inhibitory effect of cortisone on healing of open wounds in animals and man," *Annals of Surgery*, vol. 170, no. 4, pp. 633–641, 1969.

[155] J. Z. Williams and A. Barbul, "Nutrition and wound healing," *Surgical Clinics of North America*, vol. 83, no. 3, pp. 571–596, 2003.

[156] R. F. Neiva, K. Al-Shammari, F. H. Nociti Jr., S. Soehren, and H.-L. Wang, "Effects of vitamin-B complex supplementation on periodontal wound healing," *Journal of Periodontology*, vol. 76, no. 7, pp. 1084–1091, 2005.

[157] C. W. Findlay Jr., "Effect of vitamin B12 on wound healing," *Proceedings of the Royal Society Experimental Biology and Medicine*, vol. 82, no. 3, pp. 492–495, 1953.

[158] J. L. Monaco and W. T. Lawrence, "Acute wound healing: an overview," *Clinics in Plastic Surgery*, vol. 30, no. 1, pp. 1–12, 2003.

[159] E. G. Brunson, J. F. Smith, and R. Dixon, "Vitamin B12: an aid to oral mucous membrane healing," *Oral Surgery, Oral Medicine, Oral Pathology*, vol. 24, no. 1, pp. 102–112, 1967.

[160] S. Agha-Mohammadi and D. J. Hurwitz, "Potential impacts of nutritional deficiency of postbariatric patients on body contouring surgery," *Plastic and Reconstructive Surgery*, vol. 122, no. 6, pp. 1901–1914, 2008.

[161] A. C. Cepeda-Lopez, S. J. M. Osendarp, A. Melse-Boonstra et al., "Sharply higher rates of iron deficiency in obese Mexican women and children are predicted by obesity-related inflammation rather than by differences in dietary iron intake," *The American Journal of Clinical Nutrition*, vol. 93, no. 5, pp. 975–983, 2011.

[162] J. P. McClung and J. P. Karl, "Iron deficiency and obesity: the contribution of inflammation and diminished iron absorption," *Nutrition Reviews*, vol. 67, no. 2, pp. 100–104, 2009.

[163] E. M. del Giudice, N. Santoro, A. Amato et al., "Hepcidin in obese children as a potential mediator of the association between obesity and iron deficiency," *Journal of Clinical Endocrinology and Metabolism*, vol. 94, no. 12, pp. 5102–5107, 2009.

[164] A. Amato, N. Santoro, P. Calabrò et al., "Effect of body mass index reduction on serum hepcidin levels and iron status in obese children," *International Journal of Obesity*, vol. 34, no. 12, pp. 1772–1774, 2010.

[165] M. J. Jacobson and J. Van Prohaska, "The healing of wounds in iron deficiency," *Surgery*, vol. 57, no. 2, pp. 254–258, 1965.

[166] W. L. Macon and W. J. Pories, "The effect of iron deficiency anemia on wound healing," *Surgery*, vol. 69, no. 5, pp. 792–796, 1971.

[167] H. W. Trueblood, T. S. Nelsen, and H. A. Oberhelman Jr., "The effect of acute anemia and iron deficiency anemia on wound healing," *Archives of Surgery*, vol. 99, no. 1, pp. 113–116, 1969.

[168] P. Kulapongs, R. Suskind, V. Vithayasai, and R. E. Olson, "Cell mediated immunity and phagocytosis and killing function in children with severe iron deficiency anemia," *The Lancet*, vol. 2, no. 7882, pp. 689–691, 1974.

[169] E. L. Howes, H. Briggs, R. Shea, and S. C. Harvey, "Effect of complete and partial starvation on the rate of fibroplasia in the healing wound," *Archives of Surgery*, vol. 26, pp. 846–858, 1933.

[170] S. A. Localio, M. E. Morgan, and J. W. Hinton, "The biological chemistry of wound healing: the effect of di-methionine on healing of wounds in protein depleted animals," *Surgery, Gynecology & Obstetrics*, vol. 86, no. 5, pp. 582–590, 1948.

[171] J. E. Rhoads, M. T. Fliegelman, and L. M. Panzer, "The mechanism of delayed wound healing in the presence of hypoproteinemia," *The Journal of the American Medical Association*, vol. 118, pp. 21–23, 1942.

[172] M. B. Williamson and H. J. Fromm, "The incorporation of sulfur amino acids into the proteins of regenerating wound tissue," *Journal of Biological Chemistry*, vol. 212, no. 2, pp. 705–712, 1955.

[173] S. S. Malinowski, "Nutritional and metabolic complications of bariatric surgery," *American Journal of the Medical Sciences*, vol. 331, no. 4, pp. 219–225, 2006.

[174] S. L. Doyle, C. L. Donohoe, J. Lysaght, and J. V. Reynolds, "Visceral obesity, metabolic syndrome, insulin resistance and cancer," *Proceedings of the Nutrition Society*, vol. 71, no. 1, pp. 181–189, 2012.

[175] S. L. Doyle, J. Lysaght, and J. V. Reynolds, "Obesity and post-operative complications in patients undergoing non-bariatric surgery," *Obesity Reviews*, vol. 11, no. 12, pp. 875–886, 2010.

[176] S. Agha-Mohammadi and D. J. Hurwitz, "Nutritional deficiency of post-bariatric surgery body contouring patients: What every plastic surgeon should know," *Plastic and Reconstructive Surgery*, vol. 122, no. 2, pp. 604–613, 2008.

[177] S. Agha-Mohammadi and D. J. Hurwitz, "Enhanced recovery after body-contouring surgery: reducing surgical complication rates by optimizing nutrition," *Aesthetic Plastic Surgery*, vol. 34, no. 5, pp. 617–627, 2010.

[178] D. 'Ettorre M, D. Gniuli, A. Iaconelli et al., "Wound healing process in post-bariatric patients: an experimental evaluation," *Obesity Surgery*, vol. 20, no. 11, pp. 1552–1558, 2010.

[179] M. H. Shuster and J. A. Vazquez, "Nutritional concerns related to roux-en-y gastric bypass: what every clinician needs to know," *Critical Care Nursing Quarterly*, vol. 28, no. 3, pp. 227–262, 2005.

Obesity as a Consequence of Gut Bacteria and Diet Interactions

Katerina Kotzampassi,[1] Evangelos J. Giamarellos-Bourboulis,[2] and George Stavrou[1]

[1] *Department of Surgery, Medical School, Aristotle University of Thessaloniki, Thessaloniki 54006, Greece*
[2] *Fourth Department of Internal Medicine, University of Athens Medical School, Athens 12462, Greece*

Correspondence should be addressed to Katerina Kotzampassi; kakothe@yahoo.com

Academic Editors: D. Micic and E. K. Naderali

Obesity is a major public health concern, caused by a combination of increased consumption of energy-dense foods and reduced physical activity, with contributions from host genetics, environment, and adipose tissue inflammation. In recent years, the gut microbiome has also been found to be implicated and augmented research in mice and humans have attributed to it both the manifestation and/or exacerbation of this major epidemic and vice versa. At the experimental level, analysis of fecal samples revealed a potential link between obesity and alterations in the gut flora (drop in Bacteroidetes and increase in Firmicutes), the specific gut microbiome being associated with the obese phenotype. Conventionally raised mice were found to have over 40% more total body fat compared with those raised under germ-free conditions, while conventionalization of germ-free mice resulted in a significant increase in total body fat. Similarly, the sparse data in humans supports the fact that fat storage is favoured by the presence of the gut microbiota, through a multifaceted mechanism. Efforts to identify new therapeutic strategies to modulate gut microbiota would be of high priority for public health, and to date, probiotics and/or prebiotics seem to be the most effective tools.

1. Introduction

Obesity is a major public health concern, threatening both the industrialized and the developing countries, largely in parallel to the adoption of a "modern"/Western-type lifestyle. It results from a long-term disbalance between energy intake and expenditure, that is, increased consumption of more energy-dense, nutrient-poor foods containing high levels of sugar and saturated fats in combination with reduced physical activity [1]. However, the mechanisms underlying obesity seem to be far from the long-held belief in caloric intake and lifestyle factors. It is becoming evident that obesity and its causes are significantly more complex than previously thought, with contributions from host genetics, environment, diet and lifestyle, and systemic and adipose tissue inflammation [2].

Obesity is now characterized by a cluster of important chronic metabolic disorders, including insulin resistance, type 2 diabetes, fatty liver disease, atherosclerosis, hypertension, and hypercholesterolemia, and by a low grade of systemic inflammation [3], being the cause of exacerbation of all the above and leading to increased morbidity and mortality. Moreover, obesity is detrimental to the quality of life as a whole and implies high health costs as a consequence of its associated morbidities.

In recent years, augmented research worldwide has focused on the implication of intestinal microbiota in both the manifestation and exacerbation of this major epidemic and vice versa.

2. Obesity and Microbiota

Recent studies have suggested microbiota to be an environmental factor involved in the control of body weight and energy homeostasis. Experimental models using transgenic, knockout, and gnotobiotic animals, as well as human studies, provide evidence of a crucial role for intestinal microbiota in energy harvest and consequently obesity. More precisely, they show a potential link between obesity and alterations in the gut flora [4, 5], the specific gut microbiome being associated with the obese phenotype [5–10].

It is now well documented that the human gut microbiota (a total of up to 100 trillion cells), mostly Gram-positive and anaerobic [11], are unique to each individual, highly variable between persons, and remarkably stable after the first year of life [12, 13]. Despite this individual uniqueness and the high diversity in humans, there is only a small number of microbial phyla that are numerically dominant [14–16]: Firmicutes and Bacteroidetes accounting for more than 90% [17–19].

New research reveals that obese animal and human subjects have alterations in the composition of the gut microbiota compared to their leaner counterparts [20]; a greater representation of Firmicutes and fewer Bacteroidetes, as well as reduced bacterial diversity as a total [4, 5, 21, 22], the altered representation of bacterial genes being considered the cause affecting metabolic pathways [21].

In a challenge to identify more specific changes in the gut microbiota that may account for these metabolic effects, Ley et al. [5] studied genetically obese, leptin receptor-deficient (ob/ob) mice and found in the cecum biota a 50% reduction in the abundance of Bacteroidetes and a proportional increase in Firmicutes in relation to lean mice. Another researcher also found a higher proportion of Archaea microbes within the stools received from the cecum in genetically obese mice in comparison with their lean littermates [23], while diet-induced obesity in mice has also been associated with an increased proportion of *Eubacterium dolichum*, belonging to the Firmicutes division [24].

Waldram et al. [22] studied a rat obesity model, characterizing gut microbiotas in parallel with metabolites. Their results broadly support patterns of greater Firmicutes/Bacteroidetes ratios, as observed in other animal studies. Furthermore, specific bacteria were found associated with the obese phenotype (*Halomonas* and *Sphingomonas*), as were lower total bacteria counts and lower bifidobacterial counts. On the other hand, conventionally raised mice had over 40% more total body fat compared with those raised under germ-free conditions, while conventionalization of germ-free mice via colonization with cecum-derived distal microbial community resulted in a significant increase in total body fat [4].

The first study describing qualitative changes of the gut microbiota in obese human individuals over lean controls was published a few years ago [5, 9]. It analyzes the fecal gut microbiota over the course of 1 year in obese individuals participating in a weight loss programme, randomly allocated to either a fat-restricted or carbohydrate-restricted low-calorie diet. The Bacteroidetes and Firmicutes phyla were found to be the dominated microbiota, while bacterial flora showed remarkable intraindividual stability over time. At zero time-point, obese subjects had significantly fewer Bacteroidetes and more Firmicutes than lean control subjects. After weight loss, the relative proportion of Bacteroidetes increased, while Firmicutes decreased, a finding which is well correlated to the percentage of weight loss. Bacteroidetes constituted approximately 3% of the gut bacteria before diet therapy and approximately 15% after successful weight loss.

In another study on obese humans submitted to a dietary intervention of reduced carbohydrate intake and increased protein intake, Duncan et al. [25] found reductions in populations of *Bifidobacterium*, *Roseburia* spp., and *Eubacterium rectale* subgroups of clostridial cluster XIVa. Further support derived from other weight loss studies show marked and sustained changes in the microbial composition of the gut after weight loss induced by diet restriction [26, 27]. In line with these findings were those obtained from individuals subjected to weight loss surgery [28–31]. Zhang et al. [28] showed that Gamma-Proteobacteria and Verrucomicrobia were enriched after gastric bypass compared with that presenting in the stools of lean and obese controls, while Firmicutes was significantly decreased. In addition, the stomach chambers formed in Roux-en-Y gastric bypass (RYGB) surgery are colonized by bacteria to a greater extent than in the normal stomach [31].

The hypothesis of a more specific modulation of gut microbiota in obesity, far from that obtained at the phylum levels, is supported by several studies. *Bifidobacterium* spp. numbers were found higher in children who exhibited a normal weight from birth till the age of 7 years in relation to children who became overweight [32], and is it now well known that *Bifidobacterium* spp. presence is often associated with beneficial health effects [33–35]. More importantly, the authors [32] observed that the *Staphylococcus aureus* levels were lower in children who maintained a normal weight than in children who became overweight several years later and thus proposed that the protection from obesity seen with bifidobacteria may, in part, be due to its anti-inflammatory effects, whereas *S. aureus* may trigger low-grade inflammation [36], leading to the overweight status [37, 38]. Furthermore, comparable results have been found between the faecal microbiota of obese and lean twins: while a core gut microbiome exists in both subjects, obese individuals exhibit reduced diversity and an altered representation of metabolic pathways in their microbiota [39], in addition to the lower proportion of Bacteroidetes and the higher proportion of Actinobacteria associated with obesity [21].

3. What Is the Role of Food Intake?

One of the key and central questions is that whether and how diet might affect the composition of the gut microbiome. In a very recent paper Emeritus Professor Bengmark [1], well known for his extensive studies on probiotics, summarizes the role of food as follows: "The great majority of ingredients in the industrially produced foods consumed in the West are absorbed in the upper part of small intestine and thus of limited benefit to the microbiota. Lack of proper nutrition for microbiota is a major factor under-pinning dysfunctional microbiota, dysbiosis, chronically elevated inflammation, and the production and leakage of endotoxins through the various tissue barriers. Furthermore, the over-consumption of insulinogenic foods and proteotoxins, such as advanced glycation and lipoxidation molecules, gluten and zein, and a reduced intake of fruit and vegetables, are key factors behind the commonly observed elevated inflammation and the endemic of obesity and chronic diseases, factors which are also likely to be detrimental to microbiota." The fact that industrialized foods are absorbed in the upper part of the small intestine, in relation to the knowledge that lactobacilli are predominantly present in the ileum and bifidobacteria in the colon [40] would be a simplified explanation for lactobacilli overgrowth and bifidobacteria suppression in obese individuals.

On the other hand, the finding of increase in fat mass upon high-fat diet feeding in conventionalized versus germ-free animals supports the fact that the fat storage is favoured by the presence of gut microbiota [4, 7] and that carbohydrates in the diet may modulate the development of obesity upon colonization of the gut as well [41].

At experimental level, Hildebrandt et al. [42] focused on how a high-fat diet might affect the composition of the murine gut microbiome, even independently of obesity. When switching mice to a high-fat diet, they found profound changes in the gut microbiome, including a decrease in Bacteroidetes and an increase in Firmicutes and Proteobacteria. However, the main strength of their study is that they clearly show the observed changes to be independent of obesity.

In an effort to ascertain to what extent gut microbiota is an important regulator of nutrient absorption in humans, Jumpertz et al. [40] investigated the changes in the feces of 12 lean and 9 obese individuals during diets that varied in caloric content (2400 compared with 3400 kcal/d). They showed that an altered nutrient load induced rapid changes in the bacterial composition of the human gut microbiota. Moreover, these changes in the gut microbiota were directly associated with stool energy loss in lean individuals, such that a 20% increase in Firmicutes and a corresponding decrease in Bacteroidetes were associated with an increased energy harvest of about 150 kcal. They also showed that a high degree of overfeeding in lean subjects was associated with a greater fractional decrease in stool energy loss, which indicated that the degree of overnutrition relative to individual weight-maintaining energy needs may have played a role in the determination of the efficiency of nutrient absorption and may potentially explain the observation of clearer associations in lean compared with obese subjects. Thus, they suggest that the gut microbiota senses alterations in nutrient availability and subsequently modulates nutrient absorption, the difference in microbiota reflecting differences in calorie absorption. Moreover, previous studies on healthy subjects showed that about 5% of ingested calories were lost in stools [43], with those consuming high-fiber diets exhibiting a higher fecal energy loss than those consuming a low-fiber diet, although equivalent in energy content [44, 45].

The change of the composition of the upper intestine in obesity for aerobic bacteria was also confirmed in a survey of 320 patients subject to upper GI tract endoscopy. Fluid was aspirated from the lumen of the third part of the duodenum and it was quantitatively cultured. The isolation of colonic type bacteria at counts greater than 10^3 cfu/mL was considered diagnostic of the syndrome of intestinal bacterial overgrowth (SIBO). SIBO was present among 62 patients. When patients with SIBO were compared with the 258 non-SIBO patients regarding their baseline demographic characteristics, it was found that the BMI of SIBO patients was significantly greater than that of non-SIBO patients (mean 28.2 kg/m^2 versus 25.1 kg/m^2). As expected, the prevalence of type 2 diabetes mellitus was far greater among SIBO patients than among non-SIBO patients (25.5% versus 18.2%) [46].

4. Mechanisms Involved in Fat Storage

From all the above described findings, it appears clear that gut microbiota is an important environmental factor that affects energy harvest from the diet and energy storage in the host [4], through a multiple-faceted mechanism regulating the host's metabolism.

First of all, gut microbiota seems to promote fat storage by means of linking circulating triglycerides with suppression of the intestinal expression of an inhibitor of lipoprotein lipase (LPL) [4], the so-called fasting-induced adipose factor (Fiaf). This is member of the angiopoietin-like family of proteins, expressed in differentiated gut epithelial cells, as well as in the liver and the adipose tissue [47], which is considered to be a mediator of microbial regulation of energy storage [4]. Further research on germ-free and conventionalized, normal and Fiaf knockout mice has established its essential role for the microbiota-induced deposition of triglycerides in adipocytes [4, 10] by means of LPS activity. Gut microbiota-induced suppression of Fiaf leads to a higher LPL activity and as a consequence an increased cellular uptake of fatty acids and adipocyte triglyceride accumulation, that is, greater fat storage [4]. It is likely that changes in gut microbial environment prompted by Western diets may function as an "environmental" factor that affects predisposition toward energy storage and obesity [4]. On the other hand, it would appear logical to try modulating gut flora towards increasing Fiaf expression and or activity, an action that would promote leanness.

A second pathway that influences host energy storage is related to energy extraction from undigested food components. Nutrients which escape the digestion, due to host's limited capability of glycoside hydrolases to digest complex dietary plant polysaccharides, are fermented by gut microbes into monosaccharides and short-chain fatty acids (SCFAs), such as acetate, propionate, and butyrate [11, 48], representing an important energy source for the body. Normal colonic epithelia derive 60–70% of their energy supply from SCFAs, particularly butyrate [49, 50], while propionate is largely taken up by the liver for gluconeogenesis, liponeogenesis, and protein synthesis [51, 52].

Changes in the relative abundance of the two dominant bacterial phyla, the Bacteroidetes and Firmicutes, found in obese mice and humans, are associated with differences in capacity for energy harvest [4, 5]. The increase of microbiota phyla such as "obese gut microbiome" with greater energy extraction efficiency resulted in less energy left over in feces and thus greater levels of short-chain fatty acids (SCFAs) in the cecum.

Schwiertz et al. [53] found considerable differences in the stool SCFAs' concentrations between lean and obese individuals; the mean total SCFA concentration in fecal samples of obese volunteers was more than 20% higher in total than in lean volunteers ($P = 0.024$); the highest increase is seen for propionate with 41% ($P = 0.002$), followed by butyrate (28%, $P = 0.095$). In addition, this resulted in changes in the proportions of individual to total SCFA, the propionate proportion was thus higher in overweight (18.7%,

$P = 0.019$) and obese (18.3%, $P = 0.028$) than in lean subjects (15.9%).

SCFAs may also act as signalling molecules, since propionate and acetate are known ligands for 2 G-protein-coupled receptors (GPCRs), namely, the Gpr41 and Gpr43 [54, 55]. Thus, manipulation of SCFA activation of GPCRs could, theoretically, serve as a therapeutic target, modulating efficiency of caloric extraction from a polysaccharide-rich diet.

In addition to the effect on energy harvest, the bacterial microbiota can directly, via afferent nerve terminals or indirectly, via signalling peptides, modulate gut motility, alter secretion of gut hormones, and modify both gut permeability and immune function. These alterations may additionally influence the host metabolism and proinflammatory state being present in obesity [56].

A 4-week high-fat diet in a mouse model appears to increase the proportion of circulating lipopolysaccharide-(LPS-) containing microbiota [38] and thus plasma LPS levels (metabolic endotoxemia) two to threefold. Thus, a high-fat diet is thought to modulate the composition of the gut bacteria [24, 57–59] (notably by reducing bifidobacteria), leading to increase in gut permeability which allows a higher LPS plasma levels. On the other hand, greater levels of bifidobacteria have been associated with reduced gut leakiness, allowing less LPS to translocate to the serum [60].

Cani et al. [4, 59] have recently shown that an increase of LPS levels, derived from colonic Gram-negative bacteria, such as the Bacteroidetes which, in association with and/or due to changes in intestinal microbiota composition (gram-negative/gram-positive ratio), seems to be a triggering factor in chronic systemic inflammation; an increased production of proinflammatory cytokines affects negatively glucose tolerance and thus leads to insulin resistance and increase in body weight. More precisely, it is well known that LPS binding to TLR4 receptor triggers a downstream signaling cascade that encodes proinflammatory molecules. Shi et al. [61] have shown that nutritional fatty acids, whose circulating levels are often increased in obesity, activate TLR4 signaling in adipocytes and macrophages in a similar way, the chronic inflammatory state being associated with insulin resistance.

Additionally, when mice received a high-fat diet plus antibiotics, they are found to have decreased levels of endotoxin and decreased markers of inflammation, as well as reduced weight gain and improved glucose tolerance [59], a finding implying that LPS may link inflammation with the microbiota. Thus, the manipulation of the gut microbiota may provide a novel therapeutic treatment for obesity [62–64].

Another pathway of potential interaction between host and the microbiota involves the adenosine monophosphate-activated protein kinase (AMPK), a key enzyme that controls cellular energy status through stimulation of fatty acids beta-oxidation [7, 10, 65]. The gut microbiotas were found to suppress AMPK-driven fatty acid oxidation in the liver and in skeletal muscle, while germ-free mice remain lean, despite high calorie intake, due to increased activity of AMPK levels both in the liver and skeletal muscle, which stimulate fatty acid and lead to decreased glycogen levels in the liver [7].

Finally, Stappenbeck et al. [66] suggested that gut microbiota conventionalization in mice results in a doubling of the density of capillaries in the villus epithelium of the small intestine, in an effort to promote intestinal monosaccharide absorption.

5. Future Perspectives

The ability to extract energy from every kind of food and to store it as adipose tissue would be a beneficial attribute for our ancestors who had variable access to food around the year. Nowadays, in our modern, developed world, where there is ready access to inexpensive, large-portion, readily available high-calorie foods, this "benefit" becomes a disadvantage, with overweight and obesity representing major risk factors for a plethora of severe metabolic disorders, including dyslipidemia, steatosis, hypertension, insulin resistance and type 2 diabetes, cardiovascular diseases, and inflammatory bowel diseases.

However, most obese individuals have been found unable to make voluntary, lifelong changes in diet and behaviour for weight management. Moreover, very recent laboratory and clinical research has documented that excessive fat accumulation is the consequence not only of positive energy balance and decreased physical activity affected by cultural and economic factors. Major progress has been made in identifying specific nutrition components that are both directly linked to the inflammatory state of the host and dramatically shift the assemblage of gut microbiota, whichever the order of priority [67].

As has already been analyzed, at the phyla level, Firmicute dominant, "obese" microbiomes were found to contain more genes associated with lipid and carbohydrate metabolism and the breakdown of otherwise indigestible polysaccharides than Bacteroidetes dominant, the "lean" microbiomes did [37]. Therefore, efforts to identify new therapeutic strategies allowing noncognitive reduction of energy intake, energy absorption, and storage would be of high priority for public health, the most prominent target being the restoration of the gut microbiota to a healthy state. What are the next logical steps? We should search for certain dietary or pharmacological interventions to manipulate specific gut microbial species [6, 24, 55, 68].

Among the tools to modulate gut microbiota, probiotics and/or prebiotics appear to be the most important, although actual proof is still limited. The Food and Agriculture Organization of the United Nations and the World Health Organization (FAO/WHO) define probiotics as "live microorganisms that, when ingested in adequate quantities, exert a health benefit to the host," by stimulating the growth of other microorganisms, modulating mucosal and systemic immunity, and improving the nutritional and microbial balance in the intestinal tract [69]. On the other hand, prebiotics are nondigestible food ingredients that beneficially affect the host by selectively stimulating the growth and/or activity of one or a limited number of the host's gut bacteria [70].

Various probiotic strains have already been evaluated as therapeutic in animal models of obesity, such as

Bifidobacterium spp. [71, 72], *Lactobacillus paracasei* [73], and *Lactobacillus gasseri* BNR17 [74]. In humans, although actual proof is still limited, the few human trials are encouraging and seem to be very promising with regard to the efficacy of pre- and/or probiotics as antiobesity agents [75–77]. The early modulation of gut microbiota with the probiotics *Lactobacillus rhamnosus* GG and *Bifidobacterium lactis* Bb12 was found to reduce the body mass index in young children, by restraining excessive weight gain during the first 10 years of life [78]. Sixty-two obese volunteers were randomized into *Lactobacillus gasseri* BNR17 or placebo for a 12-week period, at the end of which a slight reduction in body weight and a decrease of waist and hip circumferences were noted in the BNR17 group, the nonsignificant difference being attributed to the short trial period [79]. The effect of the probiotic *Lactobacillus gasseri* SBT2055 (LG2055) was tested in 87 obese subjects, in a randomized, placebo controlled intervention which lasted 12 weeks. A significant decrease in body weight and body mass index as well as in visceral and subcutaneous fat was found, which may be linked to decreased fat absorption in relation to the control group [80].

Giving inulin-type fructooligosaccharides (FOS) as a supplement seems to stimulate the growth of *Bifidobacterium* spp. and, in some cases, *Lactobacillus* spp., which are also administrated as probiotics [81–83]. Similarly, wheat arabinoxylan was found related to consistent increases in Bacteroidetes, bifidobacteria, and *Roseburia* [84]. It is of interest to mention that the amount of Bifidobacteria found at baseline (i.e., before intervention) seems to be strongly associated with the increase achieved after treatment, indicating that preexistent gut microbiota composition enhances or possibly determines the response to the intervention [56]. Oligofructose supplementation (21 g daily) versus maltodextrin as placebo for a 12-week period in 48 healthy obese adults was found to promote weight loss and improve glucose regulation, through a modulation of satiety hormone concentrations leading to the reduction in energy intake [85].

The consumption of a symbiotic food, for one month, containing fructooligosaccharides and the probiotic strains *Lactobacillus helveticus* Bar13 and *Bifidobacterium longum* Bar33, was tested in 20 healthy subjects. The intake of the synbiotic food demonstrated no modification on the overall structure of the gut microbiome but resulted in a shift of the fecal metabolic profiles, that is, a significant increase of SCFA, ketones, carbon disulfide, and methyl acetate, suggesting potential health promoting effects [86].

In a recent randomized controlled study on 65 mechanically ventilated trauma patients it was shown that the synbiotic formula Synbiotic 2000FORTE (Medipharm, Kågeröd, Sweden), being a preparation of *Pediococcus pentosaceus* 5-33:3, *Leuconostoc mesenteroides* 32-77:1, *Lactobacillus paracasei* ssp. 19 and *Lactobacillus plantarum* 2362, plus inulin, oat bran, pectin, and resistant starch as prebiotics, administered orally for 15 days versus maltodextrin as placebo, altered the composition of gut flora in favour of anaerobes [87]. In another randomized, double-blind trial, a beverage fermented with *L. acidophilus* and *Propionibacterium freudenreichii* was given to 43 healthy female subjects in order to study the satiety-inducing effects. Subjects exhibited a nonsignificant decreasing trend in ad libitum food consumption, but felt significantly fuller ($P = 0.02$), were less hungry ($P = 0.004$) and had less desire to eat ($P = 0.006$) after consumption of the fermented dairy beverage. The appetite-decreasing effects were ascribed to the production of propionate by *P. freudenreichii* [88]. Similarly, a decrease in appetite and an increase in satiety, leading to a decrease in total energy intake, as well as a decrease in hepatic de novo lipogenesis, have been demonstrated in human volunteers fed with inulin-type prebiotics (16 g daily) versus maltodextrin as a control [89].

Finally, the success in faecal transplantation for *C. difficile* diarrhoea treatment [90, 91] gives promising results for a new era involving transplantation of stools from lean subjects to achieve weight loss.

In summary, ongoing research on human gut microbiota seems, in the short term, to allow the positive manipulation of the interior milieu of a human being by means of either the appropriate microbiome exhibiting antiobesity effects and/or the right substrate (prebiotic) to promote its growth.

Conflict of Interests

All authors disclose no financial or personal relationships with other people or organisations that could inappropriately influence the work.

References

[1] S. Bengmark, "Gut microbiota, immune development and function," *Pharmacological Research*, vol. 69, pp. 87–113, 2013.

[2] E. Maury and S. M. Brichard, "Adipokine dysregulation, adipose tissue inflammation and metabolic syndrome," *Molecular and Cellular Endocrinology*, vol. 314, no. 1, pp. 1–16, 2010.

[3] Z. Pataky, E. Bobbíoni-Harsch, A. Hadengue, A. Carpentier, and A. Golay, "Gut microbiota, responsible for our body weight?" *Revue Medicale Suisse*, vol. 5, no. 196, pp. 662–664, 2009.

[4] F. Bäckhed, H. Ding, T. Wang et al., "The gut microbiota as an environmental factor that regulates fat storage," *Proceedings of the National Academy of Sciences of the United States of America*, vol. 101, no. 44, pp. 15718–15723, 2004.

[5] R. E. Ley, F. Bäckhed, P. Turnbaugh, C. A. Lozupone, R. D. Knight, and J. I. Gordon, "Obesity alters gut microbial ecology," *Proceedings of the National Academy of Sciences of the United States of America*, vol. 102, no. 31, pp. 11070–11075, 2005.

[6] P. J. Turnbaugh, R. E. Ley, M. A. Mahowald, V. Magrini, E. R. Mardis, and J. I. Gordon, "An obesity-associated gut microbiome with increased capacity for energy harvest," *Nature*, vol. 444, no. 7122, pp. 1027–1031, 2006.

[7] F. Bäckhed, J. K. Manchester, C. F. Semenkovich, and J. I. Gordon, "Mechanisms underlying the resistance to diet-induced obesity in germ-free mice," *Proceedings of the National Academy of Sciences of the United States of America*, vol. 104, no. 3, pp. 979–984, 2007.

[8] N. M. Delzenne and P. D. Cani, "Interaction between obesity and the gut microbiota: relevance in nutrition," *Annual Review of Nutrition*, vol. 31, pp. 15–31, 2011.

[9] R. E. Ley, P. J. Turnbaugh, S. Klein, and J. I. Gordon, "Microbial ecology: human gut microbes associated with obesity," *Nature*, vol. 444, no. 7122, pp. 1022–1023, 2006.

[10] C. A. Tennyson and G. Friedman, "Microecology, obesity, and probiotics," *Current Opinion in Endocrinology, Diabetes and Obesity*, vol. 15, no. 5, pp. 422–427, 2008.

[11] F. Bäckhed, R. E. Ley, J. L. Sonnenburg, D. A. Peterson, and J. I. Gordon, "Host-bacterial mutualism in the human intestine," *Science*, vol. 307, no. 5717, pp. 1915–1920, 2005.

[12] E. K. Costello, C. L. Lauber, M. Hamady, N. Fierer, J. I. Gordon, and R. Knight, "Bacterial community variation in human body habitats across space and time," *Science*, vol. 326, no. 5960, pp. 1694–1697, 2009.

[13] C. Reinhardt, C. S. Reigstad, and F. Bäckhed, "Intestinal microbiota during infancy and its implications for obesity," *Journal of Pediatric Gastroenterology and Nutrition*, vol. 48, no. 3, pp. 249–256, 2009.

[14] E. G. Zoetendal, E. E. Vaughan, and W. M. De Vos, "A microbial world within us," *Molecular Microbiology*, vol. 59, no. 6, pp. 1639–1650, 2006.

[15] E. G. Zoetendal, M. Rajilić-Stojanović, and W. M. de Vos, "High-throughput diversity and functionality analysis of the gastrointestinal tract microbiota," *Gut*, vol. 57, no. 11, pp. 1605–1615, 2008.

[16] R. E. Ley, R. Knight, and J. I. Gordon, "The human microbiome: eliminating the biomedical/environmental dichotomy in microbial ecology," *Environmental Microbiology*, vol. 9, no. 1, pp. 3–4, 2007.

[17] P. Hugenholtz, B. M. Goebel, and N. R. Pace, "Impact of culture-independent studies on the emerging phylogenetic view of bacterial diversity," *Journal of Bacteriology*, vol. 180, no. 18, pp. 4765–4774, 1998.

[18] P. B. Eckburg, E. M. Bik, C. N. Bernstein et al., "Microbiology: diversity of the human intestinal microbial flora," *Science*, vol. 308, no. 5728, pp. 1635–1638, 2005.

[19] R. E. Ley, M. Hamady, C. Lozupone et al., "Evolution of mammals and their gut microbes," *Science*, vol. 320, no. 5883, pp. 1647–1651, 2008.

[20] P. Bercik, S. M. Collins, and E. F. Verdu, "Microbes and the gut-brain axis," *Neurogastroenterology and Motility*, vol. 24, no. 5, pp. 405–413, 2012.

[21] P. J. Turnbaugh, M. Hamady, T. Yatsunenko et al., "A core gut microbiome in obese and lean twins," *Nature*, vol. 457, no. 7228, pp. 480–484, 2009.

[22] A. Waldram, E. Holmes, Y. Wang et al., "Top-down systems biology modeling of host metabotype-microbiome associations in obese rodents," *Journal of Proteome Research*, vol. 8, no. 5, pp. 2361–2375, 2009.

[23] B. S. Samuel, E. E. Hansen, J. K. Manchester et al., "Genomic and metabolic adaptations of Methanobrevibacter smithii to the human gut," *Proceedings of the National Academy of Sciences of the United States of America*, vol. 104, no. 25, pp. 10643–10648, 2007.

[24] P. J. Turnbaugh, F. Bäckhed, L. Fulton, and J. I. Gordon, "Diet induced obesity is linked to marked but reversible alterations in the mouse distal gut microbiome," *Cell Host and Microbe*, vol. 3, no. 4, pp. 213–223, 2008.

[25] S. H. Duncan, A. Belenguer, G. Holtrop, A. M. Johnstone, H. J. Flint, and G. E. Lobley, "Reduced dietary intake of carbohydrates by obese subjects results in decreased concentrations of butyrate and butyrate-producing bacteria in feces," *Applied and Environmental Microbiology*, vol. 73, no. 4, pp. 1073–1078, 2007.

[26] A. Santacruz, A. Marcos, J. Wärnberg et al., "Interplay between weight loss and gut microbiota composition in overweight adolescents," *Obesity*, vol. 17, no. 10, pp. 1906–1915, 2009.

[27] I. Nadal, A. Santacruz, A. Marcos et al., "Shifts in clostridia, bacteroides and immunoglobulin-coating fecal bacteria associated with weight loss in obese adolescents," *International Journal of Obesity*, vol. 33, no. 7, pp. 758–767, 2009.

[28] H. Zhang, J. K. DiBaise, A. Zuccolo et al., "Human gut microbiota in obesity and after gastric bypass," *Proceedings of the National Academy of Sciences of the United States of America*, vol. 106, no. 7, pp. 2365–2370, 2009.

[29] J. P. Furet, L. C. Kong, J. Tap et al., "Differential adaptation of human gut microbiota to bariatric surgery-induced weight loss: links with metabolic and low-grade inflammation markers," *Diabetes*, vol. 59, no. 12, pp. 3049–3057, 2010.

[30] J. V. Li, H. Ashrafian, M. Bueter et al., "Metabolic surgery profoundly influences gut microbial—host metabolic cross-talk," *Gut*, vol. 60, no. 9, pp. 1214–1223, 2011.

[31] R. K. Ishida, J. Faintuch, A. M. R. Paula et al., "Microbial flora of the stomach after gastric bypass for morbid obesity," *Obesity Surgery*, vol. 17, no. 6, pp. 752–758, 2007.

[32] M. Kalliomäki, M. C. Collado, S. Salminen, and E. Isolauri, "Early differences in fecal microbiota composition in children may predict overweight," *The American Journal of Clinical Nutrition*, vol. 87, no. 3, pp. 534–538, 2008.

[33] R. J. Boesten, F. H. J. Schuren, and W. M. de Vos, "A bifidobacterium mixed-species microarray for high resolution discrimination between intestinal bifidobacteria," *Journal of Microbiological Methods*, vol. 76, no. 3, pp. 269–277, 2009.

[34] F. Turroni, J. R. Marchesi, E. Foroni et al., "Microbiomic analysis of the bifidobacterial population in the human distal gut," *ISME Journal*, vol. 3, no. 6, pp. 745–751, 2009.

[35] R. J. Boesten and W. M. de Vos, "Interactomics in the human intestine: lactobacilli and bifidobacteria make a difference," *Journal of clinical gastroenterology*, vol. 42, pp. S163–S167, 2008.

[36] A. C. Lundell, I. Adlerberth, E. Lindberg et al., "Increased levels of circulating soluble CD14 but not CD83 in infants are associated with early intestinal colonization with Staphylococcus aureus," *Clinical and Experimental Allergy*, vol. 37, no. 1, pp. 62–71, 2007.

[37] J. L. Kaplan and W. A. Walker, "Early gut colonization and subsequent obesity risk," *Current Opinion in Clinical Nutrition and Metabolic Care*, vol. 15, pp. 278–284, 2012.

[38] P. D. Cani, J. Amar, M. A. Iglesias et al., "Metabolic endotoxemia initiates obesity and insulin resistance," *Diabetes*, vol. 56, no. 7, pp. 1761–1772, 2007.

[39] H. Tilg, "Obesity, metabolic syndrome and microbiota: multiple interactions," *Journal of Clinical Gastroenterology*, vol. 44, no. 1, pp. S16–S18, 2010.

[40] R. Jumpertz, D. S. Le, P. J. Turnbaugh et al., "Energy-balance studies reveal associations between gut microbes, caloric load, and nutrient absorption in humans," *The American Journal of Clinical Nutrition*, vol. 94, no. 1, pp. 58–65, 2011.

[41] C. K. Fleissner, N. Huebel, M. M. Abd El-Bary, G. Loh, S. Klaus, and M. Blaut, "Absence of intestinal microbiota does not protect mice from diet-induced obesity," *British Journal of Nutrition*, vol. 104, no. 6, pp. 919–929, 2010.

[42] M. A. Hildebrandt, C. Hoffmann, S. A. Sherrill-Mix et al., "High fat diet determines the composition of the murine gut microbiome independently of obesity," *Gastroenterology*, vol. 137, no. 5, pp. 1716–e2, 2009.

[43] P. L. Beyer and M. A. Flynn, "Effects of high- and low-fiber diets on human feces," *Journal of the American Dietetic Association*, vol. 72, no. 3, pp. 271–277, 1978.

[44] E. Wisker, A. Maltz, and W. Feldheim, "Metabolizable energy of diets low or high in dietary fiber from cereals when eaten by humans," *Journal of Nutrition*, vol. 118, no. 8, pp. 945–952, 1988.

[45] J. Cliff Yoon, T. W. Chickering, E. D. Rosen et al., "Peroxisome proliferator-activated receptor γ target gene encoding a novel angiopoietin-related protein associated with adipose differentiation," *Molecular and Cellular Biology*, vol. 20, no. 14, pp. 5343–5349, 2000.

[46] E. Pyleris, E. J. Giamarellos-Bourboulis, D. Tzivras, V. Koussoulas, C. Barbatzas, and M. Pimentel, "The prevalence of overgrowth by aerobic bacteria in the small intestine by small bowel culture: relationship with irritable bowel syndrome," *Digestive Diseases and Sciences*, vol. 57, pp. 1321–1329, 2012.

[47] H. J. Flint, E. A. Bayer, M. T. Rincon, R. Lamed, and B. A. White, "Polysaccharide utilization by gut bacteria: potential for new insights from genomic analysis," *Nature Reviews Microbiology*, vol. 6, no. 2, pp. 121–131, 2008.

[48] K. C. Mountzouris, K. Kotzampassi, P. Tsirtsikos, K. Kapoutzis, and K. Fegeros, "Effects of Lactobacillus acidophilus on gut microflora metabolic biomarkers in fed and fasted rats," *Clinical Nutrition*, vol. 28, no. 3, pp. 318–324, 2009.

[49] E. Scarpellini, M. Campanale, D. Leone et al., "Gut microbiota and obesity," *Internal and Emergency Medicine*, vol. 5, no. 1, pp. 53–56, 2010.

[50] W. Scheppach, "Effects of short chain fatty acids on gut morphology and function," *Gut*, vol. 35, no. 1, pp. S35–S38, 1994.

[51] T. M. S. Wolever, P. Spadafora, and H. Eshuis, "Interaction between colonic acetate and propionate in humans," *The American Journal of Clinical Nutrition*, vol. 53, no. 3, pp. 681–687, 1991.

[52] M. Vernay, "Origin and utilization of volatile fatty acids and lactate in the rabbit: influence of the faecal excretion pattern," *British Journal of Nutrition*, vol. 57, no. 3, pp. 371–381, 1987.

[53] A. Schwiertz, D. Taras, K. Schäfer et al., "Microbiota and SCFA in lean and overweight healthy subjects," *Obesity*, vol. 18, no. 1, pp. 190–195, 2010.

[54] A. J. Brown, S. M. Goldsworthy, A. A. Barnes et al., "The orphan G protein-coupled receptors GPR41 and GPR43 are activated by propionate and other short chain carboxylic acids," *Journal of Biological Chemistry*, vol. 278, no. 13, pp. 11312–11319, 2003.

[55] E. le Poul, C. Loison, S. Struyf et al., "Functional characterization of human receptors for short chain fatty acids and their role in polymorphonuclear cell activation," *Journal of Biological Chemistry*, vol. 278, no. 28, pp. 25481–25489, 2003.

[56] M. Diamant, E. E. Blaak, and W. M. de Vos, "Do nutrient-gut-microbiota interactions play a role in human obesity, insulin resistance and type 2 diabetes?" *Obesity Reviews*, vol. 12, no. 4, pp. 272–281, 2011.

[57] P. D. Cani and N. M. Delzenne, "Gut microflora as a target for energy and metabolic homeostasis," *Current Opinion in Clinical Nutrition and Metabolic Care*, vol. 10, no. 6, pp. 729–734, 2007.

[58] P. D. Cani, S. Hoste, Y. Guiot, and N. M. Delzenne, "Dietary non-digestible carbohydrates promote L-cell differentiation in the proximal colon of rats," *British Journal of Nutrition*, vol. 98, no. 1, pp. 32–37, 2007.

[59] P. D. Cani, R. Bibiloni, C. Knauf et al., "Changes in gut microbiota control metabolic endotoxemia-induced inflammation in high-fat diet-induced obesity and diabetes in mice," *Diabetes*, vol. 57, no. 6, pp. 1470–1481, 2008.

[60] P. D. Cani, S. Possemiers, T. van de Wiele et al., "Changes in gut microbiota control inflammation in obese mice through a mechanism involving GLP-2-driven improvement of gut permeability," *Gut*, vol. 58, no. 8, pp. 1091–1103, 2009.

[61] H. Shi, M. V. Kokoeva, K. Inouye, I. Tzameli, H. Yin, and J. S. Flier, "TLR4 links innate immunity and fatty acid-induced insulin resistance," *Journal of Clinical Investigation*, vol. 116, no. 11, pp. 3015–3025, 2006.

[62] W. Jia, H. Li, L. Zhao, and J. K. Nicholson, "Gut microbiota: a potential new territory for drug targeting," *Nature Reviews Drug Discovery*, vol. 7, no. 2, pp. 123–129, 2008.

[63] F. A. Hoffman, "Development of probiotics as biologic drugs," *Clinical Infectious Diseases*, vol. 46, no. 2, pp. S125–S127, 2008.

[64] M. Membrez, F. Blancher, M. Jaquet et al., "Gut microbiota modulation with norfloxacin and ampicillin enhances glucose tolerance in mice," *The FASEB Journal*, vol. 22, no. 7, pp. 2416–2426, 2008.

[65] B. B. Kahn, T. Alquier, D. Carling, and D. G. Hardie, "AMP-activated protein kinase: ancient energy gauge provides clues to modern understanding of metabolism," *Cell Metabolism*, vol. 1, no. 1, pp. 15–25, 2005.

[66] T. S. Stappenbeck, L. V. Hooper, and J. I. Gordon, "Developmental regulation of intestinal angiogenesis by indigenous microbes via Paneth cells," *Proceedings of the National Academy of Sciences of the United States of America*, vol. 99, no. 24, pp. 15451–15455, 2002.

[67] E. Y. Huang, V. A. Leone, S. Devkota, Y. Wang, M. J. Brady, and E. B. Chang, "Composition of dietary fat source shapes gut microbiota architecture and alters host inflammatory mediators in mouse adipose tissue," *Journal of Parenteral and Enteral Nutrition*, vol. 37, no. 6, pp. 746–754, 2013.

[68] P. D. Cani, A. M. Neyrinck, F. Fava et al., "Selective increases of bifidobacteria in gut microflora improve high-fat-diet-induced diabetes in mice through a mechanism associated with endotoxaemia," *Diabetologia*, vol. 50, no. 11, pp. 2374–2383, 2007.

[69] K. Kotzampassi and E. J. Giamarellos-Bourboulis, "Probiotics for infectious diseases: more drugs, less dietary supplementation," *International Journal of Antimicrobial Agents*, vol. 40, pp. 288–296, 2012.

[70] G. R. Gibson, H. M. Probert, J. van Loo, R. A. Rastall, and M. B. Roberfroid, "Dietary modulation of the human colonic microbiota: updating the concept of prebiotics," *Nutrition Research Reviews*, vol. 17, no. 2, pp. 259–275, 2004.

[71] S. Kondo, J. Z. Xiao, T. Satoh et al., "Antiobesity effects of bifidobacterium breve Strain B-3 supplementation in a mouse model with high-fat diet-Induced obesity," *Bioscience, Biotechnology and Biochemistry*, vol. 74, no. 8, pp. 1656–1661, 2010.

[72] H. M. An, S. Y. Park, D. K. Lee et al., "Antiobesity and lipid-lowering effects of Bifidobacterium spp. in high fat diet-induced obese rats," *Lipids in Health and Disease*, vol. 10, article 116, 2011.

[73] L. Aronsson, Y. Huang, P. Parini et al., "Decreased fat storage by Lactobacillus paracasei is associated with increased levels of angiopoietin-like 4 protein (ANGPTL4)," *PLoS ONE*, vol. 5, no. 9, Article ID e13087, 2010.

[74] J. H. Kang, S. I. Yun, and H. O. Park, "Effects of Lactobacillus gasseri BNR17 on body weight and adipose tissue mass in diet-induced overweight rats," *Journal of Microbiology*, vol. 48, no. 5, pp. 712–714, 2010.

[75] T. Arora, S. Singh, and R. K. Sharma, "Probiotics: interaction with gut microbiome and antiobesity potential," *Nutrition*, vol. 29, pp. 591–596, 2013.

[76] V. Robles Alonso and F. Guarner, "Linking the gut microbiota to human health," *British Journal of Nutrition*, vol. 109, pp. S21–S26, 2013.

[77] N. M. Delzenne and P. D. Cani, "Nutritional modulation of gut microbiota in the context of obesity and insulin resistance: potential interest of prebiotics," *International Dairy Journal*, vol. 20, no. 4, pp. 277–280, 2010.

[78] R. Luoto, K. Laitinen, M. Nermes, and E. Isolauri, "Impact of maternal probiotic-supplemented dietary counselling on pregnancy outcome and prenatal and postnatal growth: a double-blind, placebo-controlled study," *British Journal of Nutrition*, vol. 103, no. 12, pp. 1792–1799, 2010.

[79] S. P. Jung, K. M. Lee, J. H. Kang et al., "Effect of Lactobacillus gasseri BNR17 on overweight and obese adults: a randomized, double-blind clinical trial," *Korean Journal Of Family Medicine*, vol. 34, pp. 80–89, 2013.

[80] Y. Kadooka, M. Sato, K. Imaizumi et al., "Regulation of abdominal adiposity by probiotics (Lactobacillus gasseri SBT2055) in adults with obese tendencies in a randomized controlled trial," *European Journal of Clinical Nutrition*, vol. 64, no. 6, pp. 636–643, 2010.

[81] Y. Bouhnik, L. Raskine, G. Simoneau et al., "The capacity of nondigestible carbohydrates to stimulate fecal bifidobacteria in healthy humans: a double-blind, randomized, placebo-controlled, parallel-group, dose-response relation study," *The American Journal of Clinical Nutrition*, vol. 80, no. 6, pp. 1658–1664, 2004.

[82] S. Kolida, D. Meyer, and G. R. Gibson, "A double-blind placebo-controlled study to establish the bifidogenic dose of inulin in healthy humans," *European Journal of Clinical Nutrition*, vol. 61, no. 10, pp. 1189–1195, 2007.

[83] S. Macfarlane, G. T. Macfarlane, and J. H. Cummings, "Review article: prebiotics in the gastrointestinal tract," *Alimentary Pharmacology and Therapeutics*, vol. 24, no. 5, pp. 701–714, 2006.

[84] A. M. Neyrinck, S. Possemiers, C. Druart et al., "Prebiotic effects of wheat Arabinoxylan related to the increase in bifidobacteria, roseburia and bacteroides/prevotella in diet-induced obese mice," *PLoS ONE*, vol. 6, no. 6, Article ID e20944, 2011.

[85] J. A. Parnell and R. A. Reimer, "Weight loss during oligofructose supplementation is associated with decreased ghrelin and increased peptide YY in overweight and obese adults," *The American Journal of Clinical Nutrition*, vol. 89, no. 6, pp. 1751–1759, 2009.

[86] B. Vitali, M. Ndagijimana, F. Cruciani et al., "Impact of a synbiotic food on the gut microbial ecology and metabolic profiles," *BMC Microbiology*, vol. 10, article 4, 2010.

[87] I. M. Koutelidakis, E. Bezirtzoglou, E. J. Giamarellos-Bourboulis, V. Grosomanidis, and K. Kotzampassi, "Impact of synbiotics on the intestinal flora of critically ill patients with multiple injuries," *International Journal of Antimicrobial Agents*, vol. 36, no. 1, pp. 90–91, 2010.

[88] R. M. A. J. Ruijschop, A. E. M. Boelrijk, and M. C. te Giffel, "Satiety effects of a dairy beverage fermented with propionic acid bacteria," *International Dairy Journal*, vol. 18, no. 9, pp. 945–950, 2008.

[89] P. D. Cani, E. Lecourt, E. M. Dewulf et al., "Gut microbiota fermentation of prebiotics increases satietogenic and incretin gut peptide production with consequences for appetite sensation and glucose response after a meal," *The American Journal of Clinical Nutrition*, vol. 90, no. 5, pp. 1236–1243, 2009.

[90] J. Landy, H. O. Al-Hassi, S. D. McLaughlin et al., "Review article: faecal transplantation therapy for gastrointestinal disease," *Alimentary Pharmacology and Therapeutics*, vol. 34, no. 4, pp. 409–415, 2011.

[91] T. J. Borody and J. Campbell, "Fecal microbiota transplantation: techniques, applications, and issues," *Gastroenterology Clinics of North America*, vol. 41, pp. 781–803, 2012.

15

Accuracy of Neck Circumference in Classifying Overweight and Obese US Children

Youngwon Kim,[1] Jung-Min Lee,[1] Kelly Laurson,[2] Yang Bai,[1] Glenn A. Gaesser,[3] and Gregory J. Welk[1]

[1] *Department of Kinesiology, Iowa State University, 235 Forker Building, Ames, IA 50011, USA*
[2] *School of Kinesiology and Recreation, Illinois State University, Campus Box 5120, 250 McCormick Hall, Normal, Il 61790, USA*
[3] *School of Nutrition and Health Promotion, Arizona State University, 502 East Monroe Street, Suite C 250, Phoenix, AZ 85004, USA*

Correspondence should be addressed to Youngwon Kim; youngwon@iastate.edu

Academic Editors: C. A. Gibson and H. Gordish-Dressman

Objective. To evaluate classification accuracy of NC and compare it with body mass index (BMI) in identifying overweight/obese US children. *Methods.* Data were collected from 92 children (boys: 61) aged 7 to 13 over a 2-year period. NC, BMI, and percent of body fat (BF%) were measured in each child and their corresponding cut-off values were applied to classify the children as being overweight/obese. Classification accuracy of NC and BMI was systematically investigated for boys and girls in relation to true overweight/obesity categorization as assessed with a criterion measure of BF% (i.e., Bod Pod). *Results.* For boys, Cohen's κ (0.25), sensitivity (38.1%), and specificity (85.0%) of NC were smaller in comparison with Cohen's κ (0.57), sensitivity (57.1%), and specificity (95.0%) of BMI in relation to BF% categorization. For girls, Cohen's κ (0.45), sensitivity (50.0%), and specificity (91.3%) of NC were smaller in comparison with Cohen's κ (0.52), sensitivity (50.0%), and specificity (95.7%) of BMI. *Conclusion.* NC measurement was not better than BMI in classifying childhood overweight/obesity and, for boys, NC was inferior to BMI. Pediatricians and/or pediatric researchers should be cautious or wary about incorporating NC measurements in their pediatric care and/or research.

1. Introduction

The prevalence of childhood overweight/obesity in the US has increased during the past 30 years [1]. Childhood overweight/obesity is associated with health risk factors both during childhood [2, 3] and adulthood [4, 5], and with tracking to adulthood obesity [6–8]. Consequently, identification of overweight/obese children early in life may be an important part of an overall health screening process that could be used to improve well-being in this population [9, 10].

The most commonly used screening tool for detecting childhood overweight/obesity is the body mass index (BMI; weight (kg)/height (m) squared). The standard method used in the United States relies on the use of gender and age-specific BMI growth charts from the Centers for Disease Control and Prevention (CDC) [11]. Youth above the standard 85th percentile are considered overweight while youth above the 95th percentile are considered obese.

While the BMI is widely used and accepted, there has been recent interest in the use of neck circumference (NC) as an alternative screening method. A study by Nafiu et al. [12] established age- and gender-specific cut-offs for NC using receiver operating characteristics curve (ROC curve) on a large sample of children (n = 1102, 52% boys, aged 6 to 18 yrs). The analyses were designed to maximize both sensitivity and specificity of NC cut-offs in relation to the overweight/obesity categorization using the CDC growth charts for BMI (i.e., values above the 85th percentile) [11]. This methodology resulted in a set of age- and gender-specific NC cut-offs that ranged from 28.5 cm to 39.0 cm for boys and from 27.0 cm to 34.6 cm for girls [12].

A limitation of the previous study is that it only linked NC values to BMI rather than to a more appropriate criterion. Before the NC values can be used in clinical practice, it is important to systematically validate the published NC

Table 1: Descriptive statistics of the included participants (n = 92).

Anthropometric measures	Boys (n = 61)		Girls (n = 31)	
	M	SD	M	SD
Age (yrs)	9.8	2.0	9.6	1.8
Height (cm)	146.1	14.6	140.6	10.1
Weight (kg)	40.2	15.5	34.6	8.3
Neck Circumference (cm)	30.0	3.1	28.7	2.2
Body Mass Index (BMI)	18.3	4.0	17.3	2.5
Percent body fat (%)	18.5	7.9	18.4	6.1

cut-off values in separate studies prior to its widespread use in clinical settings. To date, however, the Nafiu et al.'s NC cut-offs [12] for classifying overweight/obese children have not been evaluated using an appropriate gold standard or in an independent sample of children. Therefore, the purpose of this study was to compare the relative accuracy of the Nafiu et al.'s NC cut-offs [12] in the classification of overweight/obesity against the BMI percentiles [11] using estimates of percent of body fat (BF%) from whole body air-displacement plethysmography as a criterion measure of body composition.

2. Materials and Method

2.1. Study Design. This study was conducted as an ancillary study of a 5-year National Institute of Health-funded research Project (R01 HL910006) designed to validate varying types of accelerometer-based physical activity monitors in children. The procedures and protocol of the study were reviewed and approved by the local Institutional Review Board. Written parental consent and children's assent were obtained after informing them about the procedures and purpose of the study and prior to the participation. The data for the present study were collected in the summer of 2011 and 2012. A total of 92 children had data on the needed measures (2011: n = 60; 2012: n = 32). In Table 1, the characteristics of the included participants are summarized.

2.2. Anthropometric Measurement. Neck circumference (NC) was measured using a flexible ruler tape on the mid-point of the neck at the level of the thyroid cartilage, with a participant's body held erect, eyes facing forward, and normal breathing [12]. Standing height and body weight were measured using a wall-mounted stadiometer (*Harpenden, London, UK*) and electronic scale (*2008 Sunbeam products, Inc., Boca Raton, FL*) to the nearest 0.1 cm and 0.1 kg, respectively. BMI was calculated by dividing weight in kilograms by the square of height in meters.

BF% was measured via whole body air-displacement plethysmography with the Bod Pod (*Life Measurement, Inc., Concord, CA*), which has been considered a valid and reliable method for BF% measurement [13, 14]. The Bod Pod was calibrated according to the manufacturer's guidelines prior to each testing. Participants were wearing a tight fitting swimsuit and swim cap and were asked to sit still and not to talk in the chamber during the measurement. Body volume measurements were carried out twice and the average value of the two measurements was taken into consideration for analyses. BF% was estimated using the Lohman et al. equation [15, 16] programmed in the Bod Pod.

2.3. Data Processing/Statistical Analyses. The Nafiu et al.'s age- and gender-specific NC cut-offs [12] and the CDC growth charts for BMI [11] were applied to categorize NC and BMI values, respectively, as normal weight or overweight/obese. A set of criterion referenced health standards for BF% were used to determine the "true" classification of overweight/obesity for the participants [17, 18]. These standards (established using nationally representative data from the National Health and Nutrition Examination Survey) were found to have a sensitivity of 95.0% and specificity of 71.0% for boys and a sensitivity of 96.8% and specificity of 68.9% for girls for predicting risk of metabolic syndrome in a similarly aged population [17, 18]. Thus, they provide a defensible standard to evaluate the accuracy of these alternative screening tools available for body composition screening. The cut-off values used for NC, BMI, and BF% calculations are provided in Table 2.

All the statistical analyses were conducted using STATA/SE Version 10.0 for Windows (StataCorp LP, College Station, TX). Mean (M), standard deviations (SD), and minimum and maximum values of the anthropometric variables were calculated. Pearson correlation coefficients along with corresponding two-sided P values were obtained among NC, BMI, and BF%. A level of significance was set at 0.05. Classification accuracy of the Nafiu et al.'s NC cut-offs [12] and the CDC growth charts for BMI [11] in identifying overweight/obese children were evaluated against the standard cut-offs for BF% [17, 18] using weighted Cohen's kappa coefficient (Cohen's κ), sensitivity, specificity, positive predictive value, and negative predictive value. Cohen's κ is an index used to evaluate classification agreement between two screening tools for categorical variables, with agreement by chance corrected. Cohen's κ is categorized as "no agreement" ($\kappa \leq 0$), "slight" ($0 < \kappa \leq 0.20$), "fair" ($0.20 < \kappa \leq 0.40$), "moderate" ($0.40 < \kappa \leq 0.60$), "substantial" ($0.60 < \kappa \leq 0.80$), and "almost perfect" agreement ($0.80 < \kappa \leq 1.00$) [19]. Sensitivity refers to the ability of a certain screening method (i.e., NC or BMI in the context of the present study) to precisely detect a disease (i.e., overweight/obese) in people who indeed have the disease (i.e., as assessed with BF%), while specificity is referred to as the ability of a screening method to identify the absence of a disease (i.e., normal weight) in a population without the disease. Positive predictive value represents the proportion of people who have a disease (i.e., overweight/obese) among people who test positive. Negative predictive value is the proportion of people without a disease (i.e., normal weight) among people who test negative.

3. Results

The Nafiu et al.'s NC cut-offs [12] classified 13 (21.3%) of 61 boys and 6 (19.4%) of 31 girls as being overweight/obese.

TABLE 2: Cut-off values of neck circumference (NC), body mass index (BMI), and percent body fat (BF%) for classifying overweight/obese children.

Age (yrs)	NC (cm) by Nafiu et al. [12]		BMI[a]		BF%[b]	
	Boys	Girls	Boys	Girls	Boys	Girls
7	28.7	27.1	17.4	17.6	17.5	19.5
8	29.0	27.9	18.0	18.3	18.9	20.9
9	30.5	29.3	18.6	19.1	20.7	22.7
10	32.0	30.5	19.4	20.0	22.5	24.4
11	32.2	31.0	20.2	20.9	23.7	25.8
12	32.5	31.1	21.0	21.7	23.7	26.8
13	33.5	31.3	21.9	22.6	22.9	27.8

[a]Centers for Disease Control and Prevention growth charts (5th–85th percentile being normal weight, ≥85th percentile being overweight/obese for boys and girls).
[b]Percent body fat standards (<69th percentile being normal weight for boys, ≥69th percentile being overweight/obese for boys, <68th percentile being normal weight for girls, ≥69th percentile being overweight/obese for girls).

TABLE 3: Pearson correlation coefficients among neck circumference (NC), body mass index (BMI), and percent body fat (BF%) ($n = 92$).

	NC and BF%	BMI and BF%	NC and BMI
Boys ($n = 61$)	.44	.76	.78
Girls ($n = 31$)	.65	.74	.72

Note: all correlations were significant ($P < 0.001$).

The CDC growth charts for BMI [11] classified 14 boys (23.0%) and 5 girls (16.1%) as being overweight/obese. Twenty one boys (34.4%) and 8 girls (25.8%) were overweight/obese in accordance with the standard cut-offs for BF% [17, 18].

Table 3 shows statistically significant positive correlations among the three different measures: NC, BMI, and BF%. For boys, the correlation between NC and BF% values ($r = 0.44$, $P < 0.001$) was smaller in comparison to the correlation between BMI and BF% ($r = 0.76$, $P < 0.001$) and between NC and BMI ($r = 0.78$, $P < 0.001$). For girls, a similar pattern was observed that the correlation between NC and BF% ($r = 0.65$, $P < 0.001$) was smaller than the correlation between BMI and BF% ($r = 0.74$, $P < 0.001$) and between NC and BMI ($r = 0.72$, $P < 0.001$).

Table 4 summarized Cohen's κ, sensitivity, specificity, positive predictive value, and negative predictive value for both the Nafiu et al.'s NC cut-offs [12] and the CDC growth charts for BMI [11] in relation to the standard cut-offs for BF% [17, 18] for boys and girls. For boys, the Nafiu et al.'s NC cut-offs [12] showed "fair" classification agreement (Cohen's κ; 0.25) with the standard cut-offs for BF% [17, 18] while "moderate" classification agreement (Cohen's κ; 0.57) was observed between the CDC growth charts for BMI [11] and the standard cut-offs for BF% [17, 18]. Sensitivity (38.1%), specificity (85.0%), positive predictive value (57.1%), and negative predictive value (72.3%) of the Nafiu et al.'s NC cut-offs [12] were smaller in comparison with sensitivity (57.1%), specificity (95.0%), positive predictive value (85.7%), and negative predictive value (80.9%) of the CDC growth charts for BMI [11]. For girls, the Nafiu et al.'s NC cut-offs [12] demonstrated "moderate" classification agreement (Cohen's κ; 0.45) but was smaller than the CDC growth charts for BMI [11] (Cohen's κ; 0.52) in relation to the standard cut-offs for BF% [17, 18]. Sensitivity (50.0%), specificity (91.3%), positive predictive value (66.7%), and negative predictive value (84.0%) of the Nafiu et al.'s NC cut-offs [12] were smaller (or equivalent) in comparison with sensitivity (50.0%), specificity (95.7%), positive predictive value (80.0%), and negative predictive value (84.6%) of the CDC growth charts for BMI [11] relative to the standard cut-offs for BF% [17, 18].

4. Discussion

In the present study, classification accuracy of the recently developed set of Nafiu et al.'s NC cut-offs [12] for identifying overweight/obese children was examined in relation to the gold standard (i.e., Bod Pod) for body composition measurement. Overall, the Nafiu et al.'s NC cut-offs [12] demonstrated good classification accuracy of overweight/obesity for girls, but low for boys. However, they [12] did not prove superiority over the traditional overweight/obesity classification method, BMI assessed with the CDC growth charts [11].

Such limited classification accuracy of the Nafiu et al.'s NC cut-offs [12] appears to be due to the following two reasons. First, the CDC growth charts for BMI [11] may not be accurate enough to serve as a reference method for developing a precise set of NC cut-offs. While BMI has been considered a useful screening tool for epidemiological studies with large sample sizes [11], it tends to yield biased estimates of total fat distributions at an individual level [20], thereby limiting the practice of BMI as a "gold standard" measure in identifying overweight/obese children. This may have impaired the accuracy of the NC cut-offs developed in the Nafiu et al.'s calibration study [12]. The second potential reason is the inclusion of a large number of children (i.e., 70% of the total) in the Nafiu et al.'s calibration study [12] that were undergoing various types of outpatient surgeries at a children's hospital. Thus, the NC cut-offs [12] developed for this particular group of children appeared not to precisely classify overweight/obesity when applied for the healthy randomly selected children included in the present study. For the purpose of verifying this issue, we performed subsequent analyses (i.e., unreported herein) to obtain sensitivity and

TABLE 4: Comparisons of neck circumference (NC), body mass index (BMI), and percent body fat (BF%) in classification of overweight/obese children ($n = 92$).

	NC by Nafiu et al. [12] versus BF%		BMI versus BF%	
	Point estimate	95% CI	Point estimate	95% CI
Boys ($n = 61$)				
Weighted Cohen's kappa (κ)	.25	0, .48	.57	.30, .74
Sensitivity (%)	38.1	25.9, 50.3	57.1	44.7, 69.6
Specificity (%)	85.0	76.4, 94.0	95.0	89.5, 100
Positive predictive value (%)	57.1	44.7, 69.6	85.7	76.9, 94.5
Negative predictive value (%)	72.3	61.1, 83.6	80.9	71.0, 90.7
Girls ($n = 31$)				
Weighted Cohen's kappa (κ)	.45	.08, .73	.52	.13, .78
Sensitivity (%)	50.0	32.4, 67.6	50.0	32.4, 67.6
Specificity (%)	91.3	81.4, 100	95.7	88.5, 100
Positive predictive value (%)	66.7	50.1, 83.3	80.0	65.9, 94.1
Negative predictive value (%)	84.0	71.1, 96.9	84.6	71.9, 97.3

specificity of Nafiu et al.'s NC cut-offs [12] relative to BMI as a reference method and then to compare them with the sensitivity and specificity that were reported in the original calibration study of Nafiu et al. [12]. The present study showed lower sensitivity (i.e., 38.1% for boys and 50.0% for girls) and greater specificity (i.e., 85.0% for boys and 91.3% for girls) for Nafiu et al.'s NC cut-offs [12] in comparison with the sensitivity (i.e., 82.5% for boys and 79.7% for girls) and specificity (i.e., 83.7% for boys and 82.8% for girls) reported in the subjects studied by Nafiu et al. [12]. These differential results between the present study and that of Nafiu et al. [12] may be indicative of lower classification accuracy of NC cut-offs [12] when used in nonpatient populations.

In addition to the set of NC cut-offs by Nafiu et al. [12], other sets of NC cut-offs were independently established in an effort to identify overweight/obesity for other populations such as adults [21] and Turkish children [22]. These two studies [21, 22] also used BMI as a reference method in developing the NC cut-offs from ROC-curve analyses, thereby potentially limiting the classification accuracy of the developed NC cut-offs. Also, as discussed above, the usual practice of applying the NC cut-offs developed from patients [21] to nonpatient populations may be unwarranted. As such, the classification accuracy of NC cut-offs for patients may be maximized when applied only for specific patient populations. Moreover, all of the above-mentioned studies [12, 21, 22] advocated the use of NC measurement, primarily based on its "practicality" for clinical settings. Some of the practical features of NC measurement discussed in the studies [12, 21, 22] were as follows: easy/simple/inexpensive to use, unnecessary to remove upper clothes, and less susceptible to harsh weather than other measures (i.e., waist circumference measure). The results of the present study, however, suggest that the accuracy of NC measurement is not so reasonably high that pediatricians/pediatric educators may not be able to capitalize on the good "practicality" per se.

NC measurement may not be precise enough to serve as a stand-alone alternative to BMI. In support, in the present study, BMI showed better (or comparable) classification accuracy of overweight/obesity for boys and girls, respectively, in comparison with NC. Moreover, BMI has been recommended by numerous previous studies [9–11, 23] as a useful screening tool to identify childhood overweight/obesity. Therefore, it has become a tradition in nearly all pediatric clinical settings that height and weight are routinely measured as part of their basic check-ups for a child to yield his or her corresponding BMI value. For these reasons, unless classification accuracy of NC measurement for childhood overweight/obesity is strongly supported with scientific evidence, NC measurement may not be broadly used in clinical practice, despite its high practicality.

To date, a relatively large number of studies have been conducted to examine the associations between NC and varying health indicators in children (i.e., cardiovascular risk factors [24–26], prehypertension [27], and perioperative adverse respiratory events [28]). However, a limited body of scientific evidence has been established to determine whether or not NC measurement can serve as a useful tool for classifying childhood overweight/obesity. To our knowledge, this is the first study examining the efficacy of NC measurement in classifying childhood overweight/obesity in relation to a criterion measure of body composition in an independent sample of US children. In order for NC measurement to be widely adopted in clinical practice, therefore, additional studies are needed (1) to develop and/or (2) to evaluate a set of NC cut-offs relative to a gold-standard reference (i.e., Bod Pod, dual-energy X-ray absorptiometry) for body composition measurement with average populations of children (rather than with individuals undergoing surgeries).

Some limitations need to be taken into consideration when interpreting the results of the present study. First of all, a relatively small number of children participated in the study. Therefore, it was challenging to include a sufficient number of children in each age (i.e., 7–13 yrs), which limited the analysis and stratification of the results by age. However, since the statistical methods (e.g., Cohen's κ, sensitivity, specificity, positive predictive value, and negative predictive value) used herein are not biased with a small sample, the application of the (age-specific) NC [12], BMI [11], and %BF [17, 18] cut-offs for each age yielded unbiased estimates of classification accuracy. Another limitation was the inability to compare the accuracy of NC with other types of anthropometric measures (i.e., waist circumference, waist-to-hip ratio). However, NC was directly compared with the most commonly used classification method, BMI.

5. Conclusions

The results of this study appear not to strongly support the use of NC measurement as a useful screening tool for classifying childhood overweight/obesity. While NC measurement holds great practicality, its unsatisfactory accuracy in overweight/obesity classification may preclude the widespread use at clinical settings. Pediatricians and/or pediatric researchers should be informed of the accuracy of NC measurement in childhood overweight/obesity classification prior to incorporating it in their practical pediatric care and/or research.

Conflict of Interests

The authors declare that there is no conflict of interests regarding the publication of the paper.

Acknowledgments

The authors would like to thank all the participants and their parents for their participation in the current study and Cassie Weickert for her considerable contribution to data collection. This research was supported in part by NIH Grant R01 HL910006 to Glenn A. Gaesser.

References

[1] C. L. Ogden, M. D. Carroll, B. K. Kit, and K. M. Flegal, "Prevalence of obesity in the United States, 2009-2010," *NCHS Data Brief*, no. 82, pp. 1–8, 2012.

[2] C. Friedemann, C. Heneghan, K. Mahtani, M. Thompson, R. Perera, and A. M. Ward, "Cardiovascular disease risk in healthy children and its association with body mass index: systematic review and meta-analysis," *BMJ*, vol. 345, Article ID e4759, 2012.

[3] R. Weiss, J. Dziura, T. S. Burgert et al., "Obesity and the metabolic syndrome in children and adolescents," *The New England Journal of Medicine*, vol. 350, no. 23, pp. 2362–2374, 2004.

[4] D. S. Freedman, D. A. Patel, S. R. Srinivasan et al., "The contribution of childhood obesity to adult carotid intima-media thickness: the Bogalusa Heart Study," *International Journal of Obesity*, vol. 32, no. 5, pp. 749–756, 2008.

[5] W. Bao, S. R. Srinivasan, R. Valdez, K. J. Greenlund, W. A. Wattigney, and G. S. Berenson, "Longitudinal changes in cardiovascular risk from childhood to young adulthood in offspring of parents with coronary artery disease: the Bogalusa Heart Study," *The Journal of the American Medical Association*, vol. 278, no. 21, pp. 1749–1754, 1997.

[6] N. S. The, C. Suchindran, K. E. North, B. M. Popkin, and P. Gordon-Larsen, "Association of adolescent obesity with risk of severe obesity in adulthood," *The Journal of the American Medical Association*, vol. 304, no. 18, pp. 2042–2047, 2010.

[7] M. K. Serdula, D. Ivery, R. J. Coates, D. S. Freedman, D. F. Williamson, and T. Byers, "Do obese children become obese adults? A review of the literature," *Preventive Medicine*, vol. 22, no. 2, pp. 167–177, 1993.

[8] R. C. Whitaker, J. A. Wright, M. S. Pepe, K. D. Seidel, and W. H. Dietz, "Predicting obesity in young adulthood from childhood and parental obesity," *The New England Journal of Medicine*, vol. 337, no. 13, pp. 869–873, 1997.

[9] G. P. August, S. Caprio, I. Fennoy et al., "Prevention and treatment of pediatric obesity: an Endocrine Society clinical practice guideline based on expert opinion," *The Journal of Clinical Endocrinology and Metabolism*, vol. 93, no. 12, pp. 4576–4599, 2008.

[10] S. E. Barlow, "Expert committee recommendations regarding the prevention, assessment, and treatment of child and adolescent overweight and obesity: summary report," *Pediatrics*, vol. 120, supplement 4, pp. S164–S192, 2007.

[11] R. J. Kuczmarski, C. L. Ogden, S. S. Guo et al., "2000 CDC Growth Charts for the United States: methods and development," *Vital and Health Statistics, Series 11*, no. 246, pp. 1–190, 2002.

[12] O. O. Nafiu, C. Burke, J. Lee, T. Voepel-Lewis, S. Malviya, and K. K. Tremper, "Neck circumference as a screening measure for identifying children with high body mass index," *Pediatrics*, vol. 126, no. 2, pp. e306–e310, 2010.

[13] D. A. Fields, M. I. Goran, and M. A. McCrory, "Body-composition assessment via air-displacement plethysmography in adults and children: a review," *The American Journal of Clinical Nutrition*, vol. 75, no. 3, pp. 453–467, 2002.

[14] D. A. Fields, P. B. Higgins, and D. Radley, "Air-displacement plethysmography: here to stay," *Current Opinion in Clinical Nutrition and Metabolic Care*, vol. 8, no. 6, pp. 624–629, 2005.

[15] T. G. Lohman, K. Ring, K. Pfeiffer et al., "Relationships among fitness, body composition, and physical activity," *Medicine and Science in Sports and Exercise*, vol. 40, no. 6, pp. 1163–1170, 2008.

[16] T. G. Lohman, M. H. Slaughter, R. A. Boileau, J. Bunt, and L. Lussier, "Bone mineral measurements and their relation to body density in children, youth and adults," *Human Biology*, vol. 56, no. 4, pp. 667–679, 1984.

[17] K. R. Laurson, J. C. Eisenmann, and G. J. Welk, "Development of youth percent body fat standards using receiver operating characteristic curves," *American Journal of Preventive Medicine*, vol. 41, no. 4, supplement 2, pp. S111–S116, 2011.

[18] K. R. Laurson, J. C. Eisenmann, and G. J. Welk, "Body fat percentile curves for U.S. children and adolescents," *American Journal of Preventive Medicine*, vol. 41, no. 4, supplement 2, pp. S87–S92, 2011.

[19] J. R. Landis and G. G. Koch, "The measurement of observer agreement for categorical data," *Biometrics*, vol. 33, no. 1, pp. 159–174, 1977.

[20] S. R. Daniels, P. R. Khoury, and J. A. Morrison, "The utility of body mass index as a measure of body fatness in children and adolescents: differences by race and gender," *Pediatrics*, vol. 99, no. 6, pp. 804–807, 1997.

[21] L. Ben-Noun, E. Sohar, and A. Laor, "Neck circumference as a simple screening measure for identifying overweight and obese patients," *Obesity Research*, vol. 9, no. 8, pp. 470–477, 2001.

[22] N. Hatipoglu, M. M. Mazicioglu, S. Kurtoglu, and M. Kendirci, "Neck circumference: an additional tool of screening overweight and obesity in childhood," *European Journal of Pediatrics*, vol. 169, no. 6, pp. 733–739, 2010.

[23] W. H. Dietz and M. C. Bellizzi, "Introduction: the use of body mass index to assess obesity in children," *The American Journal of Clinical Nutrition*, vol. 70, no. 1, pp. 123S–125S, 1999.

[24] O. Androutsos, E. Grammatikaki, G. Moschonis et al., "Neck circumference: a useful screening tool of cardiovascular risk in children," *Pediatric Obesity*, vol. 7, no. 3, pp. 187–195, 2012.

[25] L. Ben-Noun and A. Laor, "Relationship between changes in neck circumference and cardiovascular risk factors," *Experimental and Clinical Cardiology*, vol. 11, no. 1, pp. 14–20, 2006.

[26] S. Kurtoglu, N. Hatipoglu, M. M. Mazicioglu, and M. Kondolot, "Neck circumference as a novel parameter to determine metabolic risk factors in obese children," *European Journal of Clinical Investigation*, vol. 42, no. 6, pp. 623–630, 2012.

[27] X. Guo, Y. Li, G. Sun et al., "Prehypertension in children and adolescents: association with body weight and neck circumference," *Internal Medicine*, vol. 51, no. 1, pp. 23–27, 2012.

[28] O. O. Nafiu, C. C. Burke, R. Gupta, R. Christensen, P. I. Reynolds, and S. Malviya, "Association of neck circumference with perioperative adverse respiratory events in children," *Pediatrics*, vol. 127, no. 5, pp. e1198–e1205, 2011.

The Relationship between High Risk for Obstructive Sleep Apnea and General and Central Obesity: Findings from a Sample of Chilean College Students

Adaeze C. Wosu,[1] Juan Carlos Vélez,[2] Clarita Barbosa,[2] Asterio Andrade,[2] Megan Frye,[2] Xiaoli Chen,[1] Bizu Gelaye,[1] and Michelle A. Williams[1]

[1] *Department of Epidemiology, Multidisciplinary International Research Training Program, Harvard School of Public Health, 677 Huntington Avenue, Kresge 500, Boston, MA 02115, USA*
[2] *Centro de Rehabilitación Club de Leones Cruz del Sur, Suiza 1441, Punta Arenas, 6211525 Magallanes, Chile*

Correspondence should be addressed to Adaeze C. Wosu; awosu@hsph.harvard.edu

Academic Editors: M. M. Al-Nozha, B. Wizner, and C. H. Wu

This cross-sectional study evaluates the prevalence and extent to which high risk for obstructive sleep apnea (OSA) is associated with general obesity and central obesity among college students in Punta Arenas, Chile. Risk for OSA was assessed using the Berlin Questionnaire and trained research nurses measured anthropometric indices. Overweight was defined as body mass index (BMI) of 25–29.9 kg/m^2 and general obesity was defined as BMI $\geq$ 30 kg/m^2. Central obesity was defined as waist circumference $\geq$ 90 centimeters (cm) for males and $\geq$ 80 cm for females. Multivariate logistic regression models were fit to obtain adjusted odds ratios (OR) and 95% confidence intervals (CI). Prevalence of high risk for OSA, general obesity, and central obesity were 7.8%, 12.8%, and 42.7%, respectively. Students at high risk for OSA had greater odds of general obesity (OR 9.96; 95% CI: 4.42–22.45) and central obesity (OR 2.78; 95% CI 1.43–5.40). Findings support a strong positive association of high risk for OSA with obesity.

1. Background

Chile, an upper middle-income country in South America, has seen increases in the prevalence of overweight and obesity, well-established risk factors for conditions such as cancer, cardiovascular disease, and diabetes [1, 2]. In 1987, the prevalence of excess weight among 6-year-olds in Chile was 13%; by 2000, it had reached 27% [3]. According to a 2012 report by the Organization for Economic Cooperation and Development (OECD), 25.1% of Chilean adults are obese and, among Chilean children aged 5–17 years, 27.1% of girls and 28.6% of boys are overweight or obese [4]. Like excess weight, sleep disorders, particularly sleep apneas, have been associated with hypertension [5, 6], coronary artery disease [7], myocardial infarction [8, 9], heart failure [10], and diabetes [9]. Although reports have been published on the prevalence of obesity and of sleep apnea in Chilean adults and young children [4, 11], few reports have focused attention on the prevalence of obesity and sleep apnea among young adults, particularly college students transitioning from adolescence into adulthood. Moreover, the college years are often characterized by insufficient sleep, increased consumption of energy drinks and caffeinated beverages, and irregular meal and sleep patterns, which can have important consequences for overall health and wellbeing [12–15]. To address the paucity of literature on the epidemiology of obstructive sleep apnea (OSA) and adiposity indices among college students in Chile, and to lay groundwork for developing health promotion and disease prevention strategies, we conducted a cross-sectional study of students at four Chilean colleges.

We investigated OSA risk and the extent to which high risk for OSA was associated with overweight, general obesity, and central obesity in this population.

2. Methods

2.1. Study Population. The study was conducted between December 2010 and June 2011 at four colleges in the Magallanes region of Chile: Universidad Tecnologica de Chile, Universidad del Mar, Universidad de Magallanes, and Universidad Santo Tomas. Detailed descriptions of the study procedures have been given previously [16]. Of the 994 full-time undergraduates who participated in the study, we excluded students who were above 35 years old or missing information on age, sleep apnea (i.e., The Berlin Questionnaire), or adiposity measures ($n = 78$). The final sample consisted of 916 students aged 18 to 35 who had complete exposure and outcome information.

2.2. Recruitment. Flyers promoting the study were posted throughout departments at the participating colleges. Interested students were invited to meet in a large room or an auditorium where they were informed about the study purpose and procedures and invited to complete anonymous questionnaires requesting demographic, lifestyle, and sleep-related information. Students who gave informed consent and completed the questionnaires were invited to participate in a brief physical examination during which trained research nurses took cardiometabolic and anthropometric measures including height, weight, blood pressure (BP), pulse rate, waist circumference (WC), and hip circumference (HC). All study procedures were approved by the institutional review boards of Centro de Rehabilitación Club de Leones Cruz del Sur, Punta Arenas, Chile, and the University of Washington, USA. The Harvard School of Public Health Office of Human Research Administration, USA, granted approval to use the anonymized dataset for analyses.

2.3. Obstructive Sleep Apnea (OSA) Risk. OSA risk was evaluated using the Berlin Questionnaire. Since it was first developed in 1996, the Berlin Questionnaire has been validated and used extensively in clinical and epidemiologic research globally including Latin America [17–23]. Numerous validation studies have reported moderate to high consistency between results of the Berlin Questionnaire and parameters of polysomnography, particularly respiratory disturbance index (RDI) > 5 and apnea-hypopnea index (AHI) ≥ 5, especially within clinical populations [24].

The questionnaire is divided into three categories [19, 25]. Category 1 evaluates snoring characteristics and how often the respondent ceases breathing during sleep. Category 2 assesses frequency of feelings of fatigue or tiredness after waking as well as sleepiness while driving. Category 3 ascertains information about obesity and hypertension [17, 19]. In the first two categories, a participant is given a positive score if he or she responds with "yes" or experiences frequent symptoms (more than 3 to 4 times per week) in two or more questions within that category. For category 3, a participant is given a positive score if he or she is obese (BMI ≥ 30 kg/m^2) or has a history of hypertension. Participants with positive scores in two or more categories are classified as having a high risk for OSA [17].

2.4. General Obesity. Body mass index (BMI) was calculated as weight in kilograms divided by height in square meters (kg/m^2). Categories of BMI were defined according to the World Health Organization (WHO) criteria (underweight: <18.5 kg/m^2; normal: 18.5–24.9 kg/m^2; overweight: 25.0–29.9 kg/m^2; and obese: ≥30.0 kg/m^2). General obesity was defined as BMI ≥ 30.0 kg/m^2 [26].

2.5. Central Obesity. Central obesity was evaluated using the International Diabetes Federation (IDF) criteria for South American men and women, that is, WC ≥ 90 cm (for men) and WC ≥ 80 cm (for women) [27]. Waist-to-hip ratio (WHR) was calculated by dividing WC by HC. WHR was further categorized by quartile distribution and central obesity defined as WHR in the top quartile. Each anthropometric measurement was taken twice, and the average was used in data analyses.

2.6. Covariates. Sociodemographic information collected included age, sex, and year in college. Lifestyle and behavioral characteristics included moderate or vigorous physical activity (yes versus no), cigarette smoking status (never, former, or current), alcohol consumption within the past year (no versus yes), and use of more than one energy or stimulant drink per week (no versus yes). Energy or stimulant drinks were defined as beverages used to boost energy levels, increase alertness, and enhance cognition and mood [16]. Examples of these beverages include coffee, yerba mate, cola, Red Bull, and Dark Dog. Other variables included self-rated health (good versus poor) and systolic and diastolic BP.

2.7. Statistical Analysis. High risk for obstructive sleep apnea (OSA), defined as described above, was the exposure and the outcomes of interest were overweight, general obesity, central obesity, BMI, WC, HC, and WHR. First, we examined the frequency distributions of sociodemographic, lifestyle, and behavioral characteristics of the students. Characteristics of participants were summarized using counts and percentages for categorical variables and mean values (± standard deviations) for continuous variables. Student's t-tests and chi-square tests were used to calculate bivariate differences for continuous and categorical variables, respectively. We examined the frequency distribution of OSA risk according to sociodemographic, lifestyle, and behavioral characteristics. Multivariate linear regression models were used to assess the associations of high OSA risk with BMI, WC, HC, and WHR. Multivariate logistic regression models were used to determine odds ratios (OR) and 95% confidence intervals (CI) of the association of high OSA risk with general obesity (BMI ≥ 30 kg/m^2), central obesity according to the IDF criteria, and WHR in the top quartile. Confounding variables were considered *a priori* on the basis of their hypothesized

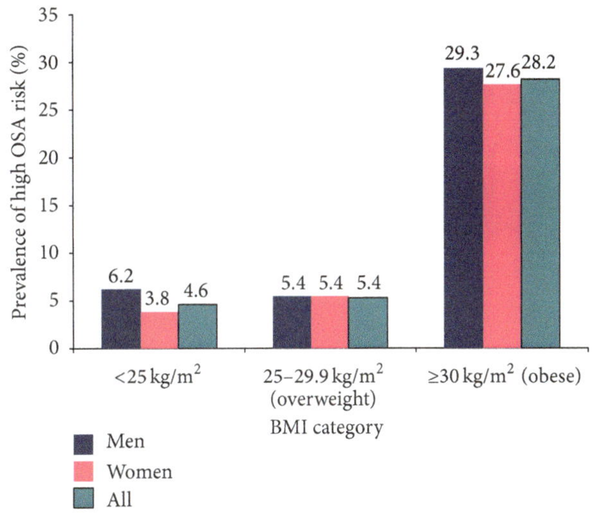

Figure 1: Prevalence of high OSA risk according to BMI category and gender.

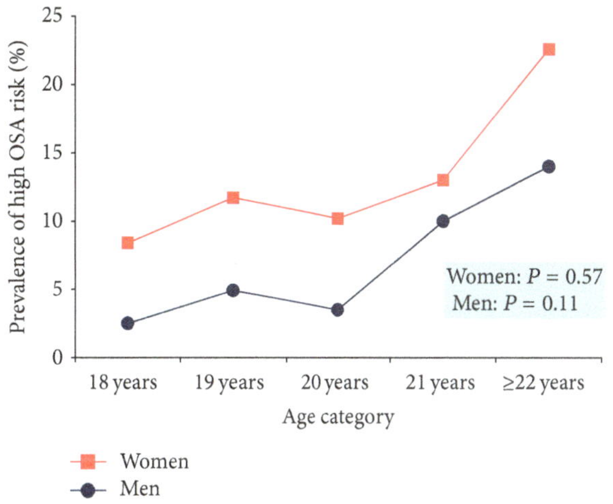

Figure 2: Prevalence of high OSA risk according to age group and gender.

relationship with OSA and adiposity. Potential confounders included age, sex, year in college, alcohol consumption, use of energy drinks, cigarette smoking status, self-rated health, BP, and participation in moderate or vigorous physical activity. We conducted stratified analyses to evaluate the extent to which, if at all, associations of high OSA risk with overweight, general obesity, and central obesity differed by sex, elevated BP, and subjects' self-rated health. All statistical analyses were performed using Statistical Analysis Software (SAS, version 9.3; SAS Institute, Cary, NC). All P values are two-sided and set at $\alpha = 0.05$.

3. Results

Of the 916 students included in the analysis, 69.5% were females and the average reported age was 21.8 (±3.3) years. Approximately 7.8% were classified as having high risk for OSA as determined using previously published scoring and classification scheme of the Berlin Questionnaire. Approximately 28.3% of students were overweight (BMI: 25–29.9 kg/m^2) and 12.8% had general obesity according to WHO criteria (BMI ≥ 30 kg/m^2). Using the IDF definition, it was determined that 42.7% of students had central obesity (WC ≥ 90 cm for men or WC ≥ 80 cm for women). High risk for OSA was associated with age, poor self-rated health, and cigarette smoking status. However, high risk for OSA was not associated with sex, year in college, systolic BP, diastolic BP, alcohol consumption, participation in moderate to vigorous physical activity, or consumption of more than one energy or stimulant drink per week (Table 1). Prevalence of high OSA risk was highest in the obese BMI category (Figure 1) and in individuals who were over 21 years old (Figure 2).

Table 2 shows the results of the fully adjusted models of the linear regression analyses. High OSA risk was statistically significantly associated with higher BMI (β: 3.25; standard error: 0.63, $P < 0.001$) and WHR (β: 0.03; standard error: 0.01, $P = 0.02$). High OSA risk was also associated with higher WC (β: 7.32; standard error: 1.54, $P < 0.001$) and HC (β: 5.00; standard error: 1.41, $P < 0.05$).

Next, we completed logistic regression analyses. In the fully adjusted models, high risk for OSA was associated with almost 10-fold increased odds of general obesity (OR 9.96; 95% CI 4.42–22.45) compared to low risk for OSA. Students with high OSA risk also had 2.78-fold odds of central obesity (OR 2.78; 95% CI 1.43–5.40). However, the odds of high risk for OSA were not elevated by overweight status (OR 0.89; 95% CI 0.35–2.23). Those with high risk for OSA were also more likely to be in the top quartile of WHR (i.e., WHR ≥ 0.8875), although statistical significance was not achieved (OR 1.45; 95% CI 0.71–2.95) (Table 3).

Similar strong positive associations between high risk for OSA and general obesity (BMI ≥ 30 kg/m^2) were evident within strata of sex (male or female), BP (nonelevated or elevated), and self-rated health (good or poor). High risk for OSA was not associated with overweight in strata of sex, BP, or self-rated health. For central obesity as defined by the IDF, the results of the stratified analyses were mixed. High risk for OSA was associated with central obesity only in men (OR 4.66; 95% CI: 1.33–16.39), in individuals with elevated BP (OR 7.34; 95% CI: 2.38–22.59), and in those with good self-rated health (OR 2.60; 95% CI 1.28–5.28) while the findings in women and those with poor self-rated health were suggestive of a positive though not statistically significant association (Table 4).

4. Discussion

In this study of Chilean college students, 7.8% were classified as having high risk for OSA as defined by the Berlin Questionnaire and there was a high prevalence of overweight (28.3%), general obesity (12.8%), and central obesity (42.7%). High OSA risk was strongly and positively associated with general obesity and central obesity, but not with overweight.

TABLE 1: Characteristics of 916 college students in Chile, according to OSA risk.

Characteristic	Overall (n = 916)	OSA risk		P value[c]
		Low (n = 845)	High (n = 71)	
Demographic characteristics				
Age, year, mean (SD)	21.8 (3.3)	21.7 (3.3)	22.5 (3.4)	0.0425
Male, %	30.5	30.0	36.6	0.2429
Education (year in college), %				
First year	37.3	37.4	35.7	0.4826
Second year	30.7	30.5	34.3	
Third year	18.5	19.0	12.9	
Fourth+ year	13.4	13.1	17.4	
Lifestyle factors				
Any physical activity participation, %	53.9	55.5	52.1	0.5811
Alcohol consumption (past year), %	80.3	80.0	85.1	0.3105
Smoking status, %				
Nonsmoker	42.7	44.2	24.6	0.0051
Current	42.4	40.9	60.0	
Former	14.9	14.9	15.4	
Use of >1 energy drinks per week, %	54.3	53.8	60.6	0.2866
Self-rated health and blood pressure				
Self-rated health[a] (poor), %	12.1	11.4	22.2	0.0183
Systolic blood pressure (mmHg)	121.5 (14.4)	121.3 (14.3)	124.6 (15.6)	0.0642
Diastolic blood pressure (mmHg)	74.2 (11.7)	74.0 (11.8)	76.5 (10.8)	0.0932
Anthropometric measurements				
BMI, kg/m^2, mean (SD)	24.9 (4.5)	24.6 (4.2)	28.6 (6.0)	<0.0001
WHO criteria of overweight and obesity (kg/m^2), %				
Underweight (BMI <18.5)	1.5	1.7	0.0	<0.0001
Normal weight (18.51–24.9)	57.4	59.4	33.8	
Overweight (BMI: 25–29)	28.3	29.0	19.7	
Obese (BMI ≥30)	12.8	9.9	46.5	
Central obesity[b], %	42.7	40.5	69.0	<0.0001
Waist circumference, cm, mean (SD)	81.9 (11.9)	81.1 (11.4)	91.0 (13.9)	<0.0001
Hip circumference, cm, mean (SD)	97.9 (10.0)	97.3 (9.7)	104.6 (11.0)	<0.0001
Waist-to-hip ratio, mean (SD)	0.84 (0.08)	0.83 (0.08)	0.87 (0.9)	0.0007
Waist-to-hip ratio, top quartile (WHR ≥ 0.8875), %	24.9	23.8	36.6	0.0162

SD: standard deviation; PA: physical activity; BP: blood pressure; BMI: body mass index.
[a]Self-rated health (SRH) was evaluated by asking, "how would you say your health compares to others your age." Poor SRH = worse than others my age. Good SRH = better or same as others my age.
[b]Based on the International Diabetes Federation (IDF) criteria for the definition of central obesity among South Americans: waist circumference ≥90 cm for men; waist circumference ≥80 cm for women.
[c]Student t-test for continuous variables; chi-square for categorical variables.

4.1. Possible Biological Mechanisms Explaining the Relationship between OSA and Obesity. Although the exact pathway linking OSA and obesity remains somewhat unclear, it is recognized that obesity contributes to airway collapse during sleep by causing increased fat deposits around the upper airway, thus narrowing it and diminishing the activity of the muscles in that region [28–31]. Conversely, sleep apnea may contribute to excess weight and obesity through sleep loss and daytime sleepiness as apneic individuals rouse often to resume breathing and reenable unobstructed air flow [29]. Moreover, insufficient sleep has been associated with increased energy need and food intake [32]. On balance, available evidence suggests mechanisms that may underlay bidirectional relationships between increased adiposity and OSA.

4.2. Association between OSA and Obesity. We found strong positive associations of high OSA risk with general obesity, central obesity, BMI, and WHR. These findings are largely consistent with findings from numerous prior studies [33–40]. In the Wisconsin Sleep Cohort Study, a 10% weight gain was associated with approximately 32% increase in AHI as assessed by polysomnography [38]. In their study of patients at primary health care centers in Dubai, Mahboub et al. found

TABLE 2: Linear regression analyses: associations of high OSA risk with anthropometric measurements among 916 college students in Chile.

Model	BMI (kg/m^2)		Waist-to-hip ratio (cm)		Waist circumference (cm)		Hip circumference (cm)	
	β (SE)	*P* value	β (SE)	*P* value	β (SE)	*P* value	β (SE)	*P* value
Model 1: unadjusted	3.93 (0.54)	<0.0001	0.034 (0.01)	0.0007	9.84 (1.43)	<0.0001	7.30 (1.21)	<0.0001
Model 2: adjusted for demographic factors[a]	3.76 (0.54)	<0.0001	0.027 (0.01)	0.0037	8.94 (1.37)	<0.0001	7.03 (1.21)	<0.0001
Model 3: adjusted for demographic & lifestyle factors[b]	4.20 (0.58)	<0.0001	0.028 (0.01)	0.0061	9.25 (1.47)	<0.0001	7.37 (1.30)	<0.0001
Model 4: Model 3 + blood pressure[c]	3.97 (0.55)	<0.0001	0.026 (0.01)	0.0101	8.59 (1.38)	<0.0001	6.83 (1.24)	<0.0001
Model 5: Model 4 + self-rated health[d]	3.25 (0.63)	<0.0001	0.028 (0.01)	0.0193	7.32 (1.54)	<0.0001	5.00 (1.41)	0.0004

[a]Demographic factors included age (continuous), sex, and education level.
[b]Lifestyle factors included any physical activity participation, alcohol consumption (within the past year—yes/no), cigarette smoking (never, former, or current), and use of energy drinks (yes/no).
[c]Continuous blood pressure variables.
[d]Self-rated health (SRH) was evaluated by asking, "how would you say your health compares to others your age." Poor SRH = worse than others my age. Good SRH = better or same as others my age.

TABLE 3: Logistic regression analyses: associations of high OSA risk with overweight and obesity among 916 college students in Chile.

Model	WHO criteria	WHO criteria		IDF criteria[f]
	BMI: 25–29 versus BMI <25	BMI ≥30 versus BMI <25	WHR ≥0.8875 versus WHR <0.8875[e]	Central obesity versus no central obesity
	OR (95% CI)	OR (95% CI)	OR (95% CI)	OR (95% CI)
Model 1: unadjusted	1.23 (0.63, 2.42)	8.45 (4.76, 15.00)	1.85 (1.11, 3.08)	3.27 (1.94, 5.51)
Model 2: adjusted for demographic factors[a]	1.09 (0.55, 2.17)	8.26 (4.59, 14.86)	1.65 (0.96, 2.86)	3.26 (1.92, 5.56)
Model 3: adjusted for demographic and lifestyle factors[b]	1.53 (0.74, 3.17)	10.24 (5.30, 19.81)	1.68 (0.93, 3.05)	3.37 (1.90, 5.97)
Model 4: Model 3 + blood pressure[c]	1.59 (0.76, 3.36)	10.92 (5.39, 22.11)	1.59 (0.87, 2.91)	3.31 (1.85, 5.95)
Model 5: Model 4 + self-rated health[d]	0.89 (0.35, 2.23)	9.96 (4.42, 22.45)	1.45 (0.71, 2.95)	2.78 (1.43, 5.40)

BMI: body mass index; WHR: waist-to-hip ratio; IDF: International Diabetes Federation; WC: waist circumference; OR: odds ratio; 95% CI: 95% confidence interval.
[a]Demographic factors included age (continuous), sex, and education level.
[b]Lifestyle factors included any physical activity participation, alcohol consumption (within the past year—yes/no), cigarette smoking (never, former, or current), and use of energy drinks (yes/no).
[c]Continuous blood pressure variables.
[d]Self-rated health (SRH) was evaluated by asking, "how would you say your health compares to others your age." Poor SRH = worse than others my age. Good SRH = better or same as others my age.
[e]WHR ≥0.8875 refers to the top quartile of WHR.
[f]Central obesity as defined by the International Diabetes Federation (IDF): WC ≥90 cm for men and WC ≥80 cm for women in South America.

that approximately 70% of those at high risk for OSA had a BMI $\geq 30\,kg/m^2$ while about 75% of the low risk group had BMI $< 30\,kg/m^2$ [41]. Likewise, Blondet et al. found in a study of middle-aged Puerto Ricans that among men with BMI $< 30\,kg/m^2$, 98% had high risk for OSA compared to 50% among nonobese men. In addition, the authors noted that 70% of women with BMI $> 28\,kg/m^2$ were at high risk for OSA compared to only 28% of those with BMI $< 28\,kg/m^2$ [42]. The prevalence of high risk for OSA among students with general obesity in our study was substantially higher (28.3%) compared to that in normal weight (4.6%) and overweight (5.4%) students. Although participants in many studies examining obesity and OSA risk are older and heavier than our population, significant positive associations between sleep apnea and obesity have also been found in pediatric and adolescent populations [43–46].

While we found no association between overweight BMI category and high risk for OSA in our sample, Peppard et al. observed a positive association between overweight BMI category and AHI in the Wisconsin Sleep Cohort Study [47]. Despite our finding of no association, overweight students should be targeted for interventions as these students are at higher risk for obesity in the near future compared to normal weight students.

TABLE 4: Stratified analysis for the association of high OSA risk with overweight, general obesity, and central obesity, by sex, blood pressure, and self-rated health[1].

Stratified variable	All participants $N = 916$	WHO criteria BMI: 25–29 versus <25 OR (95% CI)[a]	WHO criteria BMI ≥30 versus <25 OR (95% CI)[a]	IDF criteria[b] Central obesity versus no central obesity
Sex				
Male	280	0.56 (0.13, 2.47)	7.23 (1.34, 38.94)	4.66 (1.33, 16.39)
Female	636	1.16 (0.34, 3.95)	14.96 (5.40, 2.30)	2.08 (0.90, 4.81)
Elevated blood pressure[c]				
No	381	0.58 (0.12, 2.94)	8.71 (2.26, 33.59)	1.12 (0.39, 3.22)
Yes	534	1.21 (0.36, 4.09)	12.42 (4.23, 36.48)	7.34 (2.38, 22.59)
Self-rated health[d]				
Good	667	0.72 (0.25, 2.07)	8.21 (3.52, 19.16)	2.60 (1.28, 5.28)
Poor	92	3.01 (0.16, 57.86)	144.82 (2.4, ∞)	15.76 (0.93, 267.69)

BMI: body mass index; IDF: International Diabetes Federation; OR: odds ratio; 95% CI: 95% confidence interval.
[a]Except for the stratified variables, the following variables were adjusted for age (continuous), sex, education, any physical activity participation, alcohol consumption, cigarette smoking, use of energy drinks, and self-rated health.
[b]Central obesity was defined by the International Diabetes Federation (IDF) criteria for South Americans: WC ≥90 cm for men and WC ≥80 cm for women.
[c]Elevated BP defined as systolic BP ≥120 mmHg or diastolic BP ≥80 mmHg.
[d]Self-rated health (SRH) was evaluated by asking, "how would you say your health compares to others your age." Poor SRH = worse than others my age. Good SRH = better or same as others my age.

4.3. Prevalence of High Risk for OSA. The prevalence of high risk for OSA in our sample (7.8%) is higher than what is reported among US young adults. For instance, authors of a study among 1,845 students enrolled in a southeastern US college reported a prevalence of 4% as assessed using the SLEEP-50 survey [48]. However, our finding is lower than high OSA risk estimates reported for US adults (26%) who participated in the 2005 Sleep in America Poll [40]. We found no significant difference in frequency of OSA risk by sex (9.3% for men and 7.1% for women; $P = 0.25$) within our sample, although other investigators have shown that men have a higher risk for OSA compared to women—the main hypothesis being that men tend to have more fat deposits in the upper part of the body, that is, around the neck, trunk, and abdomen [49].

4.4. Prevalence of Obesity. The prevalence of general obesity in our study (12.8%) was relatively low when compared to the prevalence reported for Chilean adults by the OECD (25.1%) or that determined from a multistage cluster sampling of adults ≥40 years old in Santiago, Chile (31.7%) [4, 11]. However, the combined prevalence of overweight and obesity (i.e., BMI $\geq 25\,kg/m^2$) in our study was greater than that observed in a study of 3,461 Chilean students aged 17–24 years (41.1% versus 19%) [50]. When we examined the frequency of BMI $\geq 25\,kg/m^2$ by age within our sample, there was still a high prevalence of excess weight in the respective groups: 18–24 year-olds (39.5%) and 25–35 year-olds (48.4%); $P = 0.04$. The overall prevalence of central obesity as defined using the IDF criteria was 42.7%. These high frequencies of overweight and obesity in young adulthood are of concern as they may have implications for the development of cardiometabolic conditions in later life.

4.5. Strengths and Limitations. Our study has several strengths. First, numerous validation studies have reported moderate to high consistency between results of the Berlin Questionnaire and parameters of polysomnography, the gold-standard for diagnosing sleep disorders [24]. Second, we employed various statistical methods and assessed the relationship between high OSA risk and various indices of adiposity. Third, the likelihood for misclassification of obesity was reduced as trained research nurses used standard protocols to take anthropometric measurements, thus avoiding reliance on students' self-report.

There are some limitations that should be considered when interpreting the results of our study. Given our cross-sectional study design, we are unable to determine if high risk for OSA preceded obesity. Longitudinal studies are needed to clarify the temporal relationship between OSA and obesity. Another limitation is that participants were not sampled randomly; rather, we relied on subjects' willingness to participate. As such, our findings could be subject to volunteer bias. Approximately 8% of students were excluded because of incomplete information on sleep apnea or anthropometric data. We found no significant difference between the prevalence of poor self-rated heath among individuals in our sample and those who were excluded (12.1% versus 6.8%; $P = 0.29$) nor any significant difference in the distribution of cigarette smoking status ($P = 0.28$). However, excluded students tended to be older than those in our sample (mean ± SD age: 23.4 ± 5.0 versus 21.8 ± 3.3; $P < 0.01$). Given that OSA risk increases with age, it is possible that we missed individuals with high OSA risk among those who had incomplete sleep apnea or anthropometric information. Thus, the prevalence of high risk for OSA in our study could be an underestimate. Conversely, given the high prevalence of obesity within this sample, the use of odds ratios may give an exaggeration of the true estimate. We cannot exclude the possibility of residual confounding by unmeasured factors such as socioeconomic status, dietary intake (e.g., consumption of fruits, vegetables, or fast foods), or student's course load. Finally, due to the relatively small sample size, the 95% confidence intervals for the estimates from the logistic regression and stratified analyses are quite large and imprecise.

5. Conclusion

Our findings support significant positive associations of high OSA risk with general obesity and central obesity. Additional longitudinal evidence is needed to establish the temporal relationship of OSA and obesity. If our findings are confirmed, health care services for college students should include health promotion and disease prevention strategies about the importance of maintaining healthy weight. Strategies should also include health education modules that may be used to improve students' knowledge about sleep disorders, as prevention and control of cardiometabolic risk factors in young adulthood may have implications for preventing and mitigating chronic disease burden in later life.

Conflict of Interests

The authors declare that there is no conflict of interests regarding the publication of this paper.

Acknowledgments

This work was supported by an Award from the National Institutes of Health, National Institute on Minority Health and Health Disparities (T37-MD001449000) and Corporación de Rehabilitación Club de Leones Cruz del Sur, Punta Arenas, Chile. The authors would like to thank Universidad de Magallanes, Universidad del Mar, Instituto Profesional Santo Tomás, and INACAP Punta Arenas, for granting them permission to conduct the study on their campuses.

References

[1] L. Gitlin and P. Fuentes, "The Republic of Chile: an upper middle-income country at the crossroads of economic development and aging," *The Gerontologist*, vol. 52, no. 3, pp. 297–305, 2012.

[2] L. Aballay, A. Eynard, M. Diaz, A. Navarro, and S. Munoz, "Overweight and obesity: a review of their relationship to metabolic syndrome, cardiovascular disease, and cancer in South America," *Nutrition Reviews*, vol. 71, no. 3, pp. 168–179, 2013.

[3] T. Lobstein, "Prevalence and trends in childhood obesity," in *Obesity Epidemiology: From Aetiology to Public Health*, D. Crawford, R. Jeffery, K. Ball, and J. Brug, Eds., p. 10, Oxford University Press, New York, NY, USA, 2nd edition, 2010.

[4] F. Sassi, M. Devaux, and H. Fisher, *Obesity Update 2012*, Organization for Economic Cooperation and Development, 2012.

[5] V. Somers, D. White, R. Amin et al., "Sleep apnea and cardiovascular disease: an American Heart Association/American College of Cardiology Foundation scientific statement from the American Heart Association Council for High Blood Pressure Research Professional Education Committee, Council on Clinical Cardiology, Stroke Council, and Council on Cardiovascular Nursing. In collaboration with the National Heart, Lung, and Blood Institute National Center on Sleep Disorders Research (National Institutes of Health)," *Circulation*, vol. 118, no. 10, pp. 1080–1111, 2008.

[6] D. Silverberg, A. Oksenberg, and A. Iaina, "Sleep-related breathing disorders as a major cause of essential hypertension: fact or fiction?" *Current Opinion in Nephrology and Hypertension*, vol. 7, no. 4, pp. 353–357, 1998.

[7] Y. Peker, H. Kraiczi, J. Hedner, S. Löth, A. Johansson, and M. Bende, "An independent association between obstructive sleep apnoea and coronary artery disease," *European Respiratory Journal*, vol. 14, no. 1, pp. 179–184, 1999.

[8] J. Hung, E. Whitford, R. Parsons, and D. Hillman, "Association of sleep apnoea with myocardial infarction in men," *The Lancet*, vol. 336, no. 8710, pp. 261–264, 1990.

[9] C. Lee, S. Khoo, B. Tai et al., "Obstructive sleep apnea in patients admitted for acute myocardial infarction: prevalence, predictors, and effect on microvascular perfusion," *Chest*, vol. 135, no. 6, pp. 1488–1495, 2009.

[10] R. McEvoy, "Obstructive sleep apnea and heart failure: two unhappy bedfellows," *American Journal of Respiratory and Critical Care Medicine*, vol. 169, no. 3, pp. 329–331, 2004.

[11] L. Bouscoulet, J. Vázquez-García, A. Muiño et al., "Prevalence of sleep related symptoms in four Latin American cities," *Journal of Clinical Sleep Medicine*, vol. 4, no. 6, pp. 579–585, 2008.

[12] J. Kang and S. Chen, "Effects of an irregular bedtime schedule on sleep quality, daytime sleepiness, and fatigue among university students in Taiwan," *BMC Public Health*, vol. 9, article 248, 6 pages, 2009.

[13] A. Al-Rethaiaa, A. Fahmy, and N. Al-Shwaiyat, "Obesity and eating habits among college students in Saudi Arabia: a cross sectional study," *Nutrition Journal*, vol. 9, no. 1, article 39, 10 pages, 2010.

[14] G. Curcio, M. Ferrara, and L. de Gennaro, "Sleep loss, learning capacity and academic performance," *Sleep Medicine Reviews*, vol. 10, no. 5, pp. 323–337, 2006.

[15] V. Lohsoonthorn, H. Khidir, G. Casillas et al., "Sleep quality and sleep patterns in relation to consumption of energy drinks, caffeinated beverages, and other stimulants among Thai college students," *Sleep and Breath*, vol. 17, no. 3, pp. 1017–1028, 2013.

[16] J. Velez, A. Souza, S. Traslavina et al., "The epidemiology of sleep quality and consumption of stimulant beverages among Patagonian Chilean college students," *Sleep Disorders*, vol. 2013, Article ID 910104, 10 pages, 2013.

[17] N. Netzer, R. Stoohs, C. Netzer, K. Clark, and K. Strohl, "Using the Berlin Questionnaire to identify patients at risk for the sleep apnea syndrome," *Annals of Internal Medicine*, vol. 131, no. 7, pp. 485–491, 1999.

[18] F. Chung, B. Yegneswaran, P. Liao et al., "Validation of the Berlin questionnaire and American Society of Anesthesiologists checklist as screening tools for obstructive sleep apnea in surgical patients," *Anesthesiology*, vol. 108, no. 5, pp. 822–830, 2008.

[19] A. Vaz, M. Drummond, P. Mota, M. Severo, J. Almeida, and J. Winck, "Translation of Berlin Questionnaire to Portuguese

language and its application in OSA identifi cation in a sleep disordered breathing clinic," *Revista Portuguesa de Pneumologia*, vol. 17, no. 2, pp. 59–65, 2011.

[20] A. Saleh, M. Ahmad, and N. Awadalla, "Development of Arabic version of Berlin questionnaire to identify obstructive sleep apnea at risk patients," *Annals of Thoracic Medicine*, vol. 6, no. 4, pp. 212–216, 2011.

[21] C. Guindalini, F. Colugnati, R. Pellegrino, R. Santos-Silva, L. Bittencourt, and S. Tufik, "Influence of genetic ancestry on the risk of obstructive sleep apnoea syndrome," *European Respiratory Journal*, vol. 36, no. 4, pp. 834–841, 2010.

[22] O. Adewole, A. Hakeem, A. Fola, E. Anteyi, Z. Ajuwon, and G. Erhabor, "Obstructive sleep apnea among adults in Nigeria," *Journal of the National Medical Association*, vol. 101, no. 7, pp. 720–725, 2009.

[23] C. Moreno, F. Carvalho, C. Lorenzi et al., "High risk for obstructive sleep apnea in truck drivers estimated by the Berlin questionnaire: prevalence and associated factors," *Chronobiology International*, vol. 21, no. 6, pp. 871–879, 2004.

[24] J. Geiger-Brown, V. Rogers, K. Han, A. Trinkoff, R. Bausell, and S. Scharf, "Occupational screening for sleep disorders in 12-h shift nurses using the Berlin Questionnaire," *Sleep and Breathing*, vol. 17, no. 1, pp. 381–388, 2013.

[25] F. Kapsimalis and M. Kryger, "Sleep breathing disorders in the U.S. female population," *Journal of Women's Health*, vol. 18, no. 8, pp. 1211–1219, 2009.

[26] B. Brumpton, A. Langhammer, P. Romundstad, Y. Chen, and X.-M. Mai, "General and abdominal obesity and incident asthma in adults: the HUNT study," *European Respiratory Journal*, vol. 41, no. 2, pp. 323–329, 2013.

[27] K. Alberti, P. Zimmet, and J. Shaw, "The metabolic syndrome—a new worldwide definition," *The Lancet*, vol. 366, no. 9491, pp. 1059–1062, 2005.

[28] J. Dempsey, S. Veasey, B. Morgan, and C. O'Donnell, "Pathophysiology of sleep apnea," *Physiological Reviews*, vol. 90, no. 1, pp. 47–112, 2010.

[29] G. Pillar and N. Shehadeh, "Abdominal fat and sleep apnea: the chicken or the egg?" *Diabetes Care*, vol. 31, supplement 2, pp. S303–S309, 2008.

[30] M. Brennick, A. Pack, K. Ko et al., "Altered upper airway and soft tissue structures in the New Zealand obese mouse," *American Journal of Respiratory and Critical Care Medicine*, vol. 179, no. 2, pp. 158–169, 2009.

[31] G. Nino, M. Gutierrez, A. Ravindra, C. Nino, and C. Rodriguez-Martinez, "Abdominal adiposity correlates with adenotonsillectomy outcome in obese adolescents with severe obstructive sleep apnea," *Pulmonary Medicine*, vol. 2012, Article ID 351037, 8 pages, 2012.

[32] R. Markwald, E. Melanson, M. Smith et al., "Impact of insufficient sleep on total daily energy expenditure, food intake, and weight gain," *Proceedings of the National Academy of Sciences of the United States of America*, vol. 110, no. 14, pp. 5695–5700, 2013.

[33] N. Punjabi, J. Sorkin, L. Katzel, A. Goldberg, A. Schwartz, and P. Smith, "Sleep-disordered breathing and insulin resistance in middle-aged and overweight men," *American Journal of Respiratory and Critical Care Medicine*, vol. 165, no. 5, pp. 677–682, 2002.

[34] G. Mallory Jr., D. Fiser, and R. Jackson, "Sleep-associated breathing disorders in morbidly obese children and adolescents," *The Journal of Pediatrics*, vol. 115, no. 6, pp. 892–897, 1989.

[35] Z. Udwadia, A. Doshi, S. Lonkar, and C. Singh, "Prevalence of sleep-disordered Breathing and sleep apnea in middle-aged urban Indian men," *American Journal of Respiratory and Critical Care Medicine*, vol. 169, no. 2, pp. 168–173, 2004.

[36] O. Resta, M. Foschino-Barbaro, G. Legari et al., "Sleep-related breathing disorders, loud snoring and excessive daytime sleepiness in obese subjects," *International Journal of Obesity*, vol. 25, no. 5, pp. 669–675, 2001.

[37] A. Palla, M. Digiorgio, N. Carpenè et al., "Sleep apnea in morbidly obese patients: prevalence and clinical predictivity," *Respiration*, vol. 78, no. 2, pp. 134–140, 2009.

[38] P. Peppard, T. Young, M. Palta, J. Dempsey, and J. Skatrud, "Longitudinal study of moderate weight change and sleep-disordered breathing," *The Journal of the American Medical Association*, vol. 284, no. 23, pp. 3015–3021, 2000.

[39] N. Kim, S. Lee, C. Eun et al., "Short sleep duration combined with obstructive sleep apnea is associated with visceral obesity in Korean adults," *Sleep*, vol. 36, no. 5, pp. 723–729, 2013.

[40] D. Hiestand, P. Britz, M. Goldman, and B. Phillips, "Prevalence of symptoms and risk of sleep apnea in the US population: results from the national sleep foundation sleep in America 2005 poll," *Chest*, vol. 130, no. 3, pp. 780–786, 2006.

[41] B. Mahboub, S. Afzal, H. Alhariri, A. Alzaabi, M. Vats, and A. Soans, "Prevalence of symptoms and risk of sleep apnea in Dubai, UAE," *International Journal of General Medicine*, vol. 6, pp. 109–114, 2013.

[42] M. Blondet, P. Yapor, G. Latalladi-Ortega, E. Alicea, A. Torres-Palacios, and W. Rodriguez-Cintron, "Prevalence and risk factors for sleep disordered breathing in a Puerto Rican middle-aged population," *Sleep and Breathing*, vol. 13, no. 2, pp. 175–180, 2009.

[43] K. Kang, P. Lee, W. Weng, and W. Hsu, "Body weight status and obstructive sleep apnea in children," *International Journal of Obesity*, vol. 36, no. 7, pp. 920–924, 2012.

[44] C. Marcus, S. Curtis, C. Koerner, A. Joffe, J. Serwint, and G. Loughlin, "Evaluation of pulmonary function and polysomnography in obese children and adolescents," *Pediatric Pulmonology*, vol. 21, no. 3, pp. 176–183, 1996.

[45] S. Verhulst, N. Schrauwen, D. Haentjens et al., "Sleep-disordered breathing in overweight and obese children and adolescents: prevalence, characteristics and the role of fat distribution," *Archives of Disease in Childhood*, vol. 92, no. 3, pp. 205–208, 2007.

[46] Y. Wing, S. Hui, W. Pak et al., "A controlled study of sleep related disordered breathing in obese children," *Archives of Disease in Childhood*, vol. 88, no. 12, pp. 1043–1047, 2003.

[47] P. Peppard, T. Young, J. Barnet, M. Palta, E. Hagen, and K. Hla, "Increased prevalence of sleep-disordered breathing in adults," *American Journal of Epidemiology*, vol. 177, no. 9, pp. 1006–1014, 2013.

[48] J. Gaultney, "The prevalence of sleep disorders in college students: impact on academic performance," *Journal of American College Health*, vol. 59, no. 2, pp. 91–97, 2010.

[49] A. Schwartz, S. Patil, A. Laffan, V. Polotsky, H. Schneider, and P. Smith, "Obesity and obstructive sleep apnea: pathogenic mechanisms and therapeutic approaches," *Proceedings of the American Thoracic Society*, vol. 5, no. 2, pp. 185–192, 2008.

[50] J. Piqueras, W. Kuhne, P. Vera-Villarroel, A. van Straten, and P. Cuijpers, "Happiness and health behaviours in Chilean college students: a cross-sectional survey," *BMC Public Health*, vol. 11, article 443, 10 pages, 2011.

17

Youth, Caregiver, and Prescriber Experiences of Antipsychotic-Related Weight Gain

Andrea Lynn Murphy,[1] David Martin Gardner,[2] Steve Kisely,[3] Charmaine Cooke,[4] Stanley Paul Kutcher,[5] and Jean Hughes[6]

[1] *College of Pharmacy and Department of Psychiatry, Dalhousie University, 5968 College Street, P.O. Box 15000, Halifax, NS, Canada B3H 4R2*

[2] *Department of Psychiatry and College of Pharmacy, Dalhousie University, QEII HSC, AJLB 7517, 5909 Veterans' Memorial Lane, Halifax, NS, Canada B3H 2E2*

[3] *School of Population Health, University of Queensland, Herston, QLD 4006, Australia*

[4] *Department of Health and Wellness, Barrington Tower, P.O. Box 488, Halifax, NS, Canada B3J 2R8*

[5] *Dalhousie University, Department of Psychiatry, Dalhousie University/IWK Health Centre 5850 University Avenue, P.O. Box 9700, Halifax, NS, Canada B3K 6R8*

[6] *School of Nursing, Dalhousie University, 5869 University Avenue, P.O. Box 15000, Halifax, NS, Canada B3H 4R2*

Correspondence should be addressed to Andrea Lynn Murphy; andrea.murphy@dal.ca

Academic Editors: S. Straube and G. S. H. Yeo

Objectives. To explore the lived experience of youth, caregivers, and prescribers with antipsychotic medications. *Design.* We conducted a qualitative interpretive phenomenology study. Youth aged 11 to 25 with recent experience taking antipsychotics, the caregivers of youth taking antipsychotics, and the prescribers of antipsychotics were recruited. *Subjects.* Eighteen youth, 10 caregivers (parents), and 11 prescribers participated. *Results.* Eleven of 18 youth, six of ten parents, and all prescribers discussed antipsychotic-related weight gain. Participants were attuned to the numeric weight changes usually measured in pounds. Significant discussions occurred around weight changes in the context of body image, adherence and persistence, managing weight increases, and metabolic effects. These concepts were often inextricably linked but maintained the significance as separate issues. Participants discussed tradeoffs regarding the perceived benefits and risks of weight gain, often with uncertainty and inadequate information regarding the short- and long-term consequences. *Conclusion.* Antipsychotic-related weight gain in youth influences body image and weight management strategies and impacts treatment courses with respect to adherence and persistence. In our study, the experience of monitoring for weight and metabolic changes was primarily reactive in nature. Participants expressed ambiguity regarding the short- and long-term consequences of weight and metabolic changes.

1. Introduction

Second generation antipsychotic prescribing to young people under 25 years of age is increasing internationally [1–12]. The rise in prescription trends has generated controversy given available pediatric evidence for second generation antipsychotic effectiveness and safety data and the unknown long-term consequences with intermittent or continuous exposure [13–16]. Antipsychotic-related weight gain and changes in the metabolic profile (e.g., glucose and lipid homeostasis) that occur following, or in concert with, weight gain are frequently discussed as significant treatment-related issues. The explicit mechanisms of antipsychotic-related weight gain are not fully understood [17–24] nor are the best management approaches (e.g., lifestyle, pharmacologic), but research in these areas continues [17, 25–33].

Predictive or risk factors for antipsychotic-related weight gain are also unknown but some inferences can be made from available syntheses of the literature. These factors include lower pretreatment body mass index (BMI), triglyceride levels, more negative symptoms, polypharmacy, concomitant antidepressants, and younger age [34, 35]. Predisposing factors are similar for pediatrics and antipsychotic-naïve patients, and younger age groups appear to be at highest risk [36, 37]. Weight gain may also be more dramatic with younger patients compared to adults [36].

Given the local and international trends in utilization and controversies regarding effectiveness and safety of antipsychotics, we explored the lived experience of youth taking antipsychotics, their caregivers, and prescribers through a qualitative study using an interpretive phenomenological approach. This paper focuses on the experience of weight gain for youth taking antipsychotics, their caregivers, and the prescribers.

2. Methods

To understand the experience of antipsychotic use, we used interpretive phenomenology. Phenomenology studies the person in the situation, rather than in isolation [38]. We followed a staged approach modeled after Diekelmann et al. [39]. In stage one, all transcripts were read by AM and DG as a whole to gain a complete picture or overall understanding of the data considering weight gain. In stage two, we summarized sections of the transcripts and identified categories within weight gain. We met weekly for a month to discuss our interpretations of the categories and provided text quotes to demonstrate support. We worked to achieve consensus in the categories. In stage three, we continued with independent analysis of transcripts and compared interpretations of the categories with supporting text. In stage four, we sought to examine relational themes. Throughout the process we engaged in reflexivity through journaling. Among other strategies, our analysis process facilitated achieving credibility and dependability. We used several approaches for confirmability and transferability. Transferability may be limited to an extent as the study occurred within a Canadian province with a predominantly publically financed system (70% public, 30% private).

3. Sample and Recruitment Procedures

We recruited low income youth, defined as youth receiving government income assistance, aged 11 to 25 years, who were prescribed antipsychotics within the last two years. We also recruited their caregivers/support people. General practitioners and psychiatrists who prescribed antipsychotics to youth in the last six months and licensed to practice in Nova Scotia, a Canadian province, were eligible and were informed of the study for physician recruitment purposes and also to facilitate youth and caregiver recruitment. We advertised broadly in public places and on the Internet. All participants were offered the choice of a one time interview or focus group, and each participant was paid a one-time honorarium.

4. Data Collection

Separate interview guides (available upon request) with main and probing questions were developed for each group of participants. Youth, caregiver, and physician interviews and one physician focus group were conducted between January of 2010 and August of 2010. All interactions with participants were recorded and transcribed except one face-to-face interview (one youth refused to be recorded). All audio recordings were transcribed, and, during cleaning of transcripts by the interviewer, field notes and jottings were used to insert comments and reflections when appropriate. Responsive interviewing techniques were used with an iterative process of data analysis occurring during data collection [40]. Once cleaned, transcripts were stored and organized using Atlas.ti 6.2.

4.1. Ethical Approvals. Ethics approval was obtained from the research ethics boards (REB) of Capital District Health Authority and the IWK Health Centre given that our population spanned young people and adults. Both of these REBs have reciprocal ethical agreements with Dalhousie University REB.

4.2. Findings. The theme of weight gain emerged from an analysis of approximately 13 hours of audio from 18 youths who ranged in age from 13 to 26. Table 1 shows the range of medications and diagnoses as described by participants. The two 26-year olds were included in the analysis as their most recent antipsychotic exposures were in their 25th year of life. One youth and caregiver pair were related (i.e., mother and son) in our study, and they were interviewed separately. We collected 11 audio hours from 10 female caregivers, who will herein be referred to as "parents" given all caregivers described themselves as a "parent" and 7 audio hours from 11 prescribers ($n = 5$ prescribers in a focus group and $n = 6$ prescriber individual interviews).

Eleven of 18 youth, six of ten parents, and all prescribers discussed antipsychotic-related weight gain. Participants were highly attuned to the number in pounds as a metric for weight changes. Within the theme of weight gain, we further categorized and coded the data with body image, adherence and persistence, managing weight gain, and metabolic effects. Within the experiences of participants, these concepts were often inextricably linked, but each maintained significance as a separate concept.

4.3. Body Image. Changes in body weight affected body image and the potential to experience stigma related to weight gain. Youth were not only coping with their own emotions with weight changes but also managing the responses of others to their physical appearance. Parents and prescribers similarly discussed the concept of body image, but the concerns more shifted towards long-term implications of weight gain from a safety lens or adherence to medications. Prescribers' perceptions of the youth consciousness with weight changes were an underlying consideration in the prescriber choice of antipsychotic and anticipated adherence patterns in youth.

TABLE 1: Youth participant demographics and self-reported medications and diagnoses.

Youth	Gender	Age	Medication(s) named in participant experiences	Self-reported conditions
(1) Youth 1	Female	19	Quetiapine, Strattera, Adderall	Bipolar, depressed, mood disorder, anxiety, panic attacks
(2) Antidepressant interview				
(3) Youth 2	Female	26	Olanzapine, lorazepam, risperidone, citalopram, trazodone	Psychosis, psychosis not otherwise specified, sleep disorder
(4) Youth 3	Male	25	Risperidone, olanzapine, ziprasidone, citalopram	Psychosis
(5) Youth 4	Male	24	Paxil, lithium, "a lot of different antipsychotics"	Depression, paranoid, bipolar schizophrenia, bipolar, schizo-affective, schizophrenia with bipolar
(6) Youth 5	Female	18	Quetiapine, Cipralex, clonazepam	OCD*, anxiety
(7) Youth 6	Female	21	Quetiapine, lorazepam, Risperdal, Celexa, Effexor	Schizophrenic, bipolar
(8) Youth 7	Male	24	Risperidone	Psychosis
(9) Youth 8	Male	17	Quetiapine	Paranoia
(10) Antidepressant interview				
(11) Youth 9	Male	26	Divalproex, olanzapine, clonazepam, Dilaudid	ADHD†, "bipolar schizophrenic"
(12) Youth 10	Female	23	Cipralex, Wellbutrin, clonazepam, risperidone	Drug-induced psychosis, Paranoid schizophrenia, ADHD†, anxiety
(13) Youth 11	Female	25	Lithium, olanzapine, citalopram, Ciprolex, citalopram, Wellbutrin, zopiclone	Anxiety, depression, bipolar, manic
(14) Youth 12	Female	21	Quetiapine, Zoloft, risperidone, Prozac, Paxil, lorazepam, clonazepam, diazepam, lorazepam	Borderline personality disorder
(15) Youth 13	Female	22	Lithium, risperidone, ziprasidone, Cipralex, Epival	Bipolar, psychosis
(16) Youth 14	Male	20	Risperidone, Dexedrine, Ritalin, Wellbutrin	ADHD†, ADD‡, seizure disorder, autism
(17) Youth 15	Male	13	Biphentin, risperidone	ADHD†, anger problem, violent behaviour

*OCD: Obsessive compulsive disorder.
†ADHD: attention deficit hyperactivity disorder.
‡ADD: attention deficit disorder.

Youth 9:

> *"I don't like that I have a belly. People are like, 'Oh, you got chubby in the face.' And I'm like, 'It's because I'm taking my medication, bastard. Shut the f%$# up!'."*

Youth 11:

> *"... I've gained at least 15 pounds. And probably... I heard that usually there's a 6 month cap on it. So I'm in the clear, I guess. But I'm completely unhappy with my body."*

4.4. Managing Weight Gain. Participants in our study discussed strategies that were used in mitigating weight gain or managing potential or existing weight gain through various choices. These included consideration of the initial choice of antipsychotic in terms of its potential to cause weight gain, switching of antipsychotics, lifestyle interventions (e.g., diet, exercise), pharmacological treatments, and nonadherence or eventual antipsychotic discontinuation.

For youth, there was a frustration expressed when results of their efforts to minimize weight gain were not what they expected. Youth employed lifestyle strategies such as diet and exercise or talked about planning to initiate these strategies. Medication switches were discussed although these were initiated by prescribers. Discontinuation initiated by youth themselves was also used as an approach to stopping weight gain.

One prescriber in the focus group was the only prescriber to discuss nonswitch pharmacologic options such as metformin to manage antipsychotic induced weight gain, and other members of the group appeared unaware of this option based on the ensuing discussion. For initial antipsychotic choice, several prescribers discussed their previous experiences with patients who had gained weight and also their own values as being influential in how they made their antipsychotic choices.

Parents discussed youth engaging in behaviours to manage weight including exercising and dieting and also stopping medications. It was also evident from several parents that they made distinctions among antipsychotics, including "newer" versus "older" agents, about which were better or worse for causing weight gain, and revealing preferences for agent choice for their youth.

Youth 7:

> *"... And I was exercising, eating the same way. I find taking weight off is impossible. Weight gain, weight gain, weight gain. Big time on the weight gain on the pill."*

Youth 13:

> *"Well, I had a lot of weight gain on the Risperdal. Interviewer: And is this one supposed to be better? Youth 13: Yes, it's supposed to be better and it has been because I've actually lost weight on it since... ... Interviewer: Can you put a number on what you think you've gained? Youth 13: Overall, it was like 100 pounds."*

Parent 7:

> *"... The Seroquel is not as bad as the Risperdal. ... Yes. But the Seroquel has a weight gain thing too but it's not as bad for her anyway."*

Prescriber 4:

> *"And a situation where I have 2 parents who are [profession] [and] a child with autism. I started the child on the medication. The child started to gain weight. They were so desperate to keep him on medication because it changed his life, it changed their life. They did everything possible in the way of diet management, exercise management. Just everything possible to make sure that they minimized any metabolic effects."*

Prescriber 5:

> *"... If somebody told me, 'Take this drug. It will make you feel better but you will gain 30 pounds,' I'd say, 'no thanks'."*

4.5. Adherence and Persistence. Adherence is described as the extent that patients follow instructions provided for treatments [41] including conforming to dosing, frequency, and timing of medications [42]. Persistence is defined as the length of time that a therapy is taken from initiation to discontinuation [42]. Medication adherence and persistence are considered important components in managing symptoms of mental illness. Participants in our study discussed adherence, nonadherence, and choices made with persistence to medication directly in the context of weight gain. It seems that youth who were committed to adhering to, and persisting with, their antipsychotics had realized or perceived a benefit from treatment or understood it to be important. Youth 7 discussed exercising in response to gaining "40 pounds in nine months" after he "agreed to take" his medication and also stating, "I've got to stay on this medication and keep taking it". For one youth, she discussed discontinuing her antipsychotic due to sedation and weight gain and that this decision irreparably altered the patient-prescriber relationship.

Prescribers similarly discussed how weight gain would promote nonadherence, and this mainly centred on the belief that youth would be concerned with body image. Weight gain was generally seen as a barrier to adherence and a reason for nonadherence and lack of persistence. One prescriber's experience was that youth often withheld information about whether they persist with therapies. It also became evident that, for some prescribers, they too were challenged regarding adherence and persistence with intended treatment courses for their patient in light of weight gain. One prescriber shared information around ambivalence when weight gain occurs in the face of benefits.

Youth 2:

> *"Like January/February 2008 when I stopped taking this medication, I went to him and I was like, 'Look, I don't know why I'm taking this. It's a small dose but I'm tired all the time. I'm gaining weight.' And I'm like, 'I've actually already stopped taking it.' And he's like, 'Well, if you're not going to take the medication I prescribed you, there's nothing more I can do for you. I can have your files transferred to a different psychiatrist,' which is closer to where I live so I wouldn't have to go to [city] every time."*

Parent 8:

> *"... Then she started to gain some weight with the Invega. And my daughter is very petite and very, very conscious of her appearance and things like that. ... And gaining weight just wasn't in the cards. And she was really quite upset by that. ... The barriers really are around the weight gain and then they don't want to stay on it."*

Focus Group

Prescriber 1:

> *" So even though they may not be getting diabetic, the fact that they've gained 25 pounds on one of the antipsychotics, they may stop taking it. So that will impact. And they don't tell you."*

Prescriber 4:

> *"... Antipsychotic medications to some extent I have a little more concern about. And yet parents are a little less aware of that, unless they are well informed parents. Or until the child has been on the medication for 3 months and they start to see the child is gaining a bit more weight than they need. So we have to work to help them appreciate that this is important. But then we run into a different kind of ambivalence. The child might be functioning really well but now they are uncertain*

what to do about the weight gain, and they don't want to lose the well functioning. They feel as though they've got a child in their home for the first time. So it's a difficult situation. It's a difficult situation for us too."

4.6. Metabolic Side Effects. There was a significant discussion of "metabolic side effects", which created decisional conflicts for participants. Parents discussed concerns of the long-term consequences based on current weight or weight gain and married this information with family histories of conditions such as diabetes. One parent also discussed a concern regarding a lack of monitoring regarding cholesterol. One prescriber discussed heart disease and cholesterol whereas others that discussed metabolic side effects in the context of weight gain focused on diabetes and glucose.

Participants such as Youth 7 were concerned about diabetes in light of existing lab values, but his experience indicates he may not fully understand the possible risk or potential likelihood of having the "list" of side effects.

Prescribers expressed concern regarding the side effects, and one pleaded for judicious and rational use because of limited long-term pharmacovigilance data. Prescriber 3 through encouraging the rational use of the medications also shed light on wider systems issues. Although the medications may be viewed as a "quick fix" for some in a cost-constrained system, the potential long-term implications would not be offset by immediate gratification. They also expressed concern regarding adequacy of knowledge translation efforts regarding the use of the medications.

Youth 7:

"The only other side effect I'm worrying about actually with Risperdal... Well, one other side effect is it can cause permanent diabetes. And my blood sugar levels are a little bit high since I've been taking the pill. And the other one is the inability to conceive children. That's also a possibility. And I'm worried about that one. But I mean I get this list of side effects, and I'm like, 'Ah, what am I going to get?'."

Parent 9:

" So I had major, major concerns because he put on 70 pounds. ... I am diabetic. And weight gain is a major factor."

Parent 5:

"Yes, I do have a family doctor but she... I haven't talked to her. Because one of the things I noticed actually... I don't think [psychiatrist's name] had mentioned it, or I didn't actually pick it up, was [son's name] should probably actually have blood work done so he has a base to go by. Because if there's any problems with cholesterol or anything like that, he should kind of be watched. My doctor is not the greatest. You can get in to her right quick and she can give you a pad and then out you go. But he hasn't actually talked to her about anything."

Focus Group Discussion

Prescriber 1:

"I am seeing younger people like in the early 20s, even in late teens, where if they have a family history of diabetes as well, it's really important to get baseline blood work because it can happen."

Interview, Prescriber 2:

"I tend to stay away from olanzapine because I've had experience and ... Well, I tend to use quetiapine. That is such a crap shoot. And I don't know ... This is more like the art or the cookery, the recipe of medicine, but I've had experience with clients becoming diabetic on olanzapine."

Prescriber 3:

"... And not just a bit of change in your blood sugar but diabetes, and changes in your cholesterol, and setting people up for heart disease later on. ... ... I just don't know how widespread the caution is yet... . Like people are like for the last 5 or 6 years have been like 'okay, everybody, these drugs are scary'. Like, let's think. For some people, they need them, but let's be responsible. Let's think about who needs them, who doesn't. Let's think about how long they need them. Let's think about how we monitor when they are on it to make sure we don't cause them life-long problems... But I don't know how well that knowledge has been transmitted across the board in terms of people prescribing. And I think there are serious pressures because of resource issues, not just in [location] but everywhere in mental health, that it's easier to... that drugs are more accessible in general, ... cost being a factor. But it's easier to get a drug than to get therapies in general."

5. Discussion

Our qualitative study in the Canadian context is unique in that it gives insights into the lived experiences of three groups (youth, parents, and prescribers) with antipsychotic-related weight gain and related implications in the broader context of the lived experience of antipsychotics.

To our knowledge, this is the first study of this kind in Canada. The experiences of youth, parents, and prescribers were largely negative regarding weight gain and impacted body image and adherence and persistence with medications. Managing weight gain was a complex phenomenon, and various strategies were reported by participants. An overarching fear and concern related to metabolic side effects was evident in our data.

The rising prevalence of obesity in Canadian children and adolescents has become a public health concern [43, 44]. Ball and McCargar [43] conducted a review of prevalence and risk factor literature from studies in children and adolescents. The etiology of increasingly overweight and obese children and adolescents is thought to be multifactorial including such factors related to lifestyle (e.g., limited physical activity, rising physical inactivity), eating behaviours and nutrition, and higher height and weight subsequently leading to higher BMIs with earlier maturation [43]. Medications, including psychotropics, can also cause weight gain in children and adolescents [45, 46]. Meta-analysis data ranking antipsychotic-related weight gain are available for adults [47], and mean weight changes with antipsychotics versus placebo in children up to 18 years of age show higher increases with olanzapine at 3.47 kg (95% CI 2.94, 3.99), risperidone with 1.72 kg (95% CI 1.17, 2.26), quetiapine with 1.41 kg (95% CI 1.10, 1.81), and aripiprazole at 0.85 kg (95% CI 0.58, 1.13) [15]. The experience of weight gain with antipsychotics as discussed in our study from youth, parent, and prescriber perspectives focused heavily on numeric values in pounds of weight with wide ranges of weight gain described. An inherent limitation in our study is the inability to determine if the changes self-reported by youth and parents were abnormal. We did not explicitly link weight gain with diet, physical activity, other concomitant medications, or family histories of cardiometabolic conditions. Based on the experience of some youth and parents reporting weight gains of 70 to 100 pounds, we can infer that this would be considered abnormal and its consequences in some cases would be considered significant. There was a general concern from both the prescribers and parents that the weight gain they observed, regardless of the quantity, was a negative consequence of antipsychotics for youth.

Several anthropometric measures of body adiposity (e.g., weight, BMI, height to weight ratio, waist circumference, etc.) are available, and a standardization regarding what metrics should be used remains to be established [48]. The association of these metrics with cardiometabolic disease in adults is varied, and more research is required with the application of these metrics to long-term outcomes in children [34, 36, 43, 49–51]. The current Canadian guidelines published in 2011 on the monitoring of weight-related measures in children and adolescents taking antipsychotics recommend BMI and waist circumference measurements [52]. In our study, weight was reported as a change (i.e., increase) and in pounds. BMI and other measurements were not discussed. The Canadian guidelines were not published at the time of our interviews in 2010. The guidelines provide a good basis for clinicians to engage in monitoring practices; however, it is difficult in the context of individual patients to determine how much weight gain can be caused by individual psychotropics, the velocity at which it occurs, whether it plateaus, who is most at risk, how to manage it, and what significance is produced by the outcome given that the research in this area is limited in high quality studies of ample quantity [47, 53]. To date, studies that have examined monitoring practices show that of all parameters suggested for monitoring, weight measures are the most commonly performed [54].

A major conundrum that is apparent in the literature on the topic of antipsychotic-related weight gain in youth, or as identified in our study as "ambivalence," emerged from our data and was aptly described by a prescriber discussing weight gain occurring in concert with much anticipated and hoped for benefits of therapy. The issue of what to do in response to weight gain is especially complex when perceived positive impacts occur. Weight gain is really one of several surrogate markers of interest in relation to cardiometabolic diseases. The potential association with chronic disease (e.g., cardiovascular and endocrine) development and related morbidity and mortality is of great importance given the significant strain on population health and economic and social welfare [55]. The issue of weight gain is complicated in clinical scenarios by the fact that more than one medication in a regimen can be the cause (e.g., lithium and olanzapine used in managing bipolar disorder) or even mitigating it (e.g., stimulants). Weight changes are also set against a backdrop of physical changes occurring at developmental stages and changes in weight that may have occurred due to illness. Further, more data is needed to provide clarity regarding weight gain and cardiometabolic risks in youth taking these medications [36]. Because of these simultaneously moving targets and need for better data, making decisions regarding the appropriate course of action can be extremely complicated for youth, families, and prescribers. How these factors are prioritized in decision making within these three groups is not well known. In our study, the concerns for metabolic side effects and weight gain were apparent and influential on behaviours. Prescribers discussed their own personal values and tacit experience with treating patients and decisional dilemmas around choice of agents with one describing it as "such a crap shoot". Past experiences with patients developing diabetes steered one prescriber away from using the medications. Parents also described their knowledge of the side effects from what they observed and their concerns based on family histories of metabolic conditions (e.g., diabetes). Although the concern by parents was expressed, there was little resolution in their conflicted feelings as it appears that the youth and prescriber ultimately would be making decisions about weight management.

Interestingly, the prescribers in our study tended to be focused on glucose related complications more so than cholesterol with only one prescriber discussing "heart disease" and cholesterol. The parent and youth experience of prescriber based monitoring appeared to be variable in quantity and quality. Rates of guideline concordant monitoring of antipsychotic-related cardiometabolic side effects are often poor [54]. The approach to managing and monitoring antipsychotic-related weight gain and potential cardiometabolic effects appears mainly reactive without forethought of a larger management plan for mitigating the effects.

In addition to potential physical health concerns created by obesity, negative psychosocial consequences can result from being overweight and obese [43]. Youth in our study described impacts on body image. In adults, psychotropic related weight gain has been shown to impair quality of life proportionally with weight gain and increased feeling of hopelessness and decreased self-worth [56]. Further explication of the complex relationships with antipsychotic-related weight gain in youth and its effects on quality of life, self image, and its impact on adherence in younger people is warranted [57].

This qualitative study demonstrates that antipsychotic-related weight gain is associated with significant physical, and mental consequences and there is a shared concern regarding these sequelae among youth, parents, and prescribers. More research is needed regarding the short- and long-term implications of weight gain and cardiometabolic effects and how the risks and benefits of treatment are managed by patients and prescribers in therapeutic decision making.

List of Brand Name Medications (Alphabetical) Discussed by Participants and Their Respective Generic Names

Adderall:	Dextroamphetamine and levoamphetamine mixed salts
Biphentin:	Methylphenidate
Cipralex:	Escitalopram
Dexedrine:	Dextroamphetamine
Dilaudid:	Hydromorphone
Epival:	Divalproex sodium
Invega:	Paliperidone
Paxil:	Paroxetine
Prozac:	Fluoxetine
Risperdal:	Risperidone
Ritalin:	Methylphenidate
Seroquel:	Quetiapine
Strattera:	Atomoxetine
Wellbutrin:	Bupropion
Zoloft:	Sertraline.

Conflict of Interests

The authors declare no conflict of interests.

Acknowledgments

Funding for this research was obtained from the Nova Scotia Health Research Foundation (NSHRF). The expressed views are those of the authors and do not represent NSHRF.

References

[1] S. Alessi-Severini, R. G. Biscontri, D. M. Collins, J. Sareen, and M. W. Enns, "Ten years of antipsychotic prescribing to children: a Canadian population-based study," *Canadian Journal of Psychiatry*, vol. 57, no. 1, pp. 52–58, 2012.

[2] R. R. Aparasu and V. Bhatara, "Antipsychotic prescribing trends among youths, 1997–2002," *Psychiatric Services*, vol. 56, no. 8, article 904, 2005.

[3] W. O. Cooper, P. G. Arbogast, H. Ding, G. B. Hickson, D. C. Fuchs, and W. A. Ray, "Trends in prescribing of antipsychotic medications for US children," *Ambulatory Pediatrics*, vol. 6, no. 2, pp. 79–83, 2006.

[4] R. Goodwin, M. S. Gould, C. Blanco, and M. Olfson, "Prescription of psychotropic medications to youths in office-based practice," *Psychiatric Services*, vol. 52, no. 8, pp. 1081–1087, 2001.

[5] M. Harrison-Woolrych, J. Garcia-Quiroga, J. Ashton, and P. Herbison, "Safety and usage of atypical antipsychotic medicines in children: a nationwide prospective cohort study," *Drug Safety*, vol. 30, no. 7, pp. 569–579, 2007.

[6] M. Olfson, C. Blanco, S. M. Liu, S. Wang, and C. U. Correll, "National trends in the office-based treatment of children, adolescents, and adults with antipsychotics," *Archives of General Psychiatry*, vol. 69, no. 12, pp. 1247–1256, 2012.

[7] N. C. Patel, M. L. Crismon, K. Hoagwood et al., "Trends in the use of typical and atypical antipsychotics in children and adolescents," *Journal of the American Academy of Child and Adolescent Psychiatry*, vol. 44, no. 6, pp. 548–556, 2005.

[8] T. Pringsheim, D. Lam, and S. B. Patten, "The pharmacoepidemiology of antipsychotic medications for canadian children and adolescents: 2005–2009," *Journal of Child and Adolescent Psychopharmacology*, vol. 21, no. 6, pp. 537–543, 2011.

[9] F. Rani, M. L. Murray, P. J. Byrne, and I. C. K. Wong, "Epidemiologic features of antipsychotic prescribing to children and adolescents in primary care in the United Kingdom," *Pediatrics*, vol. 121, no. 5, pp. 1002–1009, 2008.

[10] E. Schirm, H. Tobi, J. M. Zito, and L. T. de Jong-van den Berg, "Psychotropic medication in children: a study from the Netherlands," *Pediatrics*, vol. 108, no. 2, article E25, 2001.

[11] B. Vitiello, C. Correll, B. van Zwieten-Boot, A. Zuddas, M. Parellada, and C. Arango, "Antipsychotics in children and adolescents: increasing use, evidence for efficacy and safety concerns," *European Neuropsychopharmacology*, vol. 19, no. 9, pp. 629–635, 2009.

[12] J. M. Zito, D. J. Safer, L. T. W. de Jong-van den Berg et al., "A three-country comparison of psychotropic medication prevalence in youth," *Child and Adolescent Psychiatry and Mental Health*, vol. 2, article 26, 2008.

[13] J. C. Seida, J. R. Schouten, K. Boylan et al., "Antipsychotics for children and young adults: a comparative effectiveness review," *Pediatrics*, vol. 129, no. 3, pp. e771–e784, 2012.

[14] Canadian Adverse Reaction Newsletter, "Second-generation antipsychotics and cardiometabolic adverse reactions," *Canadian Adverse Reaction Newsletter*, vol. 22, no. 1, 2012.

[15] T. Pringsheim, D. Lam, H. Ching, and S. Patten, "Metabolic and neurological complications of second-generation antipsychotic use in children: a systematic review and meta-analysis of randomized controlled trials," *Drug Safety*, vol. 34, no. 8, pp. 651–668, 2011.

[16] C. Panagiotopoulos, R. Ronsley, D. Elbe, J. Davidson, and D. H. Smith, "First do no harm: promoting an evidence-based approach to atypical antipsychotic use in children and adolescents," *Journal of the Canadian Academy of Child and Adolescent Psychiatry*, vol. 19, no. 2, pp. 124–137, 2010.

[17] T. Baptista, "Body weight gain induced by antipsychotic drugs: mechanisms and management," *Acta Psychiatrica Scandinavica*, vol. 100, no. 1, pp. 3–16, 1999.

[18] C. Deng, K. Weston-Green, and X.-F. Huang, "The role of histaminergic H1 and H3 receptors in food intake: a mechanism for atypical antipsychotic-induced weight gain?" *Progress in Neuro-Psychopharmacology and Biological Psychiatry*, vol. 34, no. 1, pp. 1–4, 2010.

[19] H. Hosojima, T. Togo, T. Odawara et al., "Early effects of olanzapine on serum levels of ghrelin, adiponectin and leptin

in patients with schizophrenia," *Journal of Psychopharmacology*, vol. 20, no. 1, pp. 75–79, 2006.

[20] D. J. Müller, C. C. Zai, M. Sicard et al., "Systematic analysis of dopamine receptor genes (DRD1-DRD5) in antipsychotic-induced weight gain," *Pharmacogenomics Journal*, vol. 12, no. 2, pp. 156–164, 2012.

[21] E. Palik, K. D. Birkás, G. Faludi, I. Karádi, and K. Cseh, "Correlation of serum ghrelin levels with body mass index and carbohydrate metabolism in patients treated with atypical antipsychotics," *Diabetes Research and Clinical Practice*, vol. 68, supplement 1, pp. S60–S64, 2005.

[22] R. Perez-Iglesias, I. Mata, J. A. Amado et al., "Effect of FTO, SH2B1, LEP, and LEPR polymorphisms on weight gain associated with antipsychotic treatment," *Journal of Clinical Psychopharmacology*, vol. 30, no. 6, pp. 661–666, 2010.

[23] G. P. Reynolds, M. J. Hill, and S. L. Kirk, "The S-HT2C receptor and antipsychotic-induced weight gain—mechanisms and genetics," *Journal of Psychopharmacology*, vol. 20, supplement 4, pp. S15–S18, 2006.

[24] M. N. Sicard, C. C. Zai, A. K. Tiwari et al., "Polymorphisms of the HTR2C gene and antipsychotic-induced weight gain: an update and meta-analysis," *Pharmacogenomics*, vol. 11, no. 11, pp. 1561–1571, 2010.

[25] L. Maayan, J. Vakhrusheva, and C. U. Correll, "Effectiveness of medications used to attenuate antipsychotic-related weight gain and metabolic abnormalities: a systematic review and meta-analysis," *Neuropsychopharmacology*, vol. 35, no. 7, pp. 1520–1530, 2010.

[26] S. K. Praharaj, A. K. Jana, N. Goyal, and V. K. Sinha, "Metformin for olanzapine-induced weight gain: a systematic review and meta-analysis," *British Journal of Clinical Pharmacology*, vol. 71, no. 3, pp. 377–382, 2011.

[27] D. B. Allison, J. L. Mentore, M. Heo et al., "Antipsychotic-induced weight gainaA comprehensive research synthesis," *American Journal of Psychiatry*, vol. 156, no. 11, pp. 1686–1696, 1999.

[28] M. Álvarez-Jiménez, O. Martínez-García, R. Pérez-Iglesias, M. L. Ramírez, J. L. Vázquez-Barquero, and B. Crespo-Facorro, "Prevention of antipsychotic-induced weight gain with early behavioural intervention in first-episode psychosis: 2-year results of a randomized controlled trial," *Schizophrenia Research*, vol. 116, no. 1, pp. 16–19, 2010.

[29] B. Parsons, D. B. Allison, A. Loebel et al., "Weight effects associated with antipsychotics: a comprehensive database analysis," *Schizophrenia Research*, vol. 110, no. 1–3, pp. 103–110, 2009.

[30] V. Simon, R. van Winkel, and M. de Hert, "Are weight gain and metabolic side effects of atypical antipsychotics dose dependent? A literature review," *Journal of Clinical Psychiatry*, vol. 70, no. 7, pp. 1041–1050, 2009.

[31] D. M. Taylor and R. McAskill, "Atypical antipsychotics and weight gain—a systematic review," *Acta Psychiatrica Scandinavica*, vol. 101, no. 6, pp. 416–432, 2000.

[32] D. K. Raynor and D. Dickinson, "Key principles to guide development of consumer medicine information—content analysis of information design texts," *Annals of Pharmacotherapy*, vol. 43, no. 4, pp. 700–706, 2009.

[33] M. Álvarez-Jiménez, S. E. Hetrick, C. González-Blanch, J. F. Gleeson, and P. D. McGorry, "Non-pharmacological management of antipsychotic-induced weight gain: systematic review and meta-analysis of randomised controlled trials," *British Journal of Psychiatry*, vol. 193, no. 2, pp. 101–107, 2008.

[34] D. L. Foley and K. I. Morley, "Systematic review of early cardiometabolic outcomes of the first treated episode of psychosis," *Archives of General Psychiatry*, vol. 68, no. 6, pp. 609–616, 2011.

[35] S. Gentile, "Contributing factors to weight gain during long-term treatment with second-generation antipsychotics. A systematic appraisal and clinical implications," *Obesity Reviews*, vol. 10, no. 5, pp. 527–542, 2009.

[36] L. Maayan and C. U. Correll, "Weight gain and metabolic risks associated with antipsychotic medications in children and adolescents," *Journal of Child and Adolescent Psychopharmacology*, vol. 21, no. 6, pp. 517–535, 2011.

[37] M. Álvarez-Jiménez, C. González-Blanch, B. Crespo-Facorro et al., "Antipsychotic-induced weight gain in chronic and first-episode psychotic disorders: a systematic critical reappraisal," *CNS Drugs*, vol. 22, no. 7, pp. 547–562, 2008.

[38] P. Benner, "Quality of life: a phenomenological perspective on explanation, prediction, and understanding in nursing science," *Advances in Nursing Science*, vol. 8, no. 1, pp. 1–14, 1985.

[39] N. Diekelmann, D. Allen, and C. Tanner, *A Hermeneutic Analysis of the NLN Criteria for the Appraisal of Baccalaureate Programs. The NLN Criteria for Appraisal of Baccaiaureate Programs: A Critical Hermeneutic Analysis*, National League for Nursing, New York, NY, USA, 1989.

[40] H. J. Streubert and D. R. Carpenter, *Qualitative Research in Nursing. Advancing the Humanistic Imperative*, Lippincott, Williams & Wilkins, Philadelphia, Pa, USA, 2003.

[41] R. B. Haynes, X. Yao, A. Degani, S. Kripalani, A. Garg, and H. P. McDonald, "Interventions to enhance medication adherence," *Cochrane Database of Systematic Rreviews*, no. 4, Article ID CD000011, 2005.

[42] J. A. Cramer, A. Roy, A. Burrell et al., "Medication compliance and persistence: terminology and definitions," *Value in Health*, vol. 11, no. 1, pp. 44–47, 2008.

[43] G. D. C. Ball and L. J. McCargar, "Childhood obesity in Canada: a review of prevalence estimates and risk factors for cardiovascular diseases and type 2 diabetes," *Canadian Journal of Applied Physiology*, vol. 28, no. 1, pp. 117–140, 2003.

[44] D. C. W. Lau, J. D. Douketis, K. M. Morrison, I. M. Hramiak, A. M. Sharma, and E. Ur, "2006 Canadian clinical practice guidelines on the management and prevention of obesity in adults and children," *Canadian Medical Association Journal*, vol. 176, supplement 8, pp. S1–S13, 2007.

[45] J. M. Jerrell and R. S. McIntyre, "Metabolic, digestive, and reproductive adverse events associated with antimanic treatment in children and adolescents: a retrospective cohort study," *Primary Care Companion to the Journal of Clinical Psychiatry*, vol. 12, no. 4, 2010.

[46] V. Hamrin, E. M. McCarthy, and V. Tyson, "Pediatric psychotropic medication initiation and adherence: a literature review based on social exchange theory," *Journal of Child and Adolescent Psychiatric Nursing*, vol. 23, no. 3, pp. 151–172, 2010.

[47] R. Dent, A. Blackmore, J. Peterson et al., "Changes in body weight and psychotropic drugs: a systematic synthesis of the literature," *PLoS One*, vol. 7, no. 6, Article ID e36889, 2012.

[48] W. V. R. Vieweg, A. B. Sood, A. Pandurangi, and J. J. Silverman, "Newer antipsychotic drugs and obesity in children and adolescents. How should we assess drug-associated weight gain?" *Acta Psychiatrica Scandinavica*, vol. 111, no. 3, pp. 177–184, 2005.

[49] A. J. Cameron, D. J. Magliano, and S. Soderberg, "A systematic review of the impact of including both waist and hip circumference in risk models for cardiovascular diseases, diabetes and mortality," *Obesity Reviews*, vol. 14, no. 1, pp. 86–94, 2013.

[50] S. Kodama, C. Horikawa, K. Fujihara et al., "Comparisons of the strength of associations with future type 2 diabetes risk among anthropometric obesity indicators, including waist-to-height ratio: a meta-analysis," *American Journal of Epidemiology*, vol. 176, no. 11, pp. 959–969, 2012.

[51] S. M. Haffner, "Relationship of metabolic risk factors and development of cardiovascular disease and diabetes," *Obesity*, vol. 14, supplement 3, pp. 121S–127S, 2006.

[52] J. Ho, C. Panagiotopoulos, B. Mccrindle, S. Grisaru, and T. Pringsheim, "Management recommendations for metabolic complications associated with second generation antipsychotic use in children and youth," *Journal of the Canadian Academy of Child and Adolescent Psychiatry*, vol. 20, no. 3, pp. 234–241, 2011.

[53] W. S. Leslie, C. R. Hankey, and M. E. J. Lean, "Weight gain as an adverse effect of some commonly prescribed drugs: a systematic review," *QJM*, vol. 100, no. 7, pp. 395–404, 2007.

[54] A. J. Mitchell, V. Delaffon, D. Vancampfort, C. U. Correll, and M. de Hert, "Guideline concordant monitoring of metabolic risk in people treated with antipsychotic medication: systematic review and meta-analysis of screening practices," *Psychological Medicine*, vol. 42, no. 1, pp. 125–147, 2012.

[55] Institute of Medicine (IOM), *Living Well with Chronic Illness: A Call for Public Health Action*, Academic Press, Washington, DC, USA, 2012.

[56] A. Mccloughen and K. Foster, "Weight gain associated with taking psychotropic medicationa: an integrative review," *International Journal of Mental Health Nursing*, vol. 20, no. 3, pp. 202–222, 2011.

[57] A. D. Vandyk and C. Baker, "Qualitative descriptive study exploring schizophrenia and the everyday effect of medication-induced weight gain," *International Journal of Mental Health Nursing*, vol. 21, no. 4, pp. 349–357, 2012.

18

Prevalence of Overweight and Obesity in Adolescents: A Systematic Review

Maria del Mar Bibiloni,[1,2] Antoni Pons,[1,2] and Josep A. Tur[1,2]

[1] *Research Group on Community Nutrition and Oxidative Stress, University of Balearic Islands, 07122 Palma de Mallorca, Spain*
[2] *CIBERobn (Fisiopatología de la Obesidad y la Nutrición CB12/03/30038), Instituto de Salud Carlos III, 15706 Santiago de Compostela, Spain*

Correspondence should be addressed to Josep A. Tur; pep.tur@uib.es

Academic Editors: G. González-Cuevas, D. Micic, E. K. Naderali, and R. Tungtrongchitr

Objective. To review the extant literature on the prevalence of overweight and obesity in adolescents (10–19 years old) of both sexes. *Design*. The search was carried out using Medline and Scopus considering articles published from the establishment of the databanks until June 7, 2012. Data on the prevalence of children being overweight and obese from the International Obesity Task Force (IOTF) website was also reviewed. Only original articles and one National Health Report were considered. Forty studies met the inclusion criteria. *Results*. Twenty-five of these studies were nationally representative, and ten countries were represented only by regional data. *Conclusions*. The prevalence of overweight and obesity among adolescents worldwide is high, and obesity is higher among boys. The IOTF criterion is the most frequently used method to classify adolescents as overweighed or obese in public health research.

1. Introduction

The prevalence of overweight and obesity among children and adolescents has widely increased worldwide [1, 2], making it one of the most common chronic disorders in this age group and in adulthood.

The use of body mass index (BMI) for age to define being overweight and obese in children and adolescents is well established for both clinical and public health applications, because of their feasibility under clinical settings and in epidemiological studies [3, 4]. In children and adolescents, the natural increases in BMI that occur with age necessitate the use of age-sex-specific thresholds. The most widely used growth charts are the Centers for Disease Control and Prevention (CDC-2000) [5], the International Task Force (IOTF) [6], and the 2007 growth references for 5 to 19 year olds produced by the World Health Organization (WHO-2007) [7].

The CDC-2000 growth charts were developed to evaluate the nutritional status of US children and were originated from five cross-sectional representative surveys carried out in the US between 1963 and 1994. These growth charts are routinely applied to identify children and adolescents with a BMI greater than the 85th or 95th percentiles following the advice of the US Expert Committee on Childhood Obesity [8]. However, the appropriateness of an American dataset for defining overweight in young people from other countries is questionable [9].

The IOTF reference also uses age-sex-specific BMI percentiles, and overweight and obesity definition corresponds to an adult BMI of 25 and 30 kg/m^2, respectively, and reflects values in children tracking to overweight and obesity in adults [6]. This reference is based on six large international cross-sectional representative datasets, identifying the BMI values that extrapolate to childhood.

The WHO-2007 growth references were created to replace the National Center for Health Statistics (NCHS) references [10, 11]. This reference was constructed using data from the 1977 NCHS/WHO growth reference (1 to 24 years old) merged with data from the 2006 WHO Child Growth Standards for preschool children (under 5 years of age) using state-of-the-art statistical methods [7].

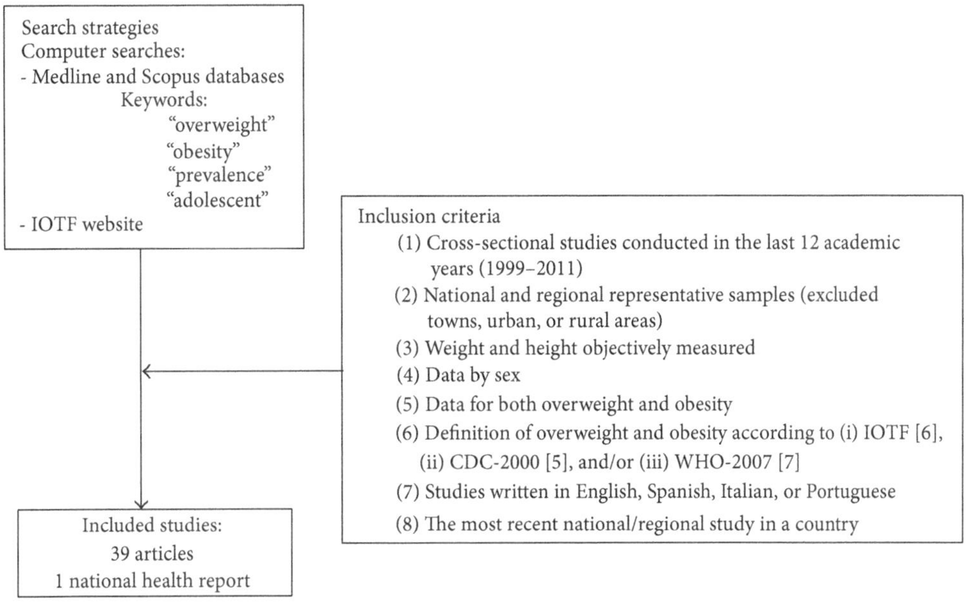

FIGURE 1: Flow diagram of study selection.

Although valuable information has been appearing in the literature or online, such as works from the Health Behaviour of School-aged Children study which is mainly related to social determinants of health and well-being among young people [12], no systematic review has been conducted to understand the worldwide magnitude of the overweight and obesity problem among the adolescent population. Thus, the objective of this study was to systematically review the literature regarding the prevalence of overweight and obesity in adolescents (10–19 years old) of both sexes published in the past 12 academic years (1999–2011).

2. Methods

A systematic literature search was performed which ended on June 7, 2012 (see Figure 1). The literature search was conducted in Medline and Scopus using the following MeSH terms: "overweight"; "obesity"; "prevalence"; "adolescent". In total, 2537 articles were selected. We also reviewed the data on the prevalence of childhood overweight and obesity on the International Obesity Task Force Website at http://www.iaso.org/iotf/. To find the articles included in this review, the following inclusion criteria were used: (1) cross-sectional studies conducted in the last 12 years (1999–2011)—when the original study did not report the survey year, it was not included; (2) national and regional representative samples, but articles published on the prevalence of overweight in towns, urban, or rural areas in a country were excluded; (3) weight and height objectively measured; (4) results presented by sex; (5) and for both overweight and obesity prevalence; (6) the definition of overweight and obesity using the (i) CDC-2000 [5], (ii) IOTF [6], and (iii) WHO-2007 [7] growth references; and (7) studies written in English, Spanish, Italian, or Portuguese. Moreover, if there were more than one national or regional study in the same country, the most recent one was included in the prevalence tables (except for USA [13] and Canada [14], countries in which the most recent data was not included in the tables due to differences in the representativeness of the samples [13] and the impossibility to calculate a single prevalence of overweight and obesity for adolescents' boys and girls [14]; however, no differences in prevalence were observed between studies as it has been indicated in the discussion). The final number of articles included in this review was 39 articles related to overweight and obesity and also a study on the latest statistics on the prevalence of overweight and obesity in South Africa [15].

Potentially relevant papers were selected by (1) screening the titles; (2) screening the abstracts, and (3) if abstracts were not available or did not provide sufficient data, the entire article was retrieved and screened to determine whether it met the inclusion criteria. Full-text articles were assessed by 2 authors (M. M. Bibiloni and J. A. Tur). Any matter of doubt was discussed by at least two of the reviewers (M. M. Bibiloni, A. Pons, and J. A. Tur).

3. Results

3.1. Literature Search. A total of thirty-nine articles and a National Health Report were eligible according to the inclusion criteria established for this review. Table 1 presents a description of the forty studies selected for this review including the continent and the country where it was performed (and region for not national studies), year of publishing, total number of participants in the study, number of adolescents, age range, proportion of girls, and number and definition for overweight and obesity classification used. All the articles were published after the year of 2002. Nationally representative data were obtained in twenty-five countries (including Northern Ireland) [15–39], and ten countries were represented only by regional data [40, 42, 44, 45, 47, 50–54].

TABLE 1: Descriptive analysis of the studies reviewed.

Area	Continent	Country, region	Date of survey	Total n of study[1]	Total n of adolescents[1]	Age (years)/school grade	Proportion of girls	Number of definition	Definition	Reference
National	Africa	Seychelles	2004	4,854	2,177	7th, 10th	51.5%	1	IOTF	Bovet et al., 2006 [16]
		South Africa	2008	9,862	9,862	13–19	50.9%	1	IOTF	Reddy et al., 2010 [15]
		Tunisia	2004	2,872	2,872	15–19	54.9%	1	IOTF	Aounallah-Skhiri et al., 2008 [17]
	America	Canada	2004	8,661	4,099	12–17	—	3	IOTF, CDC, WHO	Shields and Tremblay, 2010 [18]
		Mexico	2006	48,304	13,219	12–18	50.7%	1	IOTF	Bonvecchio et al., 2009 [19]
		USA	2007	44,101	44,101	10–17	—	1	CDC	Singh et al., 2010 [20]
	Asia	Bahrain	2000	506	506	12–17	50.8%	1	IOTF	Al-Sendi et al., 2003 [21]
		China	2002	44,880	12,475	13–17	47.7%	1	IOTF	Li et al., 2008 [22]
		Iran	2003-04	21,111	16,035	10–18	51.3%	2	IOTF, CDC	Kelishadi et al., 2008 [23]
		Israel	2003-04	5,588	5,588	11–19	55.1%	1	CDC	Nitzan Kaluski et al., 2009 [24]
		Jordan	2009	5,640	637	13–18	55.7%	1	IOTF	Khader et al., 2011 [25]
		Qatar	2003-04	3,923	3,923	12–17	49.8%	1	IOTF	Bener, 2006 [26]
		Saudi Arabia	2005	19,317	7,251	13–18	49.2%	2	CDC, WHO	El Mouzan et al., 2010 [27]
		Taiwan	2003	72,789	58,424	10–18	49.0%	1	IOTF	Liou et al., 2009 [28]
		United Arab Emirates	2009-10	1,007	276	11–18	—	1	IOTF	Ng et al., 2011 [29]
	Europe	Cyprus	1999-2000	2,467	1,694	10–17	50.7%	1	IOTF	Savva et al., 2002 [30]
		Czech Republic	2005	1,417	957	11–17	49.4%	1	IOTF	Kunesova et al., 2007 [31]
		Germany	2008	40,622	5,623	12–16	46.7%	1	IOTF	Blüher et al., 2011 [32]
		Greece	2003	14,456	14,456	13–19	53.8%	1	IOTF	Tzotzas et al., 2008 [33]
		Italy	2002	4,386	4,386	11, 13, 15	51.6%	1	IOTF	Vieno et al., 2005 [34]
		Republic of Ireland	2003	17,499	7,294	11–16	50.6%	1	IOTF	Whelton et al., 2007 [35]
		Northern Ireland	2003	2,039	964	11–15	51.5%	1	IOTF	Whelton et al., 2007 [35]
		Portugal	2008	22,048	22,048	10–18	51.5%	2	IOTF, WHO	Sardinha et al., 2011 [36]
		Sweden	2001	1,732	1,732	10, 13, 16	48.3%	1	IOTF	Ekblom et al., 2004 [37]

Table 1: Continued.

Area	Continent	Country, region	Date of survey	Total *n* of study[1]	Total *n* of adolescents[1]	Age (years)/school grade	Proportion of girls	Number of definition	Definition	Reference
	Oceania	Australia	2004	5,407	1,771	8th, 10th	45.6%	1	IOTF	Booth et al., 2007 [38]
		New Zealand	2007	8,796	8,796	13–17	45.4%	2	IOTF, WHO	Utter et al., 2010 [39]
Regional	Africa	South Africa, Eastern Cape	2008	926	926	13–19	52.1%	1	IOTF	Reddy et al., 2010 [15]
		South Africa, Free State	2008	1,236	1,236	13–19	49.1%	1	IOTF	Reddy et al., 2010 [15]
		South Africa, Gauteng	2008	931	931	13–19	52.1%	1	IOTF	Reddy et al., 2010 [15]
		South Africa, KwaZulu-Natal	2008	910	910	13–19	52.1%	1	IOTF	Reddy et al., 2010 [15]
		South Africa, Limpopo	2008	1,140	1,140	13–19	50.5%	1	IOTF	Reddy et al., 2010 [15]
		South Africa, Mpumalanga	2008	1,238	1,238	13–19	49.8%	1	IOTF	Reddy et al., 2010 [15]
		South Africa, Northern Cape	2008	1,088	1,088	13–19	48.6%	1	IOTF	Reddy et al., 2010 [15]
		South Africa, North West	2008	1,234	1,234	13–19	48.6%	1	IOTF	Reddy et al., 2010 [15]
		South Africa, Western Cape	2008	1,159	1,159	13–19	56.4%	1	IOTF	Reddy et al., 2010 [15]
	America	USA, 52 Sates[2]	2007	—	—	10–17	—	1	CDC	Singh et al., 2010 [20]
		Brazil, Pernambuco State	2006	4,210	4,210	14–19	59.8%	1	IOTF	Tassitano et al., 2009 [40]
	Asia	China, Hong Kong	2003-04	2,098	2,098	11–18	53.2%	2	IOTF, CDC	Ko et al., 2008 [41]
		India, Manipur	2005-06	3,356	3,356	12–19	56.2%	1	IOTF	Bishwalata et al., 2010 [42]
		Jordan, Irbid Governorate	2007	1,355	1,355	13–16	55.6%	1	CDC	Abu Baker and Daradkeh, 2010 [43]

Table 1: Continued.

Area Continent	Country, region	Date of survey	Total n of study[1]	Total n of adolescents[1]	Age (years)/school grade	Proportion of girls	Number of definition	Definition	Reference
Europe	Denmark, Greater Copenhagen area and 3 municipalities outside the Capital Region	2007–09	7,541	7,541	14–16	50.1%	1	IOTF	Søren and Jo, 2010 [44]
	France, Aquitaine Region	2004-05	2,385	2,385	11–18	49.1%	1	IOTF	Thibault et al., 2010 [45]
	Greece, Crete	2005-06	481	481	10–12	54.0%	1	IOTF	Manios et al., 2011 [46]
	Hungary, Szeged and Szolnok regions	2005-2006	14,290	14,290	11–16	48.1%	1	IOTF	Baráth et al., 2010 [47]
	Italy, 5 residence regions[3]	2002	4,386	4,386	11–15	51.6%	1	IOTF	Vieno et al., 2005 [34]
	Italy, Sardinia	1999–2001	3,946	3,946	11–15	49.0%	1	IOTF	Velluzzi et al., 2007 [48]
	Italy, Sicily	1999–2001	48,897	48,897	11–15	50.7%	1	CDC	Baratta et al., 2006 [49]
	Poland, Kujawsko-Pomorskie	2005	—	—	13–15	—	1	IOTF	Jodkowska et al., 2010 [50]
	Poland, Lubuskie	2005	—	—	13–15	—	1	IOTF	Jodkowska et al., 2010 [50]
	Poland, Malapolskie	2005	—	—	13–15	—	1	IOTF	Jodkowska et al., 2010 [50]
	Poland, Podlaskie	2005	—	—	13–15	—	1	IOTF	Jodkowska et al., 2010 [50]
	Poland, Pomorskie	2005	—	—	13–15	—	1	IOTF	Jodkowska et al., 2010 [50]
	Spain, Balearic Islands	2007-08	1,231	1,231	12–17	53.4%	1	WHO	Bibiloni et al., 2010 [51]
	Spain, Grand Canary	2004-05	1,002	1,002	12–14	50.0%	1	IOTF	Henríquez Sánchez et al., 2008 [52]
	Switzerland, Canton of Vaud	2005-06	5,207	5,207	10–14	49.7%	2	IOTF, CDC	Lasserre et al., 2007 [53]
	Turkey, Edirne Province	2001	989	989	12–17	48.1%	1	IOTF	Öner et al., 2004 [54]

[1]Only subjects with anthropometric measurements were included in each country.
[2]There are 52 states in the USA, but no information about total number of subjects was included in each state.
[3]Vieno et al. [34] assessed the overall overweight and obesity prevalence among Italian adolescents, and also according to the geographic region: North-West, North-East, Center, South, and Islands, but no information about total number of subjects was included in each region.
IOTF: International Obesity Task Force; CDC: Center for Disease Control and Prevention; WHO: World Health Organization.

3.2. Prevalence and Criteria for Classification. Table 2 shows overweight and obesity prevalence from the twenty-five national studies (one of them including data from Northern Ireland) that were included in this review according to the continent and the country where it was performed, year of survey, study population, age range, criteria used for classifying overweight and obesity used, and along with total data by sex. There were thirty-two different prevalence levels described in the included articles, because five countries presented data using at least two different criteria for overweight and obesity classification [18, 23, 27, 36, 39]. The IOTF cut-off was used to classify overweight and obesity in twenty-three of the twenty-five national studies considered in the present review.

There was a broad range of overweight and obesity prevalence noted. In general, the prevalence of overweight plus obesity was higher in America [18–20], Oceania [38, 39] and Europe [30–37] and lower in Africa [15–17] and certain parts of Asia [21–29] (in China [22] and Iran [23] the total prevalence was less than 10% by the IOTF cut-offs). Overall, about 30% of American adolescents and 22%–25% of European adolescents (excepting the Czech Republic and Italian adolescents' which showed a prevalence of 13.7% and 17.9%, resp.) were overweight or obese. Among Oceanian adolescents the prevalence ranged from 23.2% in Australia in 2004 to 34.2% in New Zealand in 2007. In Africa, the overall prevalence of overweight and obesity was lower than 20%. Among Asian adolescents there was a broad range of overweight plus obesity. Using IOTF cut-off, the prevalence of being overweight or obese for Asian boys and girls ranged from 5.2% in China in 2002 to 36.4% in Bahrain in 2000.

Table 3 shows regional data prevalence of overweight and obesity from fifteen countries. Specific prevalence from all the geographic regions was included in this review from three countries: South Africa (nine provinces) [15], USA (fifty two states) [20], and Italy (five regions) [34]. In Europe, data from islands of Greece (Crete) [46] and Italy (Sicily and Sardinia) [48, 49] and Spain (Balearic Islands' archipelago [51]; and the Grand Canary Island [52]) were also included. On the other hand, regional but not national data was found for eleven countries (Italy [34], Brazil [40], India [42], Jordan [43], Denmark [44], France [45], Hungary [47], Poland [48], Spain [51, 52], Switzerland [53], and Turkey [54]). The IOTF cut-off was used to classify overweight and obesity in fourteen of the eighteen selected studies that included regional data. In one study [51], data was presented using only the WHO-2007 growth charts and in two studies using only the CDC-2000 growth reference [20, 43].

In South Africa and USA, substantial geographic variations in adolescent overweight and obesity existed. In 2008, overweight and obesity prevalence varied in South Africa from 13.5% in Limpopo to 25.5% in KwaZulu-Natal. In 2007, overweight and obesity varied in USA from 23.1% in Utah and Minnesota to 44.5% in Mississippi. In 2002, the prevalence of overweight and obesity in Southern Italy and Italian islands was higher among boys. In Southern Italy, the overweight prevalence among girls also was higher than in the other geographic regions.

Comparison between the islands from Greece (Crete), Italy (Sicily and Sardinia), and Spain (Balearic Islands and Grand Canary Island) which were included in this review showed that Crete had the highest prevalence of overweight and obesity—despite data were presented using different definition. In Spain, using the IOTF cut-off (data not shown for Balearic Islands but given by authors), the prevalence of overweight plus obesity was higher in the Grand Canary Island (29.1%) than in the Balearic Islands (24.7%).

3.3. Gender Differences. According to national data, the prevalence of overweight among boys was ≥10% higher than girls in nine countries (Canada [18], Qatar [26], Taiwan [28], Cyprus [30], Czech Republic [31], Germany [32], Greece [33], Italy [34], Australia [38], Denmark [44], and Hungary [47]) and among girls ≥10% higher than boys in seven of the twenty-five countries (South Africa [15], Seychelles [16], Tunisia [17], Mexico [19], Bahrain [21], Saudi Arabia [27], and Sweden [37]). The obesity prevalence was ≥10% higher among boys in seventeen countries (Canada [18], USA [20], China [22], Iran [23], Israel [24], Qatar [26], Saudi Arabia [27], Taiwan [28], Cyprus [30], Czech Republic [31], Germany [32], Greece [33], Italy [34], Portugal [36], Sweden [37], Australia [38], New Zealand [39], Denmark [44], and Hungary [47]) and ≥10% higher among girls in four of the twenty-five countries (South Africa [14], Seychelles [16], Tunisia [17], and Bahrain [21]).

4. Discussion

The aim of this study was to review systematically the literature on overweight and obesity prevalence among adolescents worldwide. Thirty-nine articles and one National Health Report that met the inclusion criteria were considered. The overweight and obesity prevalence in the included studies ranged widely. In sixteen of the twenty-three countries with national representative data using the IOTF cut-off, overweight and obesity prevalence higher than 20% were found, five countries showed prevalence above 30%, and just in two countries prevalence was lower than 10%.

Regarding national data, when prevalence was analysed according to sex, it was observed that boys showed a higher prevalence of overweight in almost half of the countries and a higher prevalence of obesity in almost all countries. These results are consistent with previous studies that pointed out a high prevalence of abdominal obesity among boys [55]. Differences of prevalence of overweight and obesity between genders have been related to geopolitical and cultural conditions [55].

Eight articles compared data between 1980s and/or 1990s with 2000s [16, 19, 20, 22, 28, 32, 37, 50] and pointed out an increased prevalence of overweight and obesity in both sexes over this period. However, among Australian adolescents [38] the overweight and obesity prevalence increased significantly among boys but not among girls over the period 1997–2004. In the Australian National Children's Nutrition and Physical Activity Survey 2007 (NCNPAS07) [14], 25% of boys and 30% of girls aged 9- to 13-year-olds and 25% of boys and 23% of girls aged 14- to 16-year-olds were overweight or obese using

Table 2: Description of overweight and obesity prevalence (%) along with total data by sex from each national study that was included in the review according to year of survey, study population, age range, and classification criteria used.

Continent	Country	Date of survey	Study population	Age (years)/school grade	Criteria	Overweight (%)			Obesity (%)			Reference
						All	Boys	Girls	All	Boys	Girls	
Africa	Seychelles	2004	School-based survey	7th, 10th	IOTF[1]	12.0	9.5	14.3	5.1	4.2	6.0	Bovet et al., 2006 [16]
	South Africa	2008	2008 SA YRBS	13–19	IOTF[1]	14.4	7.9	20.6	5.3	3.3	7.2	Reddy et al., 2010 [15]
	Tunisia	2004	Household-based survey	15–19	IOTF[1]	12.4	11.0	14.1	2.6	1.9	3.2	Aounallah-Skhiri et al., 2008 [17]
America	Canada	2004	2004 CCHS	12–17	IOTF[1]	19.8	21.2	18.4	9.4	11.1	7.4	Shields and Tremblay, 2010 [18]
					CDC-2000[2]	15.9	17.0	14.7	12.1	14.3	9.6	
					WHO-2007[3]	20.8	21.9	19.6	12.4	15.1	9.4	
	Mexico	2006	Household-based survey	12–18	IOTF[1]	21.2	20.1	22.3	8.9	9.2	8.6	Bonvecchio et al., 2009 [19]
	USA	2007	2007 NSCH	10–17	CDC-2000[2]	15.2	15.3	15.2	16.4	19.2	13.5	Singh et al., 2010 [20]
Asia	Bahrain	2000	School-based survey	12–17	IOTF[1]	20.0	15.3	24.5	16.4	14.9	17.9	Al-Sendi et al., 2003 [21]
	China	2002	2002 CNNHS	13–17	IOTF[1]	4.6	4.6	4.6	0.6	0.7	0.5	Li et al., 2008 [22]
	Iran	2003-04	CASPIAN Study	10–18	IOTF[1]	5.9	5.7	6.0	1.3	1.5	1.1	Kelishadi et al., 2008 [23]
					CDC-2000[2]	4.5	4.3	4.7	1.9	2.3	1.6	
	Israel	2003-04	MABAT Youth Survey	11–19	CDC-2000[2]	12.9	12.7	13.0	5.6	7.4	4.1	Nitzan Kaluski et al., 2009 [24]
	Jordan	2009	Household-based survey	13–18	IOTF[1]	13.7	11.3	15.5	10.0	12.4	8.2	Khader et al., 2011 [25]
	Qatar	2003-04	School-based survey	12–17	IOTF[1]	23.8	28.6	18.9	6.3	7.9	4.7	Bener, 2006 [26]
	Saudi Arabia	2005	Household-based survey	13–18	CDC-2000[2]	17.9	16.5	19.6	7.0	8.2	5.5	El Mouzan et al., 2010 [27]
					WHO-2007[3]	16.0	13.6	18.4	10.6	11.2	10.0	
	Taiwan	2003	School-based survey	10–18	IOTF[1]	16.3	18.4	14.2	6.2	8.1	4.2	Liou et al., 2009 [28]
	United Arab Emirates	2009-10	Household-based survey	11–18	IOTF[1]	—	16.2	20.5	—	11.7	19.7	Ng et al., 2011 [29]
Europe	Cyprus	1999-00	School-based survey	10–17	IOTF[1]	18.9	21.3	16.5	5.8	7.1	4.5	Savva et al., 2002 [30]
	Czech Republic	2005	Lifestyle and Obesity Study	6–17	IOTF[1]	12.3	16.6	8.0	1.4	1.7	1.0	Kunesova et al., 2007 [31]
	Germany	2008	CrescNet database	12–16	IOTF[1]	18.2	19.3	17.0	6.2	7.6	4.6	Blüher et al., 2011 [32]
	Greece	2003	School-based survey	13–19	IOTF[1]	18.3	23.3	14.0	4.3	6.1	2.7	Tzotzas et al., 2008 [33]
	Italy	2002	HBSC Study	11, 13, 15	IOTF[1]	15.6	20.9	10.6	2.3	3.5	1.2	Vieno et al., 2005 [34]
	Republic of Ireland	2003	School-based survey	11–16	IOTF[1]	18.5	17.8	19.2	5.8	5.6	6.1	Whelton et al., 2007 [35]
	Northern Ireland	2003	School-based survey	11–15	IOTF[1]	18.2	18.5	17.8	5.9	6.0	5.7	Whelton et al., 2007 [35]
	Portugal	2008	School-based survey	10–18	IOTF[1]	17.4	17.7	17.0	5.2	5.8	4.6	Sardinha et al., 2011 [36]
					WHO-2007	21.8	20.4	23.1	9.9	10.3	9.6	
	Sweden	2001	School-based survey	10, 13, 16	IOTF[1]	15.8	14.6	16.9	4.4	5.0	3.6	Ekblom et al., 2004 [37]
Oceania	Australia	2004	2004 SPANS	8th, 10th	IOTF[1]	17.9	19.4	16.2	5.3	6.7	3.6	Booth et al., 2007 [38]
	New Zealand	2007	Youth'07 Survey	13–17	IOTF[1]	24.0	23.3	24.7	10.2	10.8	9.5	Utter et al., 2010 [39]
					WHO-2007	25.9	25.9	26.0	13.5	14.6	12.1	

[1]Overweight and obesity, all adolescents with BMI-for-age $\geq 25\,kg/m^2$ and $<30\,kg/m^2$ and $\geq 30\,kg/m^2$, respectively, according to the IOTF [6].
[2]Overweight and obesity, all adolescents with BMI-for-age ≥P85th and <P95th and ≥P95th, respectively, according to the CDC [5].
[3]Overweight and obesity, all adolescents with BMI-for-age >+1SD and <+2SD and >+2SD, respectively, according to the WHO [7].
IOTF: International Obesity Task Force; CDC: Center for Disease Control and Prevention; WHO: World Health Organization; 2008 SA YRBS: 2008 South African National Youth Risk Behaviour; 2004 CCHS: 2004 Canadian Community Health Survey; 2007 NSCH: National Survey of Children's Health; 2002 CNNHS: 2002 China National Nutrition and Health Survey; CASPIAN Study: Childhood and Adolescence Surveillance and Prevention of Adult Non-communicable disease; HBSC: Health Behaviour in School-aged Children; 2004 SPANS: 2004 NSW Schools Physical Activity and Nutrition Survey.

TABLE 3: Description of overweight and obesity prevalence (%) along with total data by sex from each regional study that was included in the review according to year of survey, study population, age range, and classification criteria used.

Continent	Country, region	Date of survey	Study population	Age (years)	Criteria	Overweight (%)			Obesity (%)			Reference
						All	Boys	Girls	All	Boys	Girls	
Africa	South Africa, Eastern Cape	2008	2008 SA YRBS	13–19	IOTF[1]	13.3	4.3	21.1	4.0	2.0	5.6	Reddy et al., 2010 [15]
	South Africa, Free State	2008	2008 SA YRBS	13–19	IOTF[1]	11.6	8.1	15.1	4.7	3.7	5.7	Reddy et al., 2010 [15]
	South Africa, Gauteng	2008	2008 SA YRBS	13–19	IOTF[1]	12.7	10.0	15.4	9.7	8.4	11.0	Reddy et al., 2010 [15]
	South Africa, KwaZulu-Natal	2008	2008 SA YRBS	13–19	IOTF[1]	20.1	8.6	31.5	5.4	3.4	7.3	Reddy et al., 2010 [15]
	South Africa, Limpopo	2008	2008 SA YRBS	13–19	IOTF[1]	10.7	6.2	15.1	2.8	1.0	4.5	Reddy et al., 2010 [15]
	South Africa, Mpumalanga	2008	2008 SA YRBS	13–19	IOTF[1]	15.5	10.0	21.1	6.1	2.3	9.9	Reddy et al., 2010 [15]
	South Africa, Northern Cape	2008	2008 SA YRBS	13–19	IOTF[1]	12.9	7.3	18.3	5.0	4.4	5.6	Reddy et al., 2010 [15]
	South Africa, North West	2008	2008 SA YRBS	13–19	IOTF[1]	11.8	7.0	16.7	3.9	2.2	5.7	Reddy et al., 2010 [15]
	South Africa, Western Cape	2008	2008 SA YRBS	13–19	IOTF[1]	14.3	9.7	18.5	5.6	2.0	8.9	Reddy et al., 2010 [15]
America	USA, Alaska	2007	2007 NSCH	10–17	CDC-2000[2]	19.8	22.7	16.7	14.1	14.6	13.7	Singh et al., 2010 [20]
	USA, Alabama	2007	2007 NSCH	10–17	CDC-2000[2]	18.2	17.6	18.9	17.9	24.4	10.9	Singh et al., 2010 [20]
	USA, Arkansas	2007	2007 NSCH	10–17	CDC-2000[2]	17.1	15.0	19.2	20.4	27.2	13.2	Singh et al., 2010 [20]
	USA, Arizona	2007	2007 NSCH	10–17	CDC-2000[2]	12.8	12.7	12.7	17.8	20.6	15.0	Singh et al., 2010 [20]
	USA, California	2007	2007 NSCH	10–17	CDC-2000[2]	15.5	13.4	17.5	15.0	17.4	12.8	Singh et al., 2010 [20]
	USA, Colorado	2007	2007 NSCH	10–17	CDC-2000[2]	13.0	17.5	8.5	14.2	17.5	10.7	Singh et al., 2010 [20]
	USA, Connecticut	2007	2007 NSCH	10–17	CDC-2000[2]	13.2	14.7	11.7	12.5	14.8	10.2	Singh et al., 2010 [20]
	USA, Washington, DC	2007	2007 NSCH	10–17	CDC-2000[2]	15.2	11.6	18.7	20.2	22.2	18.2	Singh et al., 2010 [20]
	USA, Delaware	2007	2007 NSCH	10–17	CDC-2000[2]	19.9	22.0	17.8	13.3	12.2	14.4	Singh et al., 2010 [20]
	USA, Florida	2007	2007 NSCH	10–17	CDC-2000[2]	14.8	12.7	17.1	18.3	21.5	15.0	Singh et al., 2010 [20]
	USA, Georgia	2007	2007 NSCH	10–17	CDC-2000[2]	16.0	14.4	17.7	21.3	24.7	17.7	Singh et al., 2010 [20]
	USA, Hawaii	2007	2007 NSCH	10–17	CDC-2000[2]	17.3	17.5	17.1	11.2	15.0	7.1	Singh et al., 2010 [20]
	USA, Iowa	2007	2007 NSCH	10–17	CDC-2000[2]	15.3	14.8	15.9	11.2	11.3	11.0	Singh et al., 2010 [20]
	USA, Idaho	2007	2007 NSCH	10–17	CDC-2000[2]	15.7	14.4	17.2	11.8	16.4	6.8	Singh et al., 2010 [20]
	USA, Illinois	2007	2007 NSCH	10–17	CDC-2000[2]	14.2	12.1	16.4	20.7	25.0	16.3	Singh et al., 2010 [20]
	USA, Indiana	2007	2007 NSCH	10–17	CDC-2000[2]	15.2	11.5	19.3	14.7	17.4	11.7	Singh et al., 2010 [20]
	USA, Kansas	2007	2007 NSCH	10–17	CDC-2000[2]	14.9	16.0	13.7	16.2	16.2	16.3	Singh et al., 2010 [20]
	USA, Kentucky	2007	2007 NSCH	10–17	CDC-2000[2]	16.1	17.7	14.6	21.0	22.5	19.4	Singh et al., 2010 [20]
	USA, Louisiana	2007	2007 NSCH	10–17	CDC-2000[2]	15.2	15.5	14.9	20.7	23.1	18.1	Singh et al., 2010 [20]
	USA, Massachusetts	2007	2007 NSCH	10–17	CDC-2000[2]	16.7	18.2	15.4	13.3	16.1	10.5	Singh et al., 2010 [20]
	USA, Maryland	2007	2007 NSCH	10–17	CDC-2000[2]	15.2	19.1	11.1	13.6	17.0	9.9	Singh et al., 2010 [20]
	USA, Maine	2007	2007 NSCH	10–17	CDC-2000[2]	15.3	15.6	14.9	12.9	16.0	9.8	Singh et al., 2010 [20]
	USA, Michigan	2007	2007 NSCH	10–17	CDC-2000[2]	18.1	20.4	15.8	12.5	14.3	10.5	Singh et al., 2010 [20]
	USA, Minnesota	2007	2007 NSCH	10–17	CDC-2000[2]	12.0	12.1	11.8	11.1	14.3	7.6	Singh et al., 2010 [20]
	USA, Missouri	2007	2007 NSCH	10–17	CDC-2000[2]	17.4	16.9	17.8	13.6	15.5	11.6	Singh et al., 2010 [20]
	USA, Mississippi	2007	2007 NSCH	10–17	CDC-2000[2]	22.6	21.6	23.5	21.9	25.5	18.5	Singh et al., 2010 [20]
	USA, Montana	2007	2007 NSCH	10–17	CDC-2000[2]	13.8	15.0	12.5	11.8	16.6	6.6	Singh et al., 2010 [20]
	USA, North Carolina	2007	2007 NSCH	10–17	CDC-2000[2]	14.9	13.9	16.0	18.6	19.3	17.9	Singh et al., 2010 [20]
	USA, North Dakota	2007	2007 NSCH	10–17	CDC-2000[2]	14.3	16.9	11.6	11.4	15.7	7.0	Singh et al., 2010 [20]
	USA, Nebraska	2007	2007 NSCH	10–17	CDC-2000[2]	15.7	13.9	17.5	15.8	23.0	8.1	Singh et al., 2010 [20]

Table 3: Continued.

Continent	Country, region	Date of survey	Study population	Age (years)	Criteria	Overweight (%)			Obesity (%)			Reference
						All	Boys	Girls	All	Boys	Girls	
	USA, New Hampshire	2007	2007 NSCH	10–17	CDC-2000[2]	16.6	17.1	16.2	12.8	16.3	8.8	Singh et al., 2010 [20]
	USA, New Jersey	2007	2007 NSCH	10–17	CDC-2000[2]	15.6	17.3	13.8	15.4	18.6	11.7	Singh et al., 2010 [20]
	USA, New Mexico	2007	2007 NSCH	10–17	CDC-2000[2]	16.7	15.3	18.1	16.0	20.4	11.4	Singh et al., 2010 [20]
	USA, Nevada	2007	2007 NSCH	10–17	CDC-2000[2]	19.0	21.9	16.0	15.2	19.4	10.8	Singh et al., 2010 [20]
	USA, New York	2007	2007 NSCH	10–17	CDC-2000[2]	15.8	15.1	16.5	17.1	20.3	13.8	Singh et al., 2010 [20]
	USA, Ohio	2007	2007 NSCH	10–17	CDC-2000[2]	14.8	18.7	10.9	18.5	22.9	14.2	Singh et al., 2010 [20]
	USA, Oklahoma	2007	2007 NSCH	10–17	CDC-2000[2]	13.2	18.1	8.2	16.4	17.4	15.4	Singh et al., 2010 [20]
	USA, Oregon	2007	2007 NSCH	10–17	CDC-2000[2]	14.7	16.2	13.3	9.6	11.0	8.2	Singh et al., 2010 [20]
	USA, Pennsylvania	2007	2007 NSCH	10–17	CDC-2000[2]	14.7	15.5	13.7	15.0	21.0	8.4	Singh et al., 2010 [20]
	USA, Rhode Island	2007	2007 NSCH	10–17	CDC-2000[2]	15.7	15.5	16.0	14.4	18.2	10.5	Singh et al., 2010 [20]
	USA, South Carolina	2007	2007 NSCH	10–17	CDC-2000[2]	18.5	20.8	15.9	15.3	18.4	12.0	Singh et al., 2010 [20]
	USA, South Dakota	2007	2007 NSCH	10–17	CDC-2000[2]	15.2	17.3	13.0	13.2	16.0	10.2	Singh et al., 2010 [20]
	USA, Tennessee	2007	2007 NSCH	10–17	CDC-2000[2]	15.9	14.5	17.3	20.6	23.3	17.9	Singh et al., 2010 [20]
	USA, Texas	2007	2007 NSCH	10–17	CDC-2000[2]	11.8	11.0	12.6	20.4	20.6	20.2	Singh et al., 2010 [20]
	USA, Utah	2007	2007 NSCH	10–17	CDC-2000[2]	11.7	12.1	11.2	11.4	14.7	7.9	Singh et al., 2010 [20]
	USA, Virginia	2007	2007 NSCH	10–17	CDC-2000[2]	15.8	16.1	15.4	15.2	16.6	13.9	Singh et al., 2010 [20]
	USA, Vermont	2007	2007 NSCH	10–17	CDC-2000[2]	13.8	16.4	11.1	12.9	17.0	8.4	Singh et al., 2010 [20]
	USA, Washington	2007	2007 NSCH	10–17	CDC-2000[2]	18.4	21.9	14.7	11.1	14.7	7.3	Singh et al., 2010 [20]
	USA, Wisconsin	2007	2007 NSCH	10–17	CDC-2000[2]	14.8	17.3	12.2	13.1	15.6	10.5	Singh et al., 2010 [20]
	USA, West Virginia	2007	2007 NSCH	10–17	CDC-2000[2]	16.6	16.9	16.4	18.9	21.8	15.7	Singh et al., 2010 [20]
	USA, Wyoming	2007	2007 NSCH	10–17	CDC-2000[2]	15.5	16.6	14.2	10.2	14.1	5.5	Singh et al., 2010 [20]
	Brazil, Pernambuco State	2006	GSHS	14–19	IOTF[1]	11.5	11.3	11.6	2.4	2.0	2.8	Tassitano et al., 2009 [40]
Asia	China, Hong Kong	2003-04	School-based survey	11–18	IOTF[1]	7.1	9.6	4.9	2.8	3.9	1.8	Ko et al., 2008 [41]
					CDC-2000[2]	8.3	11.3	5.8	4.1	6.0	2.4	
	India, Manipur	2005-06	School-based survey	12–19	IOTF[1]	4.4	4.1	4.7	0.7	1.0	0.4	Bishwalata et al., 2010 [42]
	Jordan, Irbid Governorate	2007	School-based survey	13–16	CDC-2000[2]	15.7	11.8	18.9	8.7	12.3	5.8	Abu Baker and Daradkeh, 2010 [43]
Europe	Denmark, Greater Copenhagen area and 3 municipalities outside the Capital Region	2007–09	School-based survey	14–16	IOTF[1]	14.0	15.2	12.9	11.2	14.1	8.2	Søren and Jo, 2010 [44]
	France, Aquitaine Region	2004-05	School-based survey	11–18	IOTF[1]	11.7	13.3	10.1	1.9	2.4	1.4	Thibault et al., 2010 [45]
	Greece, Crete	2005-06	School-based survey	10–12	IOTF[1]	28.0	30.0	27.0	13.0	15.0	10.0	Manios et al., 2011 [46]
	Hungary, Szeged and Szolnok regions	2005-06	School-based survey	11–16	IOTF[1]	16.8	17.9	15.7	6.6	7.9	5.2	Baráth et al., 2010 [47]
	Italy, North-West	2002	HBSC Study	11, 13, 16	IOTF[1]	—	18.3	7.1	—	2.5	1.1	Vieno et al., 2005 [34]
	Italy, North-East	2002	HBSC Study	11, 13, 16	IOTF[1]	—	16.5	11.7	—	0.8	1.5	Vieno et al., 2005 [34]
	Italy, Center	2002	HBSC Study	11, 13, 16	IOTF[1]	—	20.7	11.2	—	3.9	2.5	Vieno et al., 2005 [34]
	Italy, South	2002	HBSC Study	11, 13, 16	IOTF[1]	—	25.7	15.7	—	4.4	0.9	Vieno et al., 2005 [34]
	Italy, Islands	2002	HBSC Study	11, 13, 16	IOTF[1]	—	31.3	10.4	—	7.6	0.8	Vieno et al., 2005 [34]
	Italy, Sardinia	1999–2001	School-based survey	11–15	IOTF1	14.9	15.4	14.6	3.7	5.1	3.2	Velluzzi et al., 2007 [48]
	Italy, Sicily	1999–2001	Public school-based survey	11–15	CDC-2000[2]	18.3	18.8	17.8	11.8	15.1	8.5	Baratta et al., 2006 [49]

TABLE 3: Continued.

Continent	Country, region	Date of survey	Study population	Age (years)	Criteria	Overweight (%) All	Overweight (%) Boys	Overweight (%) Girls	Obesity (%) All	Obesity (%) Boys	Obesity (%) Girls	Reference
	Poland, Kujawsko-Pomorskie	2005	School based survey	13–15	IOTF[1]	10.7	12.0	9.5	1.4	1.6	1.3	Jodkowska et al., 2010 [50]
	Poland, Lubuskie	2005	School based survey	13–15	IOTF[1]	11.1	12.2	10.1	3.0	2.5	3.5	Jodkowska et al., 2010 [50]
	Poland, Malapolskie	2005	School based survey	13–15	IOTF[1]	12.7	12.8	12.6	1.6	1.9	1.3	Jodkowska et al., 2010 [50]
	Poland, Podlaskie	2005	School based survey	13–15	IOTF[1]	13.9	14.5	13.3	2.8	3.1	2.6	Jodkowska et al., 2010 [50]
	Poland, Pomorskie	2005	School based survey	13–15	IOTF[1]	13.7	13.4	13.9	2.1	2.0	2.2	Jodkowska et al., 2010 [50]
	Spain, Balearic Islands	2007-08	School-based survey	12–17	WHO-2007[3]	17.5	19.9	15.5	10.4	12.7	8.5	Bibiloni et al., 2010 [51]
	Spain, Grand Canary	2004-05	School-based survey	12–14	IOTF[1]	21.6	21.0	22.2	7.5	7.8	7.2	Henríquez Sánchez et al., 2008 [52]
	Switzerland, Canton of Vaud	2005-06	Public school-based survey	10–14	IOTF[1]	12.0	13.2	10.7	1.7	1.8	1.7	Lasserre et al., 2007 [53]
					CDC-2000[2]	10.7	11.9	9.4	3.6	4.2	3.0	
	Turkey, Edirne Province	2001	Two school-based surveys	12–17	IOTF[1]	10.9	11.3	10.6	1.9	1.6	2.1	Öner et al., 2004 [54]

[1]Overweight and obesity, all adolescents with BMI-for-age ≥25 kg/m^2 and <30 kg/m^2 and ≥30 kg/m^2, respectively, according to the IOTF [6].
[2]Overweight and obesity, all adolescents with BMI-for-age ≥P85th and <P95th and ≥P95th, respectively, according to the CDC [5].
[3]Overweight and obesity, all adolescents with BMI-for-age ≥P85th and <P95th and ≥P97th, respectively, according to the WHO [7].
IOTF: International Obesity Task Force; CDC: Center for Disease Control and Prevention; WHO: World Health Organization; 2008 SA YRBS: 2008 South African National Youth Risk Behaviour; 2007 NSCH: National Survey of Children's Health; GSHS: Global School Based Student Health Survey; HBSC: Health Behaviour in School-aged Children.

the IOTF criteria. A comparison of the 1985, 1995, and 2007 Australian national surveys of 7- to 15-year-olds indicated that Australian children are changing body shape to a more central fat distribution [14]. In USA, overweight and obesity prevalence among adolescents increased 4% in 2003 and 10% in 2007. Overweight and obesity prevalence increased by 3% and 18% among USA girls over this period. However, a cross-sectional analyses of a representative sample ($n = 4111$) of the USA child and adolescent population (birth through 19 years of age) with data from the National Health and Nutrition Examination Survey 2009-10 (NHANES) indicated a prevalence of overweight and obesity among adolescents aged 12 through 19 years of 15.2% and 18.4%, respectively. Analyses of trends in obesity prevalence for the last two NHANES surveys (2007-08 and 2009-10) indicated that the prevalence of obesity in children and adolescents has not changed in 2009-10 compared with 2007-08 [13]. On the other hand, since 2004 the overweight and obesity trends were stabilized or decreased among German adolescents [32].

In USA, substantial geographic disparities in adolescent overweight and obesity were found, with an apparent shift toward higher prevalence in 2007 for several states [20]. Generally, overweight and obesity prevalence was also higher in southern USA in 2007. Lobstein et al. [56] reported that children in Northern Europe countries generally tended to have lower overweight and obesity prevalence (10–20%) than in Southern Europe (20–35%). Also within the same country, the prevalence and trends of overweight and obesity may not be homogeneous according to different geographic regions [57]. In Italy, a north-south gradient in overweight and obesity prevalence among boys but also in overweight prevalence among girls was also reported [34]. A higher prevalence of overweight and obesity has been reported in Southern Spain in both children [58] and adults [59].

It is important to note that the choice of a reference and a cut-off point will determine the absolute prevalence of overweight and obesity and its trends, and hence different information will be obtained from the papers [60]. The IOTF classification for adolescent overweight and obesity [6] is the most frequently used. Cole et al. [6] argued that the reference they published, supported by the IOTF, is less arbitrary and more international than others and recommended its use in international comparisons. Lately, Monasta et al. [61] suggested that the IOTF reference and cut-offs could be preferable to identify overweight and obesity both at individual and population levels because they are at least based on a crude association with ill and health later in life, namely, the definition of overweight and obesity at age 18 years. However, the IOTF cut-offs have been not recommended for clinical use when assessing an individual child's growth [9, 62–64]. Furthermore, recent findings suggested that a universal BMI classification system for childhood and adolescent overweight and obesity may not correspond to a comparable level of body fatness in all populations [9]. The prevalence estimates may not accurately characterize the population groups most at risk of health disadvantages because the correlation of BMI with adiposity is highly variable and dependent on ethnic group [9, 60, 65, 66].

5. Limitations of the Study

The comparisons of overweight and obesity prevalence need interpretation with caution due to the difference in survey sampling methods, sample sizes, age range of subjects, quality of data in terms of height and weight measurement, and whether national programmes or strategies to tackle overweight and obesity are in place [57]. Even within the same country, the prevalence and trends of overweight and obesity may not be homogenous in view of different ethnicities, geographic regions, and socioeconomic status [57]. Only articles in English, Spanish, Italian, and Portuguese were included in this review.

6. Conclusions

The results of this review allow the following conclusions: (1) overweight and obesity prevalence is high; (2) obesity is higher among boys, although it is not clear which sex has a higher proportion of adolescents with overweight; (3) despite that there is no consensus about criteria to be used to classify adolescents as overweighed or obese, the most frequently used was the IOTF reference [6]. However, the international reference charts for monitoring the secular trends in childhood obesity need to be continually refined and evaluated [56]. The results of this study would contribute to guiding health planners and administrators to develop proper tools for adolescent obesity management.

Conflict of Interests

The authors state that there is no conflict of interests.

Authors' Contribution

Maria del Mar Bibiloni and Josep A. Tur contributed to the design of the strategy for the literature search and double screened and selected the retrieved documents. Antoni Pons provided previous literature searches and analysis. Maria del Mar Bibiloni and Josep A. Tur prepared the main outline of the paper and all authors contributed to the preparation of the paper.

Acknowledgments

The authors would like to thank the Spanish Ministry of Health and Consumption Affairs (Programme of Promotion of Biomedical Research and Health Sciences, Projects 05/1276 and 08/1259, and Red Predimed-RETIC RD06/0045/1004 and CIBERobn CB12/03/30038), Grant of support to research groups no. 35/2011 (Balearic Islands Government and EU FEDER funds), Spanish Ministry of Education and Science (FPU Programme, PhD fellowship to M.M.B.). The Research Group on Community Nutrition and Oxidative Stress, University of Balearic Islands belongs to the Centre Català de la Nutrició (IEC).

References

[1] C. B. Ebbeling, D. B. Pawlak, and D. S. Ludwig, "Childhood obesity: public-health crisis, common sense cure," *The Lancet*, vol. 360, no. 9331, pp. 473–482, 2002.

[2] I. Lissau, M. D. Overpeck, W. J. Ruan, P. Due, B. E. Holstein, and M. L. Hediger, "Body mass index and overweight in adolescents in 13 European Countries, Israel, and the United States," *Archives of Pediatrics and Adolescent Medicine*, vol. 158, no. 1, pp. 27–33, 2004.

[3] A. Must and S. E. Anderson, "Body mass index in children and adolescents: considerations for population-based applications," *International Journal of Obesity*, vol. 30, no. 4, pp. 590–594, 2006.

[4] J. J. Reilly, "Diagnostic accuracy of the BMI for age in paediatrics," *International Journal of Obesity*, vol. 30, no. 4, pp. 595–597, 2006.

[5] R. J. Kuczmarski, C. L. Ogden, S. S. Guo et al., "2000 CDC Growth Charts for the United States: methods and development," *Vital and Health Statistics*, no. 246, pp. 1–190, 2002.

[6] T. J. Cole, M. C. Bellizzi, K. M. Flegal, and W. H. Dietz, "Establishing a standard definition for child overweight and obesity worldwide: international survey," *British Medical Journal*, vol. 320, no. 7244, pp. 1240–1243, 2000.

[7] M. De Onis, A. W. Onyango, E. Borghi, A. Siyam, C. Nishida, and J. Siekmann, "Development of a WHO growth reference for school-aged children and adolescents," *Bulletin of the World Health Organization*, vol. 85, no. 9, pp. 660–667, 2007.

[8] S. E. Barlow and W. H. Dietz, "Obesity evaluation and treatment: expert Committee recommendations. The Maternal and Child Health Bureau, Health Resources and Services Administration and the Department of Health and Human Services," *Pediatrics*, vol. 102, no. 3, article E29, 1998.

[9] J. S. Duncan, E. K. Duncan, and G. Schofield, "Accuracy of body mass index (BMI) thresholds for predicting excess body fat in girls from five ethnicities," *Asia Pacific Journal of Clinical Nutrition*, vol. 18, no. 3, pp. 404–411, 2009.

[10] A. Must, G. E. Dallal, and W. H. Dietz, "Reference data for obesity: 85th and 95th percentiles of body mass index (wt/ht^2) and triceps skinfold thickness," *American Journal of Clinical Nutrition*, vol. 53, no. 4, pp. 839–846, 1991.

[11] A. Must, G. E. Dallal, and W. H. Dietz, "Reference data for obesity: 85th and 95th percentiles of body mass index (wt/ht^2)—a correction," *American Journal of Clinical Nutrition*, vol. 54, no. 5, article 773, 1991.

[12] "Health Behaviour of School-aged Children study," http://www.hbsc.org/.

[13] C. L. Ogden, M. D. Carroll, B. K. Kit, and K. M. Flegal, "Prevalence of obesity and trends in body mass index among US children and adolescents, 1999–2010," *Journal of the American Medical Association*, vol. 307, no. 5, pp. 483–490, 2012.

[14] "Commonwealth Scientific Industrial Research Organisation (CSIRO), University of South Australia: user Guide: 2007 Australian National Children's Nutrition and Physical Activity Survey," http://www.health.gov.au/internet/main/publishing.nsf/Content/phd-nutrition-childrens-survey-userguide.

[15] S. P. Reddy, S. James, R. Sewpaul et al., "Umthente Uhlaba Usamila—The South African Youth Risk Behaviour. South African Medical Research Council," 2010, http://www.mrc.ac.za/healthpromotion/yrbs_2008_final_report.pdf.

[16] P. Bovet, A. Chiolero, G. Madeleine, A. Gabriel, and N. Stettler, "Marked increase in the prevalence of obesity in children of the Seychelles, a rapidly developing country, between 1998 and 2004," *International Journal of Pediatric Obesity*, vol. 1, no. 2, pp. 120–128, 2006.

[17] H. Aounallah-Skhiri, H. B. Romdhane, P. Traissac et al., "Nutritional status of Tunisian adolescents: associated gender, environmental and socio-economic factors," *Public Health Nutrition*, vol. 11, no. 12, pp. 1306–1317, 2008.

[18] M. Shields and M. S. Tremblay, "Canadian childhood obesity estimates based on WHO, IOTF and CDC cut-points," *International Journal of Pediatric Obesity*, vol. 5, no. 3, pp. 265–273, 2010.

[19] A. Bonvecchio, M. Safdie, E. A. Monterrubio, T. Gust, S. Villalpando, and J. A. Rivera, "Overweight and obesity trends in Mexican children 2 to 18 years of age from 1988 to 2006," *Salud Pública de México*, vol. 51, supplement 4, pp. S586–S594, 2009.

[20] G. K. Singh, M. D. Kogan, and P. C. Van Dyck, "Changes in state-specific childhood obesity and overweight prevalence in the United States from 2003 to 2007," *Archives of Pediatrics and Adolescent Medicine*, vol. 164, no. 7, pp. 598–607, 2010.

[21] A. M. Al-Sendi, P. Shetty, and A. O. Musaiger, "Prevalence of overweight and obesity among Bahraini adolescents: a comparison between three different sets of criteria," *European Journal of Clinical Nutrition*, vol. 57, no. 3, pp. 471–474, 2003.

[22] Y. Li, E. G. Schouten, X. Hu, Z. Cui, D. Luan, and G. Ma, "Obesity prevalence and time trend among youngsters in China, 1982–2002," *Asia Pacific Journal of Clinical Nutrition*, vol. 17, no. 1, pp. 131–137, 2008.

[23] R. Kelishadi, G. Ardalan, R. Gheiratmand et al., "Thinness, overweight and obesity in a national sample of Iranian children and adolescents: CASPIAN Study," *Child*, vol. 34, no. 1, pp. 44–54, 2008.

[24] D. Nitzan Kaluski, G. Demem Mazengia, T. Shimony, R. Goldsmith, and E. M. Berry, "Prevalence and determinants of physical activity and lifestyle in relation to obesity among schoolchildren in Israel," *Public Health Nutrition*, vol. 12, no. 6, pp. 774–782, 2009.

[25] Y. S. Khader, A. Batieha, H. Jaddou, Z. Batieha, M. El-Khateeb, and K. Ajlouni, "Metabolic abnormalities associated with obesity in children and adolescents in Jordan," *International Journal of Pediatric Obesity*, vol. 6, no. 3-4, pp. 215–222, 2011.

[26] A. Bener, "Prevalence of obesity, overweight, and underweight in Qatari adolescents," *Food and Nutrition Bulletin*, vol. 27, no. 1, pp. 39–45, 2006.

[27] M. I. El Mouzan, P. J. Foster, A. S. Al Herbish et al., "Prevalence of overweight and obesity in Saudi children and adolescents," *Annals of Saudi Medicine*, vol. 30, no. 6, pp. 203–208, 2010, Erratum in: Annals of Saudi Medicine, vol. 30, 500–502, 2010.

[28] T.-H. Liou, Y.-C. Huang, and P. Chou, "Prevalence and secular trends in overweight and obese Taiwanese children and adolescents in 1991–2003," *Annals of Human Biology*, vol. 36, no. 2, pp. 176–185, 2009.

[29] S. W. Ng, S. Zaghloul, H. Ali et al., "Nutrition transition in the United Arab Emirates," *European Journal of Clinical Nutrition*, vol. 65, no. 12, pp. 1328–1337, 2011.

[30] S. C. Savva, Y. Kourides, M. Tornaritis, M. Epiphaniou-Savva, C. Chadjigeorgiou, and A. Kafatos, "Obesity in children and adolescents in Cyprus. Prevalence and predisposing factors," *International Journal of Obesity*, vol. 26, no. 8, pp. 1036–1045, 2002.

[31] M. Kunesova, J. Vignerova, A. Steflová et al., "Obesity of Czech children and adolescents: relation to parental obesity and socioeconomic factors," *Journal of Public Health*, vol. 15, no. 3, pp. 163–170, 2007.

[32] S. Blüher, C. Meigen, R. Gausche et al., "Age-specific stabilization in obesity prevalence in German children: a cross-sectional

study from 1999 to 2008," *International Journal of Pediatric Obesity*, vol. 6, no. 2, pp. e199–e206, 2011.

[33] T. Tzotzas, E. Kapantais, K. Tziomalos et al., "Epidemiological survey for the prevalence of overweight and abdominal obesity in Greek adolescents," *Obesity*, vol. 16, no. 7, pp. 1718–1722, 2008.

[34] A. Vieno, M. Santinello, and M. C. Martini, "Epidemiology of overweight and obesity among Italian early adolescents: relation with physical activity and sedentary behaviour," *Epidemiologia e Psichiatria Sociale*, vol. 14, no. 2, pp. 100–107, 2005.

[35] H. Whelton, J. Harrington, E. Crowley, V. Kelleher, M. Cronin, and I. J. Perry, "Prevalence of overweight and obesity on the island of Ireland: results from the North South Survey of Children's Height, Weight and Body Mass Index, 2002," *BMC Public Health*, vol. 7, article 187, 2007.

[36] L. B. Sardinha, R. Santos, S. Vale et al., "Prevalence of overweight and obesity among Portuguese youth: a study in a representative sample of 1018-year-old children and adolescents," *International Journal of Pediatric Obesity*, vol. 6, no. 2, pp. e124–e128, 2011.

[37] Ö. B. Ekblom, K. Oddsson, and B. T. Ekblom, "Prevalence and regional differences in overweight in 2001 and trends in BMI distribution in Swedish children from 1987 to 2001," *Scandinavian Journal of Public Health*, vol. 32, no. 4, pp. 257–263, 2004.

[38] M. L. Booth, T. Dobbins, A. D. Okely, E. Denney-Wilson, and L. L. Hardy, "Trends in the prevalence of overweight and obesity among young Australians, 1985, 1997, and 2004," *Obesity*, vol. 15, no. 5, pp. 1089–1095, 2007.

[39] J. Utter, S. Denny, S. Crengle et al., "Overweight among New Zealand adolescents: associations with ethnicity and deprivation," *International Journal of Pediatric Obesity*, vol. 5, no. 6, pp. 461–466, 2010.

[40] R. M. Tassitano, M. V. G. D. Barros, M. C. M. Tenório, J. Bezerra, and P. C. Hallal, "Prevalence of overweight and obesity and associated factors among public high school students in Pernambuco State, Brazil," *Cadernos de Saúde Pública*, vol. 25, no. 12, pp. 2639–2652, 2009.

[41] G. T. C. Ko, R. Ozaki, G. W. K. Wong et al., "The problem of obesity among adolescents in Hong Kong: a comparison using various diagnostic criteria," *BMC Pediatrics*, vol. 8, article 10, 2008.

[42] R. Bishwalata, A. B. Singh, A. J. Singh, L. U. Devi, and R. K. Bikramjit Singh, "Overweight and obesity among schoolchildren in Manipur, India," *National Medical Journal of India*, vol. 23, no. 5, pp. 263–266, 2010.

[43] N. N. Abu Baker and S. M. Daradkeh, "Prevalence of overweight and obesity among adolescents in irbid governorate, Jordan," *Eastern Mediterranean Health Journal*, vol. 16, no. 6, pp. 657–662, 2010.

[44] K. Søren and C. Jo, "The prevalence of overweight and obesity among Danish school children," *Obesity Reviews*, vol. 11, no. 7, pp. 489–491, 2010.

[45] H. Thibault, B. Contrand, E. Saubusse, M. Baine, and S. Maurice-Tison, "Risk factors for overweight and obesity in French adolescents: physical activity, sedentary behavior and parental characteristics," *Nutrition*, vol. 26, no. 2, pp. 192–200, 2010.

[46] Y. Manios, P. D. Angelopoulos, G. Kourlaba et al., "Prevalence of obesity and body mass index correlates in a representative sample of Cretan school children," *International Journal of Pediatric Obesity*, vol. 6, no. 2, pp. 135–141, 2011.

[47] Á. Baráth, K. Boda, M. Tichy, É. Károly, and S. Túri, "International comparison of blood pressure and BMI values in schoolchildren aged 11–16 years," *Acta Paediatrica, International Journal of Paediatrics*, vol. 99, no. 2, pp. 251–255, 2010.

[48] F. Velluzzi, A. Lai, G. Secci et al., "Prevalence of overweight and obesity in Sardinian adolescents," *Eating and Weight Disorders*, vol. 12, no. 2, pp. e44–e50, 2007.

[49] R. Baratta, C. Degano, D. Leonardi, R. Vigneri, and L. Frittitta, "High prevalence of overweight and obesity in 11–15-year-old children from Sicily," *Nutrition, Metabolism and Cardiovascular Diseases*, vol. 16, no. 4, pp. 249–255, 2006.

[50] M. Jodkowska, A. Oblacinska, and I. Tabak, "Overweight and obesity among adolescents in Poland: gender and regional differences," *Public Health Nutrition*, vol. 13, no. 10, pp. 1688–1692, 2010.

[51] M. M. Bibiloni, E. Martinez, R. Llull, M. D. Juarez, A. Pons, and J. A. Tur, "Prevalence and risk factors for obesity in Balearic Islands adolescents," *British Journal of Nutrition*, vol. 103, no. 1, pp. 99–106, 2010.

[52] P. Henríquez Sánchez, J. Doreste Alonso, P. Laínez Sevillano et al., "Prevalence of obesity and overweight in adolescents from Canary Islands, Spain. Relationship with breakfast and physical activity," *Medicina Clínica*, vol. 130, pp. 606–610, 2008.

[53] A. M. Lasserre, A. Chiolero, F. Cachat, F. Paccaud, and P. Bovet, "Overweight in Swiss children and associations with children's and parents' characteristics," *Obesity*, vol. 15, no. 12, pp. 2912–2919, 2007.

[54] N. Öner, Ü. Vatansever, A. Sari et al., "Prevalence of underweight, overweight and obesity in Turkish adolescents," *Swiss Medical Weekly*, vol. 134, no. 35-36, pp. 529–533, 2004.

[55] A. C. F. De Moraes, R. P. Fadoni, L. M. Ricardi et al., "Prevalence of abdominal obesity in adolescents: a systematic review," *Obesity Reviews*, vol. 12, no. 2, pp. 69–77, 2011.

[56] T. Lobstein, L. Baur, and R. Uauy, "Obesity in children and young people: a crisis in public health," *Obesity Reviews*, vol. 5, supplement 1, pp. 4–85, 2004.

[57] S. Low, M. C. Chin, and M. Deurenberg-Yap, "Review on epidemic of obesity," *Annals of the Academy of Medicine Singapore*, vol. 38, no. 1, pp. 57–59, 2009.

[58] L. Serra Majem, L. Ribas Barba, J. Aranceta Bartrina, C. Pérez Rodrigo, P. Saavedra Santana, and L. Peña Quintana, "Childhood and adolescent obesity in Spain. Results of the enKid study (1998–2000)," *Medicina Clinica*, vol. 121, no. 19, pp. 725–732, 2003.

[59] J. Aranceta, C. Pérez Rodrigo, L. Serra Majem et al., "Prevalencia de la obesidad en España: resultados del estudio SEEDO, 2000," *Medicina Clínica*, vol. 120, pp. 608–612, 2003.

[60] J. Kain, R. Uauy, F. Vio, and C. Albala, "Trends in overweight and obesity prevalence in Chilean children: comparison of three definitions," *European Journal of Clinical Nutrition*, vol. 56, no. 3, pp. 200–204, 2002.

[61] L. Monasta, T. Lobstein, T. J. Cole, J. Vignerová, and A. Cattaneo, "Defining overweight and obesity in pre-school children: IOTF reference or WHO standard?" *Obesity Reviews*, vol. 12, no. 4, pp. 295–300, 2011.

[62] L. A. Moreno, M. G. Blay, G. Rodríguez et al., "Screening performances of the International Obesity Task Force body mass index cut-off values in adolescents," *Journal of the American College of Nutrition*, vol. 25, no. 5, pp. 403–408, 2006.

[63] M. De Onis and T. Lobstein, "Defining obesity risk status in the general childhood population: which cut-offs should we use?" *International Journal of Pediatric Obesity*, vol. 5, no. 6, pp. 458–460, 2010.

[64] J. J. Reilly, J. Kelly, and D. C. Wilson, "Accuracy of simple clinical and epidemiological definitions of childhood obesity: systematic review and evidence appraisal," *Obesity Reviews*, vol. 11, no. 9, pp. 645–655, 2010.

[65] D. S. Freedman, J. Wang, J. C. Thornton et al., "Racial/ethnic differences in body fatness among children and adolescents," *Obesity*, vol. 16, no. 5, pp. 1105–1111, 2008.

[66] J. J. Reilly, "Obesity in childhood and adolescence: evidence based clinical and public health perspectives," *Postgraduate Medical Journal*, vol. 82, no. 969, pp. 429–437, 2006.

19

From Passive Overeating to "Food Addiction": A Spectrum of Compulsion and Severity

Caroline Davis

Kinesiology & Health Sciences, Faculty of Health, York University, 343 Bethune College, 4700 Keele Street, Toronto, ON, Canada M3J 1P3

Correspondence should be addressed to Caroline Davis; cdavis@yorku.ca

Academic Editors: H. Gordish-Dressman, E. K. Naderali, S. J. Pintauro, S. Straube, S. Weitzman, and J. Zempleni

A psychobiological dimension of eating behaviour is proposed, which is anchored at the low end by energy intake that is relatively well matched to energy output and is reflected by a stable body mass index (BMI) in the healthy range. Further along the continuum are increasing degrees of overeating (and BMI) characterized by more severe and more compulsive ingestive behaviours. In light of the many similarities between chronic binge eating and drug abuse, several authorities have adopted the perspective that an apparent dependence on highly palatable food—accompanied by emotional and social distress—can be best conceptualized as an addiction disorder. Therefore, this review also considers the overlapping symptoms and characteristics of binge eating disorder (BED) and models of food addiction, both in preclinical animal studies and in human research. It also presents this work in the context of the modern and "toxic" food environment and therein the ubiquitous triggers for over-consumption. We complete the review by providing evidence that what we have come to call "food addiction" may simply be a more acute and pathologically dense form of BED.

Nothing would be more tiresome than eating and drinking if God had not made them a pleasure as well as a necessity.
(Voltaire)

1. Introduction

By many accounts, obesity now ranks as one of the greatest and most preventable global threats to public health [1, 2]. Furthermore, as a result of fetal programming, it will likely gather momentum and become a self-perpetuating problem as a form of "inheritance of acquired characteristics" from one generation to the next [3–5]. Currently, more than half the adult population is described as overweight or obese, (Implied in the terms overweight and obese is an excess in one's level of adiposity or percentage of body fat, not in other components of the mass that comprises their body weight such as muscle or bone density. In other words, body weight (typically expressed as body mass index (BMI): (weight kg/height metres2)) is typically and conveniently used as a surrogate for adiposity—although as an estimate of fatness, it has a considerable margin of error at the individual level.) marking the first time in human evolutionary history that the number of people with excess body weight has surpassed those who are underweight [6, 7]. Indeed, in the United States alone, as many as one in three adult women now have a BMI greater than 30 [8]. Moreover, and on a similar trajectory, estimates of the global prevalence of this condition in children increased from 42% in 1990 to 67% in 2010 [9]. During the same time period, both mean maternal weight at delivery and mean offspring birth weight were steadily increasing [10]. These are important issues since maternal obesity is a strong predictor of fetal insulin resistance [11] and childhood obesity [12, 13].

Reflecting the obesity "pandemic"—with its prodigious economic burden on societies worldwide [14]—has been the relatively sudden and very pronounced global increase in obesity-related research since the end of the 20th century [15]. While several factors coalesced to serve as catalysts, what largely prompted this research focus was the powerful evidence, which had steadily accumulated since the 1930s, of a broad range of health risks associated with possessing too much fatness, including links to metabolic, cardiovascular, and oncological disease, as well as to orthopedic complications and psychiatric disturbances [16, 17].

At the beginning of the 21st century, there was a noticeable migration from the earlier research emphasis on health-related *outcomes* of obesity to an emerging focus on the *causes* of, and *antecedent factors* leading to, obesity. This new endeavor was prompted, in part, by several important scientific developments such as the discovery of leptin [18], technological advances in genetic research including the sequencing the human genome [19], and the burgeoning field of neuroscience with its sophisticated neuroimaging techniques [20]. At about the same time, political influences also played an important role in bringing about a new direction in research. Public health officials and advocates began a relentless exposition of the dramatically changed food environment and of the food and beverage industry's powerful role in promoting poor nutrition policies [21–23].

Some of the 'highlight' observations and conclusions from the resulting body of research were that most animals, including *homo sapiens*, are biologically predisposed to overeat when energy resources are available and that we do this with alacrity when foods are of a particularly appealing composition [24, 25]. This once adaptive biological drive is now contributing to widespread overnutrition in a fundamental way, especially because economic growth in capitalist cultures began to switch from a demand for cheap labour to an emerging emphasis on consumption and how best to drive consumer behavior [5].

1.1. Evolution and Energy Resources. These events raise the interesting and topical question: *why* are individuals prone to eat, often voraciously, beyond caloric need and to store an excess of adipose tissue when the long-term consequences of these inherent strategies are so remarkably deleterious? A biocultural viewpoint, highlighting co-evolutionary processes, is, undoubtedly, the best viewpoint for understanding these issues [26]. Since such a rapid and recent change in the population phenotype could not be genetic, one must assume that our current environment interacts with our evolved biology, in some complex way, to give rise to the situation where a substantial proportion of the population are prone to persistent weight gain [4].

Evolutionary theory pivots on the fundamental premise that most characteristics we possess resulted largely from natural selection such that gene frequencies of alleles increase across generations because they confer reproductive success, that is, more progeny are produced who survive until they are procreant. And energy availability is the most important environmental factor for sustainable reproduction [27]. The crux of the issue, however, is that in most environments, and for most species, energy availability has been historically inconsistent and unpredictable. In other words, it has typically been difficult to obtain even ample resources let alone a surplus of food—at least until modern times during which there have been dramatic changes to the food environment. In many parts of the world, the industrialization of food processing and the advanced technology to enlarge food supplies have created an ubiquitous, greatly available, and inexpensive source of energy-dense (high sugar and fats) food, and concomitantly, pronounced reductions in the need for energy expenditure to secure this food [26].

Another basic tenet of evolutionary biology is that even though a gene ultimately decreases the lifespan, if it increases the ability to produce offspring and raise them to maturity, that gene will be selected. Schneider [28] argues that, historically, the mechanisms that prioritized eating or copulating were very successful at perpetuating our species. In other words, the tendency to engage in these behaviours evolved in an environment where there was typically a choice between time spent foraging and feeding, and time spent courting and mating. A compelling body of recent and related animal research has demonstrated that leptin increases sexual motivation in females independent of the effects of the estrous cycle [29], and that in males it also increases the relative motivation to engage in sexual activity rather than in eating behaviours [30]. In modern times, these same mechanisms have likely contributed to increases in obesity because leptin levels increase as weight is gained. Specifically, obesity is a highly transmissible condition (~.6 to .8) suggesting a mainly genetic influence on population variation in BMI [31, 32]. Heritability estimates for obesity are also greater in women than in men [33, 34]. Since obese mothers tend to have significantly more children than their lean counterparts, obesity is therefore likely to increase from generation to generation for purely genetic reasons [35].

1.2. Overconsumption and Weight Gain. While the population prevalence of obesity has doubled in the past few decades, its morbid form (BMI > 40) has seen an alarming 4-fold increase compared to cohorts with lower BMI values [36]. These findings suggest that, on average, the more weight one gains, the easier or more likely it is that the process will escalate over time. The issue of "overeating sensitization" will be discussed in greater detail in a later section of this paper.

At a basic physiological level, the only way to accumulate body fat is by a sustained state of positive energy balance. A question that continues to be debated, however, amongst scientists trying to explain the rise in obesity rates is the relative contribution of chronic increases in energy intake on the one hand, as against chronic decreases in energy expenditure on the other [37]. In a sense, this is a question without a clear answer because, in the context of energy balance, the two contributing factors are rather difficult to uncouple. Nevertheless, some related evidence seems rather indisputable. For instance, data from a variety of sources have consistently demonstrated an increasing trend in daily calorie intake in most developed countries over the past few generations [14, 38]. Also, in most high-income countries, energy expenditure has been decreasing since the beginning of the 20th century—to the very low levels we see today—largely because of mechanization, urbanization, and computerization [14].

In a well-modulated biological system we would expect decreases in physical activity to be matched by decreases in food intake, as was generally seen in the first half of the 20th century. Swinburn et al. [14] have described the "energy balance flipping point" (pg 807), a phenomenon which occurred around 1960, when population energy intake no longer matched output. This, he argued, occurred almost entirely because of the emergence, and great availability, of highly caloric and very tasty processed foods whose characteristics disrupted the homeostatic mechanisms that had evolved to keep intake and expenditure roughly in balance, except, of course, in times of unavoidable energy scarcity such as seasonal food shortages and periods of drought or botanical pestilence.

This singular shift in the direction of weight gain in the past several decades inspired a novel research focus on the issue of *nonhomeostatic* drivers of food intake. There was a pressing need to better understand the universal human tendency to eat beyond caloric need—and in the absence of physiological signals of hunger—when individuals are in the presence of a rich variety of highly palatable and visually attractive food. Descriptively, the term "hedonic hunger" has been used to depict the imaginative cravings associated with these foods, and the motivational drive which fosters eating primarily because of the gustatory rewarding properties of the cuisine [39]. In an environment where hyperpalatable foods are abundant and proliferate, hedonic hunger contributes in a powerful way to patterns of overeating such as frequent snacking [40] and larger portion sizes [41], and the consequential weight gain that can lead to obesity.

While the physiological mechanisms regulating homeostatic hunger are generally well understood [42–44], a clear understanding of the neural and peripheral brain pathways driving hedonically-based eating is only beginning to emerge. For example, it is now recognized that highly palatable foods activate the mesocorticolimbic reward circuits of the brain by the release of dopamine, as well as other neurotransmitters and hormones like the endogenous opiates [45]. Indeed, after a period of food deprivation any wholesome food will activate the reward pathway, which evolved to regulate the experience of pleasure from behaviours that are essential for our survival, and to enhance the motivation to seek out these rewards in our environment. The important distinction, however, is that delicious foods activate the neurochemical signals more reliably and more potently than less tasty substances.

Recent experimental findings also indicated that when the motivation to eat is activated by highly palatable food such as pastries and cakes, and there is no prior and extended period of energy deprivation, activation of two other rewarding chemical signals—endocannabinoids and ghrelin—occurs [46]. Importantly, this hedonic response was not generated when bland foods like dry bread and milk were offered to participants under the same laboratory conditions.

2. The Modern Food Environment

The dramatic rise in obesity rates in the past few generations can mostly be explained by pronounced changes in the physical environment and in people's personal economic environment [47]. In particular, a reduction in the time-cost of food across the global food system has been a major contributor to recent population weight gain [14]. What has been described as a markedly "toxic" food environment is also exemplified by the increased prevalence of chemical additives and flavor enhancers in the food supply [48]. Some have even suggested that the highly processed foods we eat would be more correctly labeled "food-like products" to distinguish them from the natural sources of energy like fruits and vegetables that comprised the diet of our ancestral predecessors [49].

The marketing power of palatable foods is not only seen by the high consumer demand for these products and the double-digit growth of goods like luxury chocolate, but by the invocation of food images to sell a host of other nonedible products. For example, the odorants currently used to sell bath and beauty products, and perfumes and colognes, now regularly imitate the scents and aromas of tasty and beloved foods, rather than the floral and botanical alternatives like lavender and gardenia that were traditionally used. A poignant illustration is the spring 2013 Special Promotion, by a very successful fragrance manufacturer, of their *Sugar and Spice* collection inspired by "delectable ingredients" that are "decadently tempting." Their items bear names such as "Lemon Tart," "Bitter Orange and Chocolate," and "Ginger Biscuit."

Given the profound alterations to modern life on many parts of the globe, there has been much speculation about a current "mismatch" between our evolved human propensity to consume good tasting food when it is available—even in the absence of hunger—and the much-altered food environment where high-energy resources are prodigiously and excessively available [50–53]. Research has also focused on the complex interaction between the "human epigenome" and the modern food supply. For instance, there is accumulating evidence that maternal body weight and diet may work, via *in utero* placental signaling, to alter her offspring's future eating behavior and risk for obesity [4].

Globally, the prevalence of obesity is greater in women than men [54]; similar data were also found in those of African descent and in Hispanics in the United States, but for some reason, not among American Caucasians [8]. In a recent study, and using as evidence 20th century famines that occurred around the world, it was shown that the female offspring of women whose diets were nutritionally restricted during their pregnancy, and who later found themselves raised in an environment with an abundance of calorie-rich food, were at greater risk of obesity than their male counterparts [55]. Interestingly, this phenomenon is most visible in moderately developed countries where the economy has expended rapidly in recent years, illustrating the strength of the *in utero* or perinatal nutritional environment in altering risk for obesity. These findings also provide some insight into factors contributing to global sex differences in obesity prevalence. Since the modern food environment also increases the likelihood that some individuals will develop a compulsive pattern of overeating and show signs of dependence on sugary and fatty substances (to be discussed later in this review), it may be that women are also more prone to "food addiction" than men.

2.1. Brain Reward Mechanisms and Food Consumption. For at least half a century, we have known that dopamine neural circuitry in the midbrain modulates the reinforcing properties of addictive drugs like alcohol, psychomotor stimulants ("speed"), and nicotine [56]. Surprisingly, however, the regulatory role of these same pathways in relation to food consumption—especially when the diet is highly palatable—has only been investigated systematically for a few decades [57]. Somehow, the chronology of these respective scientific "discoveries" seems rather upturned—like the proverbial "cart before the horse." In other words, the time sequence implies that the human brain somehow evolved to find drugs of abuse highly reinforcing, and that coincidentally, these same brain regions are activated, albeit less potently (It has been estimated, for instance, that the dopamine release from psychomotor stimulant drugs is about 10-fold greater than to a normal meal when one is hungry [58].), by a wide variety of tasty foods.

Anthropological evidence indicates that human beings shared a co-evolutionary relationship with psychotropic plant substances, such as the coca leaf and the poppy, in prehistory for millennia. Indeed, they frequently ate them as food because their ingestion solved a recurrent problem faced by our ancestors [59]. Due to famines and seasonal food shortages, people experienced deficits in the brain's "chemical messengers" (e.g., dopamine and serotonin) with considerable regularity—depletions which can adversely affect critical behaviours and emotions like motor activities, cognitive abilities, and mood [60]. Because these plant-based "neurotransmitter analogues" prevented fatigue, diminished appetite, and increased tolerance for hunger when they were eaten, they helped to counteract the deleterious consequences of stress if adequate food sources were challenged [59]. In other words, plant substances served the dual purpose of substituting for more costly energy and of buffering against the biological ravages of prolonged strain and tension.

It is well established that the mesocorticolimbic dopamine system, and its neurophysiological connections, evolved to subserve primitive and necessary biological functions long before the concept of addiction was relevant and even considered [61]. These neural pathways originate in the ventral tegmental area, which sends projections to the limbic structures, including the amygdala, and to the striatal regions of the basal ganglia. There are also afferent and efferent connections between these subcortical structures and parts of the prefrontal cortex [62]. Collectively this brain circuitry is also known as the *common reward pathway* because we experience pleasure and an enhanced sense of well-being from its activation, which occurs when we engage in a wide variety of activities, like eating, sex, and maternal behaviours, that are essential for our continued existence. More broadly, these midbrain pathways comprise both a survival and a reproductive regulatory system because they respond to perceived threats against our reproductive fitness, as well as to the positive behaviours we find rewarding [63].

Substance abuse is a relatively recent phenomenon in the history of our species and occurs largely because we learned to purify and synthesize potent drugs from plant materials and because their routes of administration to the brain have become more direct [64, 65]. In other words, it is the concentrated doses of these substances, and their ubiquity, that have contributed to wide-spread human drug addictions. Consequently, it seems reasonable to conclude that organic compounds in our environment—whether they derive from psychotropic plant substances or from edible energy resources—can only be viewed as *beneficial* or *harmful* when we take account of their potency, the frequency of their consumption, and the relevant characteristics of those who partake of them [66].

2.2. Some Foods as Addictive Substances. Of all the macronutrients, carbohydrates—and in particular disaccharides like table sugar (sucrose)—have been ascribed the greatest, potentially addictive, properties [67]. It is hardly surprising, therefore, that sweet-tasting foods are the ones we most prefer to eat, and that this preference is especially enhanced when foods contain fat and salt in addition to sugar. It appears, however, that in the quantities we currently consume these highly palatable ingredients, they have a capacity for abuse similar to other addictive drugs [67–71]. The poignant observation that most rats show a stronger preference for a sweet solution than for cocaine—even in animals with an extensive history of drug use—is a strong testament to the powerful effects of sugar and its great reinforcing value [72].

As we have seen, a substance's addictive potential is increased both by its potency and by its rapid absorption into the bloodstream [71, 73]. Relevantly, sugar is quickly absorbed and thereby substantially more reinforcing than many other foods. As foods became more processed and altered by the manufacturing industry, they began to take on more and more properties of addictive drugs, largely because of the ingredients that were added to enhance the taste of food [70]. A particularly powerful example is the evolution of corn in the human diet. For generations, it was a staple and frequently consumed source of complex carbohydrate. Due, however, to advanced technological and subsidies to the corn farmers in the United States in the 1960s and 1970s, this crop was refined into high fructose corn syrup (HFCS), an exceedingly concentrated and very sweet simple carbohydrate. Otherwise fructose is found only in small amounts and in a few of the natural foods that comprised most traditional diets [74]. Over the past 40 years or so, the abundance of HFCS—added as a sweetener to a large variety of processed foods such as soft drinks, breakfast cereals, and desserts—has been a powerful contributor to the greatly enhanced palatability of many of the foods we eat regularly. Indeed, our consumption of this inexpensive simple sugar has increased substantially in a few generations from about 4% to 12% of our daily caloric intake [75].

The special physiological properties of fructose render it very similar to substances like alcohol because the two are biochemically congruent; ethanol is simply the fermented byproduct of fructose [76]. When taken in large quantities, both substances can promote neurobiological changes that encourage further problematic use such as excessive overconsumption. As with all addictive drugs, excessive consumption causes a dampening of the brain's "pleasure" signal, which can foster increased intake of the substance, pronounced cravings, continued use despite negative consequences, and withdrawal symptoms during periods of abstinence [77].

The metabolic impact of fructose also differs substantially from other sugars like glucose because it blunts leptin signaling, thereby promoting sensations of hunger and activation of the reward pathways creating a desire for consumption independent of energy needs [78]—a phenomenon that is directly comparable to what occurs when alcohol is used [76]. In other words, while glucose stimulates the release of insulin, decreasing the desire to eat, fructose and ethanol produce this effect to a very weak degree. Interestingly, etiologic links between overeating and alcohol use have also been demonstrated in a recent study. Women with a family history of alcoholism (i.e., a biological parent or sibling) had almost double the odds of being obese compared to those without a family history—a statistical association that remained robust after controlling for a number of well-established covariates of obesity [79]. While this relationship was seen in men as well, it was not as strong as in women.

Diets high in concentrated fats and sugars are not only dense in calories, but metabolically efficient because they provide a large proportion of daily energy requirements. They also tend to elevate mood by releasing neuropeptides which reinforce their selective preference [80]. Although hyperpalatable foods differ in some ways from the key characteristics of traditional addictive drugs, they also have many features in common [70]. For instance, highly processed foods and drugs of abuse are both capable of triggering cravings [81, 82]. Biologists believe that "cravings" for sugar and fat evolved to enhance human energy intake in unpredictable nutritional environments [66]. Consumption of highly processed foods and drugs of abuse are also both associated with compulsive overuse even in the face of severely adverse consequences [83]. And finally, the loss-of-control over intake and the inability to cut down consumption of both substances are additional characteristics they have in common [83]. In summary, while highly processed foods do not cause the intoxication of alcohol or the euphoria produced by some stimulant drugs like cocaine, there are nevertheless significant areas of overlap with conventional addictive drugs [70].

2.3. Compulsive Overeating as an Addictive Behaviour. The parallels between compulsive overeating and drug abuse have been recognized by clinicians for decades, albeit mostly in anecdotal reports, and with particular reference to the pronounced cravings and the mood-enhancing effects they produce [70, 84–90]. Among the general public, the notion that overeating can be an addictive behavior has also been widely accepted for many years—as seen, for instance, by the many 12-Step treatment programs (e.g., *Overeaters Anonymous* founded in 1960; *Food Addicts Anonymous* founded in 1987) established for those who suffer from an apparent loss-of-control over food intake [91]. Interestingly, however, a recent study, using both surveys and an experimental paradigm, found that the public perception of "food addiction" was more favourable than it was for other addictions like drug and nicotine abuse, and alcoholism [92]. Consequently, this putative condition may be less vulnerable than other addiction disorders to the ill effects of social stigma.

Although there are no formal or agreed-upon diagnostic criteria, the notion of an addiction to hyperpalatable food is also receiving widespread and increased attention from the popular media. It is only very recently, however, that the term "food addiction" has gained any scientific credibility. For instance, according to the Web of Science data base, there has been a steeply exponential increase in the number of scientific publications devoted to this topic, from 3 in 2008 to 34 in 2012, and only two publications between 2000 and 2007. An important catalyst for the renewed interest in food addiction is the very convincing and accumulating evidence—illustrated in the previous section—that highly palatable foods rich in sugar, fat, and salt have an abuse potential similar to addictive drugs like cocaine and alcohol [67, 70, 71]. In addition, evidence of the biological parallels between drug and food abuse, as demonstrated by preclinical experiments and behavior genetic research, has further strengthened the credibility of the food-addiction construct [93, 94]. Functional neuroimaging studies have also demonstrated that pleasant looking, smelling, and tasting foods have reinforcing properties similar to drugs of abuse [95].

Drug addiction is a dynamic behavioural disorder progressing from intermittent to regular use, and eventually to excessive and intractable intake. Evidence from population-based transmission studies also suggests that *common* biological influences contribute to the abuse of a broad range of addictive substances and that these factors are of equal importance in men and women [96]. While natural and pharmacologic reinforcers activate both limbic and cortical structures and connections known collectively as the mesocorticolimbic dopamine pathway (described in a previous section) [97], the pleasure experienced from either tasty foods or addictive drugs correlates positively with the amount of dopamine released specifically in the striatum [98, 99]. Not surprisingly, individual differences affecting the responsiveness of the dopamine system have been a major target for investigating vulnerability to drug abuse [100] and more recently, risk for compulsive overeating [94, 101, 102].

One source of evidence for a common biological connection between overeating and drug taking comes from a converging body of human and animal research demonstrating that excessive food consumption and drug self-administration are closely related genetically [103, 104]. For example, in a study of female twins, there was a moderate to large degree of overlap in additive genetic factors between alcohol use and binge eating, and no overlap in environmental effects [105]. Rats selectively bred for high sweet preference also represent a robust (drug) addiction-prone phenotype compared to the low sweet-preference group who appear to be an addiction-resistant animal model [103]. Similarly the inverse also obtains. Sugar preference is also greater in animals with high alcohol responsiveness compared to their low-responsive counterparts [106].

2.3.1. The Development of Tolerance. Regulatory or homeostatic systems evolved to respond to challenges to the normal "evolutionary experience" of the organism and to make suitable compensatory adjustments [4]. When any homeostatic system remains chronically activated, or activated to a level outside its norm due to persistent external pressures, it will eventually sustain damage or long-lasting alterations in the related physiology [4].

Following chronic exposure to a potent addictive substance, the original response to the drug tends to diminish so that more, or more frequent, exposure is required to elicit the strength of the initial reaction. This process—the development of *tolerance*—is a cardinal characteristic of drug addiction. The neuro-adaptive changes in the brain's reward pathways that give rise to this phenomenon only occur when levels of reward stimulation by addictive drugs, or other dopamine agonists, become excessive. Specifically, the neuro-adaptation that occurs is a postsynaptic downregulation, which results in the reactivity of the reward pathway becoming desensitized [107]. For instance, reductions of striatal dopamine receptor levels, and of dopamine signaling strength, have been observed in response to repeated psychomotor stimulant administration [108–111]. There is also evidence of decreased brain cannabinoid receptor levels in human subjects who chronically smoke cannabis [112]. Consequently, as a result of the high and sustained levels of reward stimulation in substance abusers, and the subsequent downregulation, a pronounced decrease occurs in the individual's sensitivity or responsiveness to any kind of reward—a motivational and mood state known as *anhedonia*.

Preclinical research has also demonstrated downregulation of dopamine receptor availability in rodents following chronic exposure to high fat foods [113], as well as markedly reduced basal levels of dopamine in the nucleus accumbens (assessed by microdialysis procedures) after 5-day access to a high-fat diet in obese-prone compared to obese-resistant animals [114]. Other evidence of downregulated striatal dopamine signaling has also been found in some groups of adults with obesity. For example, using positron emission tomography (PET), a group of morbidly obese adults were found to have significantly lower D2 receptor densities in the striatum compared to a group of nonobese controls [115]. These findings were replicated in more recent study of obese women and nonobese controls using SPECT imaging [116]. There are, however, important caveats to consider when drawing conclusions from these particular results.

Neuroimaging studies simply illustrate the current state of brain-circuitry activation, and they have mostly used case-control designs in addiction-risk research, constraining the ability to separate *causal* factors from *consequences* of the addictive behavior [117]. Self-report measures of reward sensitivity are also limited by the incapacity to distinguish antecedents from outcomes in those with addiction disorders. In other words, the evidence indicating a dampened down dopamine signal in some cases of obesity could simply be a reflection of the neuro-adaptation to excessive brain stimulation from potent dopamine activators like foods high in sugar and fat. By contrast, the study of genetic variation underlying addictions is able to address causality and is grounded on the premise that exposure to various environmental influences—in combination with one's inherent biology—determines the initial response to drugs as well as the neuro-adaptations that contribute to the transition from casual use to the addicted state [118].

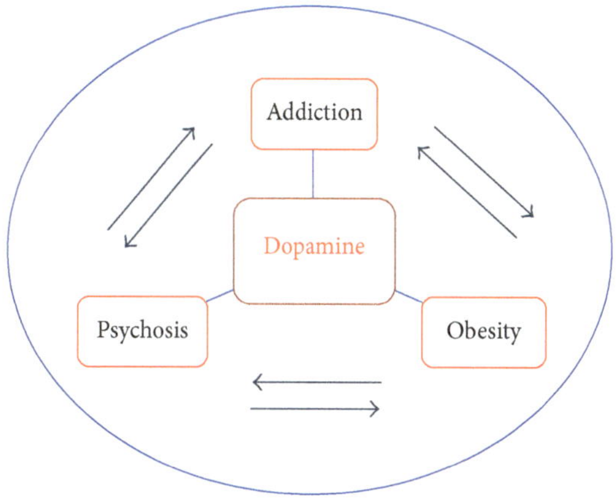

FIGURE 1: Comorbid interconnections among psychotic, addictive, and compulsive disorders and their biological links to dopamine regulatory brain pathways.

2.3.2. Escalation of Intake and Binge Consumption. While there is debate about precise mechanisms, another hallmark of addiction is that extended access to, and use of, drugs can precipitate a rapid escalation of intake, often in the form of binge-like consumption [119–122]. A similar response has been seen in animals exposed to high fat/sugar diets [93]. Based on sound theory and good empirical evidence, Alsio and colleagues [123] have proposed a "feed-forward" system involving neural adaptations in both the regulation of homeostatic and of hedonic hunger to explain the development of this behavioural pattern. Specifically, diets that are persistently high in fat and sugar promote a positive feedback signal that is experienced as an elevated or sensitized preference for, and consumption of, palatable foods, which in turn contributes to increased tendencies to overeat. The result can be a vicious cycle of craving and compulsive overeating, which is relatively resistant to change and highly prone to relapse after attempts to restrict palatable food intake. Such a pattern is clearly very similar to the psycho-behavioural blueprint that defines drug addiction.

Not only does dopamine play a pivotal role in the compulsive nature of addiction disorders and overeating, but it is strongly associated with the pathophysiology of *psychosis*, all of which are themselves interconnected [124], as depicted graphically in Figure 1. Evidence for the associated network among these conditions comes not only from clinical practice but also from a growing body of research findings. For example, some Parkinson's patients treated with L-dopa experience episodes of drug-induced psychosis, especially when the drug is given at high doses [125, 126]. This is very similar to the dose-dependent, transient psychotic/paranoid symptoms associated with cocaine, cannabis, and methamphetamine abuse [127–129]. Compulsive behaviours such as excessive spending/shopping, binge eating, and hypersexuality can also be provoked by longstanding exposure to dopamine replacement therapy in Parkinson's patients [130, 131].

Considered from the "flip-side" perspective, the neuroleptic drugs used to treat psychosis dampen down dopamine signaling and, as a consequence, tend to foster symptoms of Parkinsonism, as well as obesity, in some vulnerable individuals [132, 133]. There is also a close relationship between psychotic disorders and a host of addictions such as to cigarette smoking, alcoholism, and opiate abuse [134–136]. And finally, there is substantial evidence that obese individuals are more likely to engage in a variety of addictive behaviours compared to their lean counterparts [137]. For instance, in a sample of almost 200 adults, we have recently found that those with obesity were significantly more likely to smoke cigarettes ($p = 0.026$), to engage in excessive spending ($p < 0.0001$), and to have episodes of binge eating ($p < 0.0001$) compared to their normal weight counterparts [138].

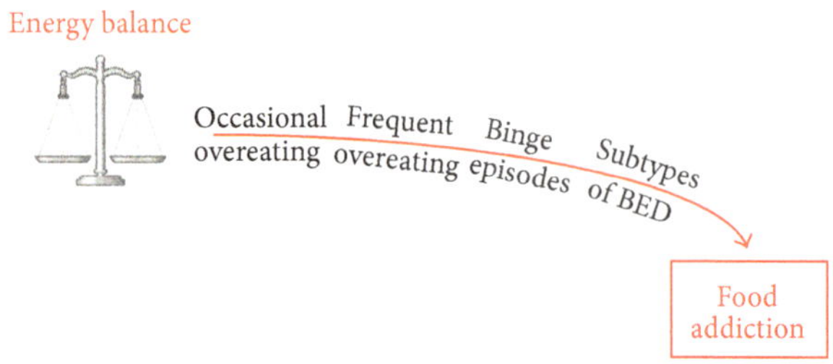

FIGURE 2: A downwardly escalating dimension of (over)eating and behaviours reflecting increased severity and compulsiveness.

3. A Dimensional View of Overeating

Most overweight and obese individuals do not display any distinctive, or especially aberrant, patterns of food consumption, nor do they typically suffer from clinically significant psychopathology or other behavioural disturbances. Some individuals overeat because the supreme self-regulation required to exercise dietary restraint is very difficult to muster in our obesogenic food environment [139]. Others may overeat because they are highly sensitivity or responsive to rewarding stimuli, of which palatable food is a primary target [140, 141]. Still others may use food to "self-medicate" a negative affect because sweet tastes have well-known mood-elevating, and pain-suppressing, properties [142]. However, a smaller proportion of individuals do show signs of disordered or dysregulated overeating, in varying degrees of severity, which are typically characterized by episodes of compulsive intake and/or nocturnal hyperphasia, and are associated with a range of psychiatric co-morbidities like depression, attention deficit/hyperactivity disorder (ADHD), and psychosis [143]. Despite some earlier suggestions to the contrary [144] obesity itself is not a mental disorder. There may, however, be some individuals, whose overeating and weight gain are caused by a psychiatric disturbance like depression [145], and others where the cause relates to their treatment, as seen in the case of neuroleptic-induced weight gain [124].

In the following sections of this review, the primary aim is to consider theoretical arguments and related evidence for the proposed view that *overeating* is a dimensional prototype reflecting collectively its severity, its degree of compulsiveness, and its clinically significant level of personal impairment, as presented in Figure 2. It will also be argued that chronic overeating—irrespective of the motivational factors that may have prompted this behaviour—increases the risk that over time food consumption will become more uncontrollable and intractable to change. Eventually, and in certain susceptible individuals, the nature of the behaviour will closely resemble a drug-addiction disorder [146].

At the beginning of the "eating continuum" is what we might call "homeostatic eating" reflected largely by a stable body weight falling within the "healthy range" (BMI between 18.5 and 25) according to regulatory institutions like the World Health Organization [147]. This state does not reflect any particular daily calorie intake, but rather that the energy consumed matches the energy expended in the form of physical activity and one's metabolic requirements. Further along the gamut we have "passive overeating", but with little or no concomitant psychopathology. The majority of individuals whose weight increases slowly over time, are largely unaware of living in a chronic state of positive energy balance. We live in an environment where it is enormously difficult for even the most restrained individuals to eat a diet sufficiently reduced in calories to match their energy expenditure. The proliferation of high-calorie fast food outlets and the convenience and low cost they provide, the increased portion sizes served in grocery stores and restaurants, the vast array and constant availability of food, and the enhanced taste experience of eating due to the sweeteners added to many foods and beverages, have created a collective inertia that is difficult to escape.

Still further along the eating continuum we see mild and intermittent "loss-of-control" eating, which manifests as episodic binges that tend to become more compulsive and more frequent in some individuals over time. When these behaviours become severe—as reflected by the downward curve displayed in Figure 2—a diagnosis of binge eating disorder (BED) may be warranted. Like virtually all psychiatric disturbances, despite a uniform clinical label, there is considerable heterogeneity in symptomatology, aetiology, and outcome in BED. Its heritability is also well established, with estimates suggesting that the genetic contribution is about 50%, and that its prevalence is significantly greater in women [148–150]. However, the quest for specific risk-markers for this disorder has been obstructed considerably by the complexity of the phenotype.

Although BED research is still relatively limited compared to more established disorders, it is important to identify and understand subtypes of BED with specific psychobiological profiles that may convey different vulnerabilities to environmental risk factors and therefore indicate different targets for intervention. Such an approach will better inform personalized treatment strategies for those who struggle with overeating and weight gain. For example, some individuals with BED have a BMI in the normal healthy range, and in many cases, are difficult to distinguish from normal-weight adults with nonpurging bulimia nervosa.

Among overweight adults with BED—a group who comprise the large majority of individuals with this disorder—some manifest virtually no psychopathological or behaviourally-aberrant differences from overweight adults without BED *except* for their binge eating and their elevated responsiveness to highly palatable food. Others, however, express significantly more severe and compulsive symptomatology and more psychopathological characteristics. They also display a clinical profile strongly akin to individuals with conventional drug-addiction disorders. In these individuals it seems eminently more appropriate to describe their condition as a "food addiction" and to recognize the biological state of dependence and the downwardly spiraling *pathophysiology* propelling the behaviours, rather than viewing it as a condition where *psychopathological* factors are largely driving the chaotic episodes of loss-of-control eating.

To recapitulate briefly, near the low end of the (over) eating continuum are those who—despite excessive calorie intake and weight gain—display little or no behavioural pathology and psychiatric disturbances, followed by those with a similar lack of pathology except in relation to their compulsive binge eating. At the higher end of the continuum are those with BED who display significant psychopathology and strong addictive tendencies towards food—indeed meeting the diagnostic criteria proposed for "food addiction" [151] based on the DSM-IV criteria for substance dependence. In particular, these individuals are highly impulsive, manifest significant mood disturbances, and display emotionally-driven bouts of overeating.

The following sections will provide a psychobiological discussion of BED followed by a detailed discussion of the evidence supporting the concept of food addiction. Arguments will then be presented, with supporting research evidence, that food addiction is largely a severe and compulsive form of BED rather than a clinically distinct condition with a unique aetiology and clinical course.

3.1. Bingeing and Binge Eating Disorder (BED). BED is an overeating syndrome seen much more frequently in those who are substantially overweight [152–154]. Frequent bingeing can also occur episodically in those who do not meet the criteria for an eating disorder according to the DSM [155]. The cardinal features of BED are recurrent binge eating without compensatory weight control behaviour such as self-induced vomiting, diuretic use, and excessive levels of physical activity (DSM-IV). The disorder is also associated with eating large amounts of food in the absence of hunger, eating alone because one is embarrassed, and feeling guilty, depressed, and disgusted after the binge episode.

BED also appears to be a behaviourally distinct subtype of obesity with an unique risk profile reflecting a heightened response to rewarding stimuli. In particular, individuals with this disorder display a hyperreactivity to the hedonic properties of food as seen by greater food cravings, preoccupation with thoughts of food, emotionally-induced overeating, and a greater preference for sweet and fatty foods [102, 156]. Moreover, it is no longer seen as a syndrome exclusive to adulthood as it once was. In recent years, bingeing or "loss-of-control" eating has also become prevalent in middle childhood and early adolescence [157]. Also pertinent to the theme of the current review is the observation that the 12-month prevalence of binge eating and illicit drug dependence occurs at roughly the same rate—in about 2% to 3% of the population [158].

3.1.1. Animal Studies of Binge Eating. Using animal paradigms to model psychological disorders is challenging and inevitably cannot represent the complexities seen in the human condition, nor the intricate factors that give rise to their development. On the other hand, animal models provide the opportunity to manipulate conditions, induce behavioural or physiological changes, and thereby isolate important causal factors that would be impossible to do in human research where studies are typically carried out in those with preexisting conditions.

Although several animal models of binge eating have been developed in recent years, the *limited access* paradigm is one of the most rigorously tested and is based on relevant DSM-IV criteria for binge eating [158]. In the typical protocol, one group of rats is given limited and intermittent access to fatty and/or sugary foods 3 times a week while the control group has access to the same foods every day of the week. Neither group is food deprived. Over a period of several weeks, the "intermittent" group shows increased intake of the palatable food at a significantly greater degree than the daily access group. In a brief period of time, they also eat larger amounts of the palatable food than is considered normal [159].

Similar findings have been observed in nonhuman primates who were given limited access to chocolate candy [160]. While excessive eating was clearly based on the palatability of the food in this paradigm, it was also moderated by social factors since the submissive animals—both male and female—ate more palatable food than their dominant counterparts [160, 161]. Interestingly these findings mesh with evidence that submissive primates also self-administered more cocaine than their dominant counterparts [162]. In summary, the *limited access* model has good clinical validity because many people who binge eat try to limit their access to sweet and fatty foods, and then typically binge on the very foods they have unsuccessfully tried to restrict [163, 164].

Another theory of binge eating with good face validity is the *maternal separation* animal model, which implicates stressful experiences occurring in childhood with behavioural abnormalities later in life [165]. Specifically, neonatal maternal separation or isolation is associated with the development of binge-related eating if the animal is confronted with social or metabolic stressors later in life. Many studies have demonstrated that traumatic events early in life form a major risk factor for developing subsequent depressive disorders [166, 167]. We also know that individuals with compulsive, binge-like overeating frequently have cooccurring symptoms of depression and anxiety that predate the eating disturbances [168, 169].

3.1.2. Biological Underpinnings of Binge Eating. The research has consistently demonstrated that repeated consumption of highly palatable food can produce dopamine signaling changes in the brain, which promote an escalation of intake

[170]. It also appears that intermittently restricted access to highly palatable foods results in sustained stimulation of the reward system, which in turn fosters chronic overeating and binge-eating susceptibility [171]. In this regard, it is relevant that individuals with BED tend to under-eat during the mornings [172], but show a propensity for high-calorie nocturnal eating [173], and do greater snacking in the evenings [174] compared to weight-matched adults who do not binge eat.

Neuro-scientific evidence of high reward responsiveness in BED is seen by the greater medial orbitofrontal cortex reactivity to food cues in people with this disorder relative to comparison groups [175]—a finding which accords with the important role of this brain area in drug cravings, and which confirms the significance of dopaminergic mechanisms in the aetiology of BED [176, 177]. Larger brain-activation differences in the amygdala and ventral striatum have also been found in obese adults with BED compared to weight-matched controls, suggesting a greater motivational sensitivity to, and visual processing of, palatable food cues in the former group [178]. The finding that obese binge eaters have greater increases in extracellular dopamine levels in the caudate nucleus, when presented with tasty food compared to nonbinge eating controls, provides further evidence of a *hyper-responsiveness* to reward in BED [179]. Additionally, a recent study has shown that exposure to personally relevant, high-calorie food cues elicited hyper-responsive fMRI BOLD reactions in overweight adults with binge-eating behaviour, and importantly, that the magnitude of these responses increased as the binge-eating symptoms increased in frequency [180]. Finally, and again in response to food cues, binge eating women showed hyper-responsiveness and increased neural communication between the ventral striatum and a widespread network involved in reward and action planning compared to weight-matched controls [181].

In accord with the evidence described above—that BED reflects a heightened responsiveness to reward—we recently reported that genetic markers reflecting enhanced dopaminergic signaling were positively related to the food-related sub-phenotypes of BED such as binge eating, food cravings, and emotional eating [94]. In addition, a multilocus genetic profile score—indicative of stronger dopamine responsiveness imparted by cumulative functional genotypic influences [182]—was significantly higher in a group of obese adults with BED compared to their age- and BMI-matched counterparts [101].

3.1.3. Emotional Dysregulation in Binge Eating. In clinical practice, stress, depressed mood, anger, and irritability are the most commonly reported triggers of binge eating [183]. Negative "everyday" emotions are also more prominent in those with BED compared to obese control participants [184, 185]. Such findings have prompted efforts to better understand the possible causal mechanisms for these associations. An important target is the role of stress responsiveness as a moderating factor in the development of binge eating. For instance, obese patients with BED appear to have significantly higher than expected co-morbid rates of posttraumatic stress disorder (PTSD) than weight-matched controls—a relationship that was also characterized by eating-related psychopathology [186]. Other related research has demonstrated a greater cortisol response to stress in this group compared to obese controls [183].

These findings have also been corroborated by experimental stress-induction laboratory studies. In one such paradigm, obese BED participants in the stress condition demonstrated a stronger motivation to eat and a weaker satiety perception compared to those without BED and who were not in the stress condition, suggesting that BED is more affected by stress than is seen in weight-matched controls [187]. There is other evidence of increased cardiovascular activity, and a greater sadness and insecurity response to stress induction in BED participants compared to their controls [188].

Preclinical evidence also supports this conclusion. Socially-isolated female rats (single-caged housing is an established stressor in these animals) showed a greater intake of cookies (when they had access to this food) compared to their standard chow, and they demonstrated more depression-like behaviours than the controls who were housed in group cages [189]. In addition, and not unexpectedly, basal levels of plasma corticosterone were elevated in the stressed animals. Previous research has clearly demonstrated that administration of glucocorticoids and corticosterone leads to hyperphasia and weight gain [183].

Findings such as those described above have generally been interpreted as an indication that the excessive ingestion of palatable food is largely a form of "self-medication" to restore or improve a disturbed affect. What has not been considered, however, is that the more sustained negative affect in those with BED could be a response to pronounced withdrawal symptoms as defined by the diagnostic criteria for drug addictions. Withdrawal symptoms include anhedonic mood, irritability, and a variety of somatic symptoms. The return to substances relieves this discomfort and therefore the behaviour is maintained through a negative reinforcement process whereby continued use avoids the unpleasant symptoms. Indeed, the same mood improvement is seen following a binge in those with BED [185]. It has also been found that negative mood tended to improve just prior to the binge [185]—a finding that is reminiscent of the cue-induced neural activation of striatal brain regions that occurs even before the drug is administered [190]. In other words, while the frequent eating of highly palatable foods may be initiated by a high sensitivity to rewarding stimuli, over time attempts to refrain from binge eating are followed by withdrawal symptoms in the form of depressed and irritable mood, which then restores the overeating to calm the distress. Like other addiction disorders, the cycle becomes increasingly compulsive and results in repeated failures to refrain from the behaviour.

3.2. Food Addiction. While "behavioral addictions" have been recognized by scientists and clinicians for many years [191], they have only recently been endorsed by the American Psychiatric Association with the proposed classification of Addiction and Related Disorders in the forthcoming *Diagnostic and Statistical Manual[DSM]-5* [192]. The DSM diagnostic shift is timely in light of growing evidence that excessive consumption of hyper-palatable food is an identifiable clinical entity with striking biobehavioral parallels to drug abuse [60, 193, 194]. Indeed, as we have seen in Section 2.3 above, the concept of food addiction has recently generated a strong public interest as well as an increased research focus.

3.2.1. Animal Models of Food Addiction. The food-addiction construct earned its scientific credibility largely from evidence that some aspects of this syndrome can be very successfully modeled in animals. Rodent models of food addiction have typically used behavioral paradigms based on experimentally inspired analogues of the *Diagnostic and Statistical Manual* (DSM-IV-TR) [195] criteria for substance dependence. For example, "tolerance" has been operationalized as an increase in brain-stimulation reward (BSR) thresholds following extended exposure to addictive drugs [196]. The inference is that stronger excitation is required because the sensitivity of the organism has been de-sensitized by chronic drug use. When extrapolating this principle to eating behaviors, rats with 18–23 hours/day access to palatable energy-dense food displayed a worsening deficit in brain reward function, as seen by their progressively elevated BSR thresholds across days, compared to rats on a standard chow diet [196].

Escalation of intake over time has been used as a marker of the substance-dependence criterion "taking the substance in larger amounts than was intended" [197]. In this regard, there is reliable evidence that rats, fed an intermittent diet of sugar, develop a pattern of copious consumption resembling human cases of binge eating [93, 198]. These studies show that a sugar-enhanced diet increases daily food intake over time, and that following its removal, the animals show aggression, anxiety, teeth-chattering, and head-shaking—all symptoms associated with "withdrawal" from drugs like heroin. Similar increased intake has been found when animals were given high-fat [45] or other highly palatable diets [196]. Evidence of withdrawal has also been observed in animals showing depressive-like symptoms after access to highly palatable food for 7 weeks, as indicated by increased immobility in the forced-swim test and decreased intake in the sucrose consumption test [199]. Interestingly, some of the depressive symptoms were abolished in these animals when they were given renewed access to the palatable diet, suggesting that high-calorie food can relieve withdrawal-induced negative effect, as well as fostering its onset. Recent evidence also indicates that rises in extracellular acetylcholine and decreases in dopamine in the striatal area contribute to the aversive state which characterizes both drug and palatable food withdrawal [200].

It also seems that compulsive patterns of palatable food intake only require a short time to develop, and that rats rapidly display a lack of flexibility in their food choices by rejecting standard chow even when the greatly preferred rich "cafeteria diet" is only intermittently available [201]. Even very limited (10 min) daily access to high sugar/fat diets can cause binge-like eating patterns and excessive weight gain in rats. Interestingly, however, this occurs without the physical and emotional withdrawal responses seen in rats with access to sugar-rich diets [202]—a finding which adds to the growing evidence that only minimal withdrawal symptoms are associated with diets rich in fat, or a combination of sugar and fat, compared to the very pronounced withdrawal symptoms following removal from a high-sugar diet [203, 204]. Various explanations have been proposed for these differences including the greater hedonic intensity of sugar relative to fat [202], and the more pronounced opioid-activating potential of sugar [203]. In general, it seems that a high-fat diet is largely responsible for weight gain while sugar may be mainly responsible for producing addictive-like behaviour including explicit withdrawal symptoms [194].

Another diagnostic criterion for addiction is the unremitting continuation of the behaviour in the face of unpleasant consequences. There are several examples of such compulsive food seeking and food intake in animals. For instance, binge-prone female rats tend, on average, to tolerate significantly higher levels of foot shock for access to Oreo cookies than their binge-resistant counterparts, confirming the "continued use despite negative consequences" criteria for substance dependence [205]. Other evidence of abnormal motivation for sweet and fatty foods has been demonstrated in paradigms where rats with extended exposure to a highly palatable cafeteria diet continued to eat even when the food was laced with quinine to produce an unpleasant bitter taste [201]. Preliminary data also confirm that compulsive eating in response to a highly palatable diet emerges only in a subset of animals with a genetically determined susceptibility [206].

Finally, while numerous studies have found behavioral and consummatory cross-sensitization from one addictive drug to another [93]—and between drugs and responsiveness to stress [30]—there is now good evidence that sugar intake also cross-sensitizes to drugs of abuse, and *vice versa* [198, 207, 208]. Interestingly, however, a recent study has shown that uncertain reinforcement with a sweet solution produced an enhanced locomotor cross-sensitization response to amphetamine compared to animals exposed to a predictable sweet reinforcement [209]. In other words, gambling-like reinforcement promotes more pronounced cross-sensitization to psychomotor stimulant effects—supporting the evidence that pathological gambling and compulsive/binge-eating disorder are regulated by similar brain substrates. Given the strong taste-appeal preference of salty foods, it is also important to note that animals pretreated with cocaine show a stronger salt appetite, and that these two substances show reciprocal behavioural cross-sensitization [210].

In conclusion, in any model of addiction it is fundamentally important to recognize the great variability in proneness to its development [211]. Only a subgroup of animals and people who are exposed to drugs of abuse, or highly-palatable food, seem to develop full-blown symptoms of dependence and loss-of-control over their intake [212, 213]—an observation that has galvanized attention on identifying the important risk factors, and the biological mechanisms underlying vulnerability [214]. One emerging area of interest stems from evidence that early-life stressors, and various dietary differences that arise from these stressors, are influential in the susceptibility to compulsive intake of palatable foods [211].

When assessing animal paradigms that support the food-addiction construct, an important consideration is that a pattern of compulsive intake—behaviourally similar to what we call *binge eating* in the human condition—is a universal feature of all models [211, 215]. In other words, animals do not display symptoms of withdrawal, tolerance, or any of the other analogue criteria for substance abuse, without also showing binge-like consumption of the experimental food. Moreover, all animal models require the introduction of highly palatable foods—typically those that are sugary or fatty—and sometimes a combination of both. Pivotally, compulsive intake does not occur in response to tasteless foods that comprise the chow that is typically fed to laboratory animals.

3.2.2. Human Studies of Food Addiction. Despite the persuasive evidence of sugar/fat dependence in rodents, there are limited parallel findings in human research except for anecdotal reports and various qualitative clinical accounts [68, 151, 216, 217]. Recently, researchers at Yale University advanced the field with their development of a measure which operationalizes "food addiction" using the DSM-IV-TR diagnostic criteria for substance dependence [218]. Their preliminary findings suggested that the *Yale Food Addiction Scale* (YFAS) has high convergent validity with other measures of eating pathology, especially binge eating, and may therefore be a useful tool for identifying individuals with compulsive and addictive tendencies towards food. In a more recent YFAS validation study, the high symptom group demonstrated faster reaction times in response to food cues versus neutral cues and reported higher attentional impulsivity, compared to the low symptom group—similar to findings in those with other addiction disorders [219].

Our group published the first case-control study of food addiction in obese men and women using the YFAS diagnostic criteria for classification [218]. The results provided very good evidence that food addiction is a discernible clinical syndrome characterized by psychiatric co-morbidities and a psycho-behavioural profile with strong similarities to those found in conventional addiction disorders like alcoholism and drug abuse. For example, those who met the diagnostic criteria for YFAS food addiction had a significantly greater prevalence of BED, of severe depression, and reported more pronounced symptoms of ADHD compared to their obese counterparts. In addition, they reported more intense food cravings and greater emotional overeating. They were also more impulsive than the obese controls.

3.2.3. Neurobiological Evidence. The last point (above) is particularly relevant given that hypo-functioning of prefrontal cortical systems—cognitive processes, known broadly as "executive functions" and regulated largely by dopaminergic circuitry—may be a cardinal feature of addiction disorders, especially as it contributes to proneness to relapse and poor success in recovery [220]. Moreover, as addictive behaviours escalate there appear to be growing deficits in the individual's ability to exert "self-control" and to resist engaging in excessive behaviours [146]. In other words, decreased activity in the prefrontal cortex has been consistently associated with relatively high levels of impulsive behaviours, and these findings relate both to the abuse of drugs [221] as well as to an overindulgence in palatable foods [222, 223]. There is, however, some evidence that drug-related cues are more potent triggers of drug-seeking behaviour than food-related cues are to eating, although the differences appear to be more a matter of magnitude than of quality [224].

Low brain serotonin function has also been widely associated with impaired emotional regulation, impulsivity, and impulse control disorders [225]. Based on experimental evidence that tryptophan (a precursor amino acid for serotonin) depletion tends to foster high consumption of sweet/fatty foods, and that it can also trigger depressive episodes, some have argued that overeating of highly palatable foods is fundamentally a form of *self-medication* to ameliorate dysphoric mood [226]. In light of the significantly more severe levels of depression in those with food addiction, and their reported proneness to emotionally-driven eating, these interrelationships may well explain a downwardly spiraling cycle whereby a biological predisposition to negative mood (e.g., low serotonin availability) could foster a voracious appetite for sugary and fatty foods. In our highly obesogenic environment with its proliferation of processed foods, this hungriness can easily be satisfied, in turn causing down-regulated brain reward pathways and further contributing to dysphoria and its consequences on eating behaviours.

Currently there has only been one neuroimaging study designed to assess biological correlates of food addiction [227]. Reward circuitry activation in the caudate and amygdala, in response to the anticipated receipt of food, was positively associated with YFAS-symptom scores. This study was, however, rather limited by a small all-female sample, and because only two participants met the diagnostic criteria for food addiction. However, in a recent study—and the first to provide genetic support for the food-addiction construct—our findings meshed well with these neuroimaging data [228]. A multilocus genetic index score, which reflected the cumulative effect of several functional markers on striatal dopamine signaling strength, was significantly higher in a group of overweight adults with YFAS food addiction compared to their weight-, age- and gender-matched counterparts. This relationship was also mediated by greater food cravings, bingeing, and emotional eating. Together, these findings support the view that, like BED, food addiction is a high reward-responsive phenotype of obesity. They also suggest a reward-based process model whereby a biologically based vulnerability contributes to increased risk for overeating, which in turn tends to promote addictive tendencies towards highly palatable foods.

3.3. Food Addiction as a Severe Form of Binge Eating Disorder. As we have seen, the available research—albeit still very limited as it pertains to the human condition—consistently endorses the view that food addiction is an identifiable clinical entity with many similarities to drug addictions. At the same time, however, these investigations, and related work, have implicitly raised the question of whether the YFAS-inspired definition of food addiction simply reflects a more severe sub-type of BED. This issue is especially germane given the clear overlap in the proposed diagnostic criteria for the two conditions. They also share substantial symptom overlap [218, 229], they have many co-morbidities in common [218], and they appear to share similar biological underpinnings [101, 228].

The studies by Davis et al. [218] and Gearhardt et al. [229] found that about 50% of obese adults diagnosed with YFAS food addiction also met criteria for BED. Moreover, in an earlier study [230], using structured telephone interviews in women diagnosed with BED, the investigators found that 92% of their sample met the DSM-IV-TR [195] criteria for substance dependence when the word "food" was substituted for "drug" in the interview questions. Clarifying whether the two conditions are sufficiently different in aetiology and clinical course to warrant classification as separate pathological phenotypes of overeating is an important next-step in eating disorder and addiction research. Resolution will also help guide personalized treatment strategies for those who struggle with intractable and excessive food consumption [91].

As an initial attempt to assess our continuum hypothesis, we examined group differences on several variables related to demographic characteristics (age and BMI), patterns of overeating, personality risk factors, and co-morbid clinical symptoms [91]. In the first set of analyses, we compared two equivalent groups of overweight men and women who met DSM-IV-TR criteria for BED: one *with* co-occurring YFAS-diagnosed food addiction and the other *without*. Results indicated that the two BED groups were equivalent in age and BMI. On almost all other variables, however, the differences were highly statistically significant. Those with food addiction were much more likely to overeat for emotional and cue-driven reasons, they had more severe binge eating and food cravings, and they were more responsive to the rewarding properties of food. This group also had more addictive personality traits, was more impulsive, and had greatly elevated symptoms of depression compared to their non-food addict BED counterparts. While the food-addict group also reported greater ADHD symptoms, both currently and in childhood, these differences only approached statistical significance. Collectively, these findings mesh well with a related study of food addiction in BED patients where the number of YFAS *symptoms* (scores ranging from 0–7) was shown to correlate positively with Beck depression ratings, poor self-esteem, and difficulties in emotion regulation, as well as with certain measures of eating pathology including frequency of binge episodes [229]. Similarly, in a recent study of weight-loss treatment-seeking adults, YFAS symptom scores related significantly to increased depression, emotional eating, and binge eating [231]. In this study, increased symptomatology was also related to less weight loss after several weeks of treatment, suggesting that food addiction, with related signs of tolerance and withdrawal, may undermine efforts to lose weight in those trying to adopt better eating habits.

In the second analysis we carried out to test the continuum hypothesis [91], we compared the BED group *without* food addiction to a weight- and age-matched group of adults *without* BED and *without* food addiction on the same variables described in the first set of analyses. By contrast to the earlier comparisons, these two groups were very similar to each other and demonstrated only a few significant differences. For instance, and hardly surprisingly, the BED group had higher binge-eating scores and reported more hedonic eating and elevated food cravings than the non-BED controls.

Despite the novel and interesting findings from our preliminary investigation, it is important to acknowledge that the results are based on a relatively small sample of participants with BED. Nevertheless, the highly statistically significant findings from the first set of analyses suggest that the sample was not under-powered since the mean differences were sufficiently large, relative to their standard errors, to demonstrate strong effect sizes. Unfortunately, however, in the total sample of mainly overweight adults, there were only a few individuals without a diagnosis either of BED or of food addiction, precluding a full factorial 2-way analysis of the data. Unfortunately such a skewed distribution is liable to be a problem for all future comparative research in this area because of the well-established associations between psychopathology and BMI in overeating disorders.

Although *normal-weight* adults only account for a small proportion of those with BED, they appear to be another distinct subset of the BED population, suggesting that body weight is also an important feature or correlate of the overeating spectrum. For instance, some studies have found that normal-weight BED adults are younger [232, 233], and that their binge episodes are less frequent [233] and of shorter duration than their overweight/obese counterparts [232]. Particularly relevant are the findings that those with normal-weight BED report a greater "drive for thinness" [234], more pronounced cognitive and dietary restraint [235], and significantly greater and more extreme compensatory weight-control behaviors like skipping meals, exercising excessively, and restricting their food intake [232].

Not surprisingly, a diagnosis of BED has been shown to predict weight gain over time [236, 237]. Indeed it is physiologically self-evident that chronic episodes of binge eating in the absence of any compensation for the excessive ingestion of energy substantially increase the risk for obesity as individuals grow older. Therefore—and because one of the diagnostic criteria for BED is the absence of "inappropriate compensatory behaviors like purging, fasting, and excessive exercise"—the boundary between normal-weight BED and nonpurging bulimia nervosa is clearly blurred, and their differences seem to be largely a matter of calorie-sparing severity.

4. Summary and Conclusions

In the upcoming May 2013 release of DSM-5, there will be a number of notable changes to the status of BED. First, it will move from the Appendix of the previous DSM and be included as a free-standing disorder in the new version of this manual. The criteria for diagnosis have also been relaxed in that the required duration of symptoms has reduced from 6 months to 3 months, and the frequency criterion for binge episodes has dropped from at least twice a week to at least once a week, on average [238]. Together these changes should capture a greater number of individuals suffering from a clinically significant impairment in their compulsive overeating. It has been estimated, however, that while the point prevalence of BED will naturally increase with the more liberal criteria, the lifetime prevalence is unlikely to increase markedly [239]. Another important change in DSM-5 is the addition of severity ratings based on the number of weekly binge episodes—an index also of the compulsiveness of the behaviour.

It is anticipated that the inclusion of more individuals with debilitating BED-like symptoms, without compromising the validity of the BED diagnosis, will allow future researchers to assess the hypothesis presented in this paper, that "food addiction" is not a separable entity from BED but rather that it reflects—at least in most case—a more severe and more compulsive subtype of BED. In proposing a continuum hypothesis of overeating it is also important to acknowledge that at the extreme of some dimensions, a sort of "chaos" ensues rather than an orderly progression of the underlying or defining characteristics in degrees of magnitude. In other words, there may be a qualitative difference as well as a quantitative difference in the clinical picture at the high (food addiction) end of the overeating continuum such as can be seen, for example, in the case of Obsessive Compulsive Disorder. In that condition, the obsessive-compulsive personality traits not only manifest as severe, rigid, and debilitating characteristics, but there is the emergence of associated cognitions and behaviours that are chaotic, aberrant, and often discernibly unrelated to features of the personality.

In conclusion, as we have seen in this review, an increasing number of scientists and clinicians subscribe to the view that compulsive overeating—a quintessentially defining feature of BED—shares pronounced similarities with conventional addictions like substance abuse [60, 211, 240, 241]. Not surprisingly, such discussions have inspired cautious conclusions that *some* forms of excessive overeating are most appropriately viewed as an addiction disorder. While evidence for the validity of the food-addiction construct is rapidly gaining ground, it is inevitable that this perspective has also found its detractors [242]. Unfortunately, some of those participating on the negative side of the debate have conflated obesity and overeating with "food addiction," in presenting their arguments—an issue which has clouded the possible distinctiveness of the concept and muddled efforts to properly assess its diagnostic utility.

It is clearly a misinterpretation of the research for anyone to perceive that supporters are claiming that *all* cases of overeating—even prodigious overeating—reflect an "addiction to food," in the same way as it would be illogical to maintain that all heavy drinkers are alcoholics. In other words, there are no explicit assertions from advocates of the food-addiction concept that more than a subset of the population could, or would, be affected by this condition. Like virtually all psychiatric disorders, including drug abuse and behavioral addictions such as pathological gambling, there is a relatively low base rate in the population, even though the related symptoms and endo-phenotypes exist in the general population along a continuum of varying magnitude or severity. Most individuals who use addictive substances—drugs or highly palatable food—do not develop dependence. Many contributing elements explain an individual's propensity to these disorders. Moreover, it is highly unlikely that a homogeneous set of risk factors pertains to all phases of their development [243].

References

[1] B. Caballero, "The global epidemic of obesity: an overview," *Epidemiologic Reviews*, vol. 29, no. 1, pp. 1–5, 2007.

[2] A. H. Mokdad, J. S. Marks, D. F. Stroup, and J. L. Gerberding, "Actual causes of death in the United States, 2000," *Journal of the American Medical Association*, vol. 291, no. 10, pp. 1238–1264, 2004.

[3] H. A. de Boo and J. E. Harding, "The developmental origins of adult disease (Barker) hypothesis," *Australian and New Zealand Journal of Obstetrics and Gynaecology*, vol. 46, no. 1, pp. 4–14, 2006.

[4] M. Power, "The human obesity epidemic, the mismatch paradigm, and our modern "captive" environment," *American Journal of Human Biology*, vol. 24, pp. 116–122, 2012.

[5] J. C. K. Wells, "Obesity as malnutrition: the role of capitalism in the obesity global epidemic," *American Journal of Human Biology*, vol. 24, pp. 261–276, 2012.

[6] K. M. Flegal, M. D. Carroll, B. K. Kit et al., "Prevalence of obesity and trends in the distribution of body mass index among US adults, 1999–2010," *Journal of the American Medical Association*, vol. 307, pp. 491–497, 2012.

[7] H. L. Walls, D. J. Magliano, C. E. Stevenson et al., "Projected progression of the prevalence of obesity in Australia," *Obesity*, vol. 20, pp. 872–878, 2012.

[8] K. M. Flegal, M. D. Carroll, C. L. Ogden, and L. R. Curtin, "Prevalence and trends in obesity among US adults, 1999—2008," *Journal of the American Medical Association*, vol. 303, no. 3, pp. 235–241, 2010.

[9] M. de Onis, M. Blössner, and E. Borghi, "Global prevalence and trends of overweight and obesity among preschool children," *American Journal of Clinical Nutrition*, vol. 92, no. 5, pp. 1257–1264, 2010.

[10] P. M. Catalano, A. Thomas, L. Huston-Presley, and S. B. Amini, "Phenotype of infants of mothers with gestational diabetes," *Diabetes Care*, vol. 30, supplement 2, pp. S156–S160, 2007.

[11] P. M. Catalano, L. Presley, J. Minium, and S. H. D. Mouzon, "Fetuses of obese mothers develop insulin resistance in utero," *Diabetes Care*, vol. 32, no. 6, pp. 1076–1080, 2009.

[12] A. E. Frias and K. L. Grove, "Obesity A transgenerational problem linked to nutrition during pregnancy," *Seminars in Reproductive Medicine*, vol. 30, pp. 472–478, 2012.

[13] J. J. Reilly, J. Armstrong, A. R. Dorosty et al., "Early life risk factors for obesity in childhood: cohort study," *British Medical Journal*, vol. 330, no. 7504, pp. 1357–1359, 2005.

[14] B. A. Swinburn, G. Sacks, K. D. Hall et al., "The global obesity pandemic: shaped by global drivers and local environments," *The Lancet*, vol. 378, pp. 804–814, 2011.

[15] L. H. Epstein, "Commentary: future research directions in pediatric obesity research," *Journal of Pediatric Psychology*, vol. 24, no. 3, pp. 251–252, 1999.

[16] A. G. Dulloo, J. Jacquet, G. Solinas, J. P. Montani, and Y. Schutz, "Body composition phenotypes in pathways to obesity and the metabolic syndrome," *International Journal of Obesity*, vol. 34, supplement 2, pp. S4–S17, 2010.

[17] M. A. Kalarchian and M. D. Marcus, "Psychiatric comorbidity of childhood obesity," *International Review of Psychiatry*, vol. 24, pp. 241–246, 2012.

[18] F. Rohner-Jeanrenaud and B. Jeanrenaud, "The discovery of leptin and its impact in the understanding of obesity," *European Journal of Endocrinology*, vol. 135, no. 6, pp. 649–650, 1996.

[19] A. Paoloni-Giacobino, "Post-genomic decade—the epigenome and exposure challenges," *Swiss Medical Weekly*, vol. 141, article w13245, 2011.

[20] M. T. Neary and R. L. Batterham, "Gaining new insights into food reward with functional neuroimaging," in *Frontiers in Eating and Weight Regulation.*, W. Langhans and N. Geary, Eds., vol. 63 of *Forum of Nutrition*, pp. 152–163, Karger, Basel, Switzerland, 2010.

[21] J. L. Pomeranz and K. D. Brownell, "Portion sizes and beyond—government's legal authority to regulate food-industry practices," *The New England Journal of Medicine*, vol. 367, pp. 1383–1385, 2012.

[22] N. L. Novak and K. D. Brownell, "Taxation as prevention and as a treatment for obesity: the case of sugar-sweetened beverages," *Current Pharmaceutical Design*, vol. 17, no. 12, pp. 1218–1222, 2011.

[23] A. H. Gearhardt, M. A. Bragg, R. L. Pearl et al., "Obesity and public policy," *Annual Review of Clinical Psychology*, vol. 8, pp. 405–430, 2012.

[24] E. A. Brown, "Genetic explorations of recent human metabolic adaptations: hypotheses and evidence," *Biological Reviews*, vol. 87, pp. 838–855, 2012.

[25] J. V. Neel, "The "thrifty genotype" in 1998," *Nutrition Reviews*, vol. 57, pp. S2–S9, 1999.

[26] G. J. Armelagos, "The Omnivore's Dilemna. The evolution of the brain and determinants of food choice," *Journal of Anthropological Research*, vol. 66, pp. 161–186, 2010.

[27] F. H. Bronson, "Climate change and seasonal reproduction in mammals," *Philosophical Transactions of the Royal Society B*, vol. 364, no. 1534, pp. 3331–3340, 2009.

[28] J. E. Schneider, "Metabolic and hormonal control of the desire for food and sex: implications for obesity and eating disorders," *Hormones and Behavior*, vol. 50, no. 4, pp. 562–571, 2006.

[29] J. E. Schneider, J. F. Casper, A. Barisich et al., "Food deprivation and leptin prioritize ingestive and sex behavior without affecting estrous cycles in Syrian hamsters," *Hormones and Behavior*, vol. 51, no. 3, pp. 413–427, 2007.

[30] A. A. Ammar, F. Sederholm, T. R. Saito, A. J. W. Scheurink, A. E. Johnson, and P. Södersten, "NPY-leptin: opposing effects on appetitive and consummatory ingestive behavior and sexual behavior," *American Journal of Physiology*, vol. 278, no. 6, pp. R1627–R1633, 2000.

[31] H. Choquet and D. Meyre, "Molecular basis of obesity: current status and future prospects," *Current Genomics*, vol. 12, no. 3, pp. 154–168, 2011.

[32] C. Nan, B. Guo, C. Warner et al., "Heritability of body mass index in pre-adolescence, young adulthood and late adulthood," *European Journal of Epidemiology*, vol. 27, pp. 247–253, 2012.

[33] Y. M. Hur, "Sex difference in heritability of BMI in South Korean adolescent twins," *Obesity*, vol. 15, no. 12, pp. 2908–2911, 2007.

[34] K. Schousboe, G. Willemsen, K. O. Kyvik et al., "Sex differences in heritability of BMI: a comparative study of results from twin studies in eight countries," *Twin Research*, vol. 6, no. 5, pp. 409–421, 2003.

[35] L. Ellis and D. Haman, "Population increases in obesity appear to be partly due to genetics," *Journal of Biosocial Science*, vol. 36, no. 5, pp. 547–559, 2004.

[36] R. Sturm, "Increases in clinically severe obesity in the United States, 1986–2000," *Archives of Internal Medicine*, vol. 163, no. 18, pp. 2146–2148, 2003.

[37] N. M. Byrne and A. P. Hills, "Biology or behavior: which is the strongest contributor to weight gain?" *Current Obesity Reports*, vol. 2, pp. 65–76, 2013.

[38] B. M. Popkin, S. J. Nielsen, and A. M. Siega-Riz, "Trends in energy intake in U.S. between 1977 and 1996: similar shifts seen across age groups," *Obesity Research*, vol. 10, no. 5, pp. 370–378, 2002.

[39] M. R. Lowe, M. L. Butryn, E. R. Didie et al., "The power of food scale. A new measure of the psychological influence of the food environment," *Appetite*, vol. 53, no. 1, pp. 114–118, 2009.

[40] J. G. Thomas, S. Doshi, R. D. Crosby, and M. R. Lowe, "Ecological momentary assessment of obesogenic eating behavior: combining person-specific and environmental predictors," *Obesity*, vol. 19, no. 8, pp. 1574–1579, 2011.

[41] P. J. Allen, P. Batra, B. M. Geiger et al., "Rationale and consequences of reclassifying obesity as an addictive disorder: neurobiology, food environment and social policy perspectives," *Physiology & Behavior*, vol. 107, pp. 126–137, 2012.

[42] V. Drapeau and A. R. Gallant, "Homeostatic and circadian control of food intake: clinical strategies to prevent overconsumption," *Current Obesity Reports*, vol. 2, no. 1, pp. 93–103, 2013.

[43] S. Gahagan, "Development of eating behavior: biology and context," *Journal of Developmental & Behavioral Pediatrics*, vol. 33, pp. 261–271, 2012.

[44] T. F. Gamage and A. H. Lichtman, "The endocannabinoid system: role in energy regulation," *Pediatric Blood & Cancer*, vol. 58, pp. 144–148, 2012.

[45] M. Lutter and E. J. Nestler, "Homeostatic and hedonic signals interact in the regulation of food intake," *Journal of Nutrition*, vol. 139, no. 3, pp. 629–632, 2009.

[46] P. Monteleone, F. Piscitelli, P. Scognamiglio et al., "Hedonic eating is associated with increased peripheral levels of ghrelin and the endocannabinoid 2-arachidonoyl-glycerol in health humans: a pilot study," *The Journal of Clinical Endocrinology and Metabolism*, vol. 97, pp. E917–E924, 2012.

[47] A. Drewnowski and N. Darmon, "The economics of obesity: dietary energy density and energy cost," *The American Journal of Clinical Nutrition*, vol. 82, supplement 1, pp. 265S–273S, 2005.

[48] K. B. Horgen and K. D. Brownell, "Comparison of price change and health message interventions in promoting healthy food choices," *Health Psychology*, vol. 21, no. 5, pp. 505–512, 2002.

[49] M. Pollan, "In defence of food," *New Scientist*, vol. 197, article 50, 2008.

[50] K. Boekelheide, B. Blumberg, R. E. Chapin et al., "Predicting later-life outcomes of early-life exposures," *Environmental Health Perspectives*, vol. 120, pp. 1353–1361, 2012.

[51] P. D. Gluckman and M. A. Hanson, "Developmental and epigenetic pathways to obesity: an evolutionary-developmental perspective," *International Journal of Obesity*, vol. 32, supplement 7, pp. S62–S71, 2008.

[52] D. Okin and R. Medzhitov, "Evolution of inflammatory diseases," *Current Biology*, vol. 22, pp. R733–R740, 2012.

[53] J. R. Speakman, "Obesity: the integrated roles of environment and genetics," *Journal of Nutrition*, vol. 134, supplement 8, pp. 2090S–2105S, 2004.

[54] J. C. Lovejoy, C. M. Champagne, L. de Jonge, H. Xie, and S. R. Smith, "Increased visceral fat and decreased energy expenditure during the menopausal transition," *International Journal of Obesity*, vol. 32, no. 6, pp. 949–958, 2008.

[55] W. R. Robinson, "Gender-specific effects of early nutritional restriction on adult obesity risk: evidence from quasi-experimental studies," *Obesity*, vol. 20, pp. 2464–2466, 2012.

[56] J. M. van Rossum and J. A. T. M. Hurkmans, "Mechanism of action of psychomotor stimulant drugs. Significance of dopamine in locomotor stimulant action," *Neuropharmacology*, vol. 3, no. 2, pp. 227–239, 1964.

[57] G. P. Smith and L. H. Scheider, "Relationships between mesolimbic dopamine function and eating behavior," *Annals of the New York Academy of Sciences*, vol. 537, pp. 254–261, 1988.

[58] N. D. Volkow and R. A. Wise, "How can drug addiction help us understand obesity?" *Nature Neuroscience*, vol. 8, no. 5, pp. 555–560, 2005.

[59] R. J. Sullivan and E. H. Hagen, "Psychotropic substance-seeking: evolutionary pathology or adaptation?" *Addiction*, vol. 97, no. 4, pp. 389–400, 2002.

[60] C. Davis and J. C. Carter, "Compulsive overeating as an addiction disorder. A review of theory and evidence," *Appetite*, vol. 53, no. 1, pp. 1–8, 2009.

[61] R. A. Wise, "The role of reward pathways in the development of drug dependence," *Pharmacology and Therapeutics*, vol. 35, no. 1-2, pp. 227–263, 1987.

[62] M. Morales and V. M. Pickel, "Insights to drug addiction derived from ultrastructural views of the mesocorticolimbic system," in *Addiction Reviews*, G. R. Uhl, Ed., vol. 1248, pp. 71–88, Annals of the New York Academy of Sciences, New York, NY, USA, 2012.

[63] D. B. Newlin, "The self-perceived survival ability and reproductive fitness (SPFit) theory of substance use disorders," *Addiction*, vol. 97, no. 4, pp. 427–445, 2002.

[64] R. M. Nesse, "An evolutionary perspective on substance abuse," *Ethology and Sociobiology*, vol. 15, no. 5-6, pp. 339–348, 1994.

[65] T. G. Smith and A. Tasnádi, "A theory of natural addiction," *Games and Economic Behavior*, vol. 59, no. 2, pp. 316–344, 2007.

[66] L. M. Gerber, G. C. Williams, and S. J. Gray, "The nutrient-toxin dosage continuum in human evolution and modern health," *Quarterly Review of Biology*, vol. 74, no. 3, pp. 273–289, 1999.

[67] B. Spring, K. Schneider, M. Smith et al., "Abuse potential of carbohydrates for overweight carbohydrate cravers," *Psychopharmacology*, vol. 197, no. 4, pp. 637–647, 2008.

[68] J. R. Ifland, H. G. Preuss, M. T. Marcus et al., "Refined food addiction: a classic substance use disorder," *Medical Hypotheses*, vol. 72, no. 5, pp. 518–526, 2009.

[69] J. A. Cocores and M. S. Gold, "The salted food addiction hypothesis may explain overeating and the obesity epidemic," *Medical Hypotheses*, vol. 73, no. 6, pp. 892–899, 2009.

[70] A. N. Gearhardt, C. Davis, R. Kuschner et al., "The addiction potential of hyperpalatable foods," *Current Drug Abuse*, vol. 4, pp. 140–145, 2011.

[71] P. J. Kenny, "Reward mechanisms in obesity: new insights and future directions," *Neuron*, vol. 69, no. 4, pp. 664–679, 2011.

[72] L. Cantin, M. Lenoir, E. Augier et al., "Cocaine is low on the value ladder of rats: possible evidence for resilience to addiction," *PLoS ONE*, vol. 5, no. 7, Article ID e11592, 2010.

[73] J. E. Henningfield and R. M. Keenan, "Nicotine delivery kinetics and abuse liability," *Journal of Consulting and Clinical Psychology*, vol. 61, no. 5, pp. 743–750, 1993.

[74] G. A. Bray, "Fructose: should we worry?" *International Journal of Obesity*, vol. 32, supplement 7, pp. S127–S131, 2008.

[75] M. B. Vos, J. E. Kimmons, C. Gillespie, J. Welsh, and H. M. Blank, "Dietary fructose consumption among US children and adults: the Third National Health and Nutrition Examination survey CME," *MedGenMed Medscape General Medicine*, vol. 10, no. 7, article 160, 2008.

[76] R. H. Lustig, "Fructose: metabolic, hedonic, and societal parallels with ethanol," *Journal of the American Dietetic Association*, vol. 110, no. 9, pp. 1307–1321, 2010.

[77] M. Melis, G. Pillolla, S. Perra, G. Colombo, A. L. Muntoni, and M. Pistis, "Electrophysiological properties of dopamine neurons in the ventral tegmental area of Sardinian alcohol-preferring rats," *Psychopharmacology*, vol. 201, no. 4, pp. 471–481, 2009.

[78] S. J. Haring and R. B. S. Harris, "The relation between dietary fructose, dietary fat, and leptin responsiveness in rats," *Physiology & Behavior*, vol. 104, pp. 914–922, 2011.

[79] R. A. Grucza, R. F. Krueger, S. B. Racette, K. E. Norberg, P. R. Hipp, and L. J. Bierut, "The emerging link between alcoholism risk and obesity in the United States," *Archives of General Psychiatry*, vol. 67, no. 12, pp. 1301–1308, 2010.

[80] A. E. Kelley, B. A. Baldo, and W. E. Pratt, "A proposed hypothalamic-thalamic-striatal axis for the integration of energy balance, arousal, and food reward," *Journal of Comparative Neurology*, vol. 493, no. 1, pp. 72–85, 2005.

[81] M. L. Pelchat, A. Johnson, R. Chan, J. Valdez, and J. D. Ragland, "Images of desire: food-craving activation during fMRI," *NeuroImage*, vol. 23, no. 4, pp. 1486–1493, 2004.

[82] M. A. White, B. L. Whisenhunt, D. A. Williamson, F. L. Greenway, and R. G. Netemeyer, "Development and validation of the food-craving inventory," *Obesity Research*, vol. 10, no. 2, pp. 107–114, 2002.

[83] A. N. Gearhardt, W. R. Corbin, and K. D. Brownell, "Food addiction: an examination of the diagnostic criteria for dependence," *Journal of Addiction Medicine*, vol. 3, no. 1, pp. 1–7, 2009.

[84] J. C. Kayloe, "Food addiction," *Psychotherapy*, vol. 30, no. 2, pp. 269–275, 1993.

[85] M. McDowell, "Compulsive eating as a non-neurotic food addiction phenomenon," *Obesity and Bariatric Medicine*, vol. 7, article 140, 1978.

[86] T. G. Randolph, "Food allergy and food addiction," *Journal of the American Medical Association*, vol. 153, article 821, 1953.

[87] T. G. Randolph, "The descriptive features of food addiction: addictive eating and drinking," *Quarterly Journal of Studies on Alcohol*, vol. 17, no. 2, pp. 198–224, 1956.

[88] T. G. Randolph, "Food addiction, (chronic food allergy)—apparent basis of other addictions," *Clinical Research*, vol. 26, article A700, 1978.

[89] P. J. Rogers and H. J. Smit, "Food craving and food "addiction": a critical review of the evidence from a biopsychosocial perspective," *Pharmacology Biochemistry and Behavior*, vol. 66, no. 1, pp. 3–14, 2000.

[90] T. Tuomisto, M. M. Hetherington, M. F. Morris et al., "Psychological and physiological characteristics of sweet food 'addiction'," *International Journal of Eating Disorders*, vol. 25, pp. 169–175, 1999.

[91] C. Davis, "Compulsive overeating as an addictive behavior: overlap between food addiction and binge eating disorder," *Current Obesity Reports*, 2013.

[92] J. A. DePierre, R. M. Puhl, and J. Luedicke, "A new stigmatized identity? Comparisons of a "food addict" label with other stigmatized health conditions," *Basic and Applied Social Psychology*, vol. 35, pp. 10–21, 2013.

[93] N. M. Avena, P. Rada, and B. G. Hoebel, "Evidence for sugar addiction: behavioral and neurochemical effects of intermittent, excessive sugar intake," *Neuroscience and Biobehavioral Reviews*, vol. 32, no. 1, pp. 20–39, 2008.

[94] C. Davis, R. D. Levitan, Z. Yilmaz et al., "Binge eating disorder and the dopamine D2 receptor: genotypes and subphenotypes," *Progress in Neuro-Psychopharmacology and Biological Psychiatry*, vol. 38, pp. 328–335, 2012.

[95] Y. Zhang, K. M. von Deneen, J. Tian, M. S. Gold, and Y. Liu, "Food addiction and neuroimaging," *Current Pharmaceutical Design*, vol. 17, no. 12, pp. 1149–1157, 2011.

[96] A. Agrawal and M. T. Lynskey, "Are there genetic influences on addiction: evidence from family, adoption and twin studies," *Addiction*, vol. 103, no. 7, pp. 1069–1081, 2008.

[97] V. Bassareo and G. Di Chiara, "Modulation of feeding-induced activation of mesolimbic dopamine transmission by appetitive stimuli and its relation to motivational state," *European Journal of Neuroscience*, vol. 11, no. 12, pp. 4389–4397, 1999.

[98] D. M. Small, M. Jones-Gotman, and A. Dagher, "Feeding-induced dopamine release in dorsal striatum correlates with meal pleasantness ratings in healthy human volunteers," *NeuroImage*, vol. 19, no. 4, pp. 1709–1715, 2003.

[99] W. C. Drevets, C. Gautier, J. C. Price et al., "Amphetamine-induced dopamine release in human ventral striatum correlates with euphoria," *Biological Psychiatry*, vol. 49, no. 2, pp. 81–96, 2001.

[100] B. Le Foll, A. Gallo, Y. L. Strat, L. Lu, and P. Gorwood, "Genetics of dopamine receptors and drug addiction: a comprehensive review," *Behavioural Pharmacology*, vol. 20, no. 1, pp. 1–17, 2009.

[101] C. Davis, R. D. Levitan, J. C. Carter et al., "Binge eating disorder and "food addiction": a multi-locus genetic-profile study," in *Proceedings of the Annual conference of the Eating Disorder Research Society*, Porto, Portugal, 2012.

[102] C. Davis, R. D. Levitan, J. C. Carter et al., "Dopamine for "wanting"and opioids for "liking": a comparison of overweight/obese adults with and without binge eating disorder," *Obesity*, vol. 17, pp. 1220–1225, 2009.

[103] M. E. Carroll, A. D. Morgan, J. J. Anker, J. L. Perry, and N. K. Dess, "Selective breeding for differential saccharin intake as an animal model of drug abuse," *Behavioural Pharmacology*, vol. 19, no. 5-6, pp. 435–460, 2008.

[104] E. J. Nestler, "Is there a common molecular pathway for addiction?" *Nature Neuroscience*, vol. 8, no. 11, pp. 1445–1449, 2005.

[105] J. D. Slane, S. A. Burt, and K. L. Klump, "Bulimic behaviors and alcohol use: shared genetic influences," *Behavior Genetics*, vol. 42, no. 4, pp. 603–613, 2012.

[106] J. E. Woods, P. F. McKay, J. Masters et al., "Differential responding for brain stimulation reward and sucrose in high-alcohol-drinking (HAD) and low-alcohol-drinking (LAD) rats," *Alcoholism*, vol. 27, no. 6, pp. 926–936, 2003.

[107] G. F. Koob and M. Le Moal, "Plasticity of reward neurocircuitry and the "dark side" of drug addiction," *Nature Neuroscience*, vol. 8, no. 11, pp. 1442–1444, 2005.

[108] R. H. Mach, M. A. Nader, R. L. Ehrenkaufer et al., "Persistent downregulation of dopamine D2 receptors in a rhesus monkey model of cocaine abuse and withdrawal," *Journal of Nuclear Medicine*, vol. 38, article 300, 1997.

[109] D. Thompson, L. Martini, and J. L. Whistler, "Altered ratio of D1 and D2 dopamine receptors in mouse striatum is associated with behavioral sensitization to cocaine," *PLoS ONE*, vol. 5, no. 6, Article ID e11038, 2010.

[110] M. A. Nader, D. Morgan, H. D. Gage et al., "PET imaging of dopamine D2 receptors during chronic cocaine self-administration in monkeys," *Nature Neuroscience*, vol. 9, no. 8, pp. 1050–1056, 2006.

[111] N. D. Volkow, L. Chang, G. J. Wang et al., "Low level of brain dopamine D2 receptors in methamphetamine abusers: association with metabolism in the orbitofrontal cortex," *American Journal of Psychiatry*, vol. 158, no. 12, pp. 2015–2021, 2001.

[112] J. Hirvonen, R. S. Goodwin, C. T. Li et al., "Reversible and regionally selective downregulation of brain cannabinoid CB1 receptors in chronic daily cannabis smokers," *Molecular Psychiatry*, vol. 17, pp. 642–649, 2012.

[113] E. van de Giessen, S. E. la Fleur, K. de Bruin et al., "Free-choice and no-choice high-fat diets affect striatal dopamine D-2/3 receptor availability, caloric intake, and adiposity," *Obesity*, vol. 20, pp. 1738–1740, 2012.

[114] P. Rada, M. E. Bocarsly, J. R. Barson, B. G. Hoebel, and S. F. Leibowitz, "Reduced accumbens dopamine in Sprague-Dawley rats prone to overeating a fat-rich diet," *Physiology & Behavior*, vol. 101, no. 3, pp. 394–400, 2010.

[115] G. J. Wang, N. D. Volkow, J. Logan et al., "Brain dopamine and obesity," *The Lancet*, vol. 357, no. 9253, pp. 354–357, 2001.

[116] B. A. de Weijer, E. van de Giessen, T. A. van Amelsvoort et al., "Lower striatal dopamine D2/3 receptor availability in obese compared with non-obese subjects," *EJNMMI Research*, vol. 1, article 37, 2011.

[117] D. W. Hommer, J. M. Bjork, and J. M. Gilman, "Imaging brain response to reward in addictive behaviors," *Annals of the New York Academy of Sciences*, vol. 1216, pp. 50–61, 2011.

[118] I. Maze and E. J. Nestler, "The epigenetic landscape of addiction," *Annals of the New York Academy of Sciences*, vol. 1216, no. 1, pp. 99–113, 2011.

[119] J. J. Anker, T. R. Baron, N. E. Zlebnik et al., "Escalation of methamphetamine self-administration in adolescent and adult rats," *Drug and Alcohol Dependence*, vol. 124, pp. 149–153, 2012.

[120] M. Lenoir, K. Guillem, G. F. Koob et al., "Drug specificity in extended access cocaine and heroin self-administration," *Addiction Biology*, vol. 17, pp. 964–976, 2012.

[121] M. A. Parvaz, N. Alia-Klein, P. A. Woicik et al., "Neuroimaging for drug addiction and related behaviors," *Reviews in the Neurosciences*, vol. 22, pp. 609–624, 2011.

[122] G. Zernig, S. H. Ahmed, R. N. Cardinal et al., "Explaining the escalation of drug use in substance dependence: models and appropriate animal laboratory tests," *Pharmacology*, vol. 80, no. 2-3, pp. 65–119, 2007.

[123] J. Alsiö, P. K. Olszewski, A. S. Levine et al., "Feed-forward mechanisms: addiction-like behavioral and molecular adaptations in overeating," *Frontiers in Neuroendocrinology*, vol. 33, pp. 127–139, 2012.

[124] S. Thornley, B. Russell, and R. Kydd, "Carbohydrate reward and psychosis: an explanation for neuroleptic induced weight gain and path to improved mental health?" *Current Neuropharmacology*, vol. 9, no. 2, pp. 370–375, 2011.

[125] J. G. Goldman, C. L. Vaughan, and C. G. Goetz, "An update expert opinion on management and research strategies in Parkinson's disease psychosis," *Expert Opinion on Pharmacotherapy*, vol. 12, pp. 2009–2024, 2011.

[126] S. Aarons, C. Peisah, and C. Wijeratne, "Neuropsychiatric effects of Parkinson's disease treatment," *Australasian Journal on Ageing*, vol. 31, pp. 198–202, 2012.

[127] J. B. Listman, C. Ittiwut, J. F. Cubells et al., "Association between polymorphisms in Catechol-O-methyltransferese (COMT) and cocaine-induced paranoia in European-American and African-American populations," *American Journal of Medical Genetics B*, vol. 156, pp. 651–660, 2011.

[128] F. Vorspan, V. Bloch, G. Brousse et al., "Prospective assessment of transient cocaine-induced psychotic symptoms in a clinical setting," *American Journal on Addictions*, vol. 20, pp. 535–537, 2011.

[129] A. Gururajan, E. E. Manning, M. Klug et al., "Drugs of abuse and increased risk for psychosis development," *Australian and New Zealand Journal of Psychiatry*, vol. 46, pp. 1120–1135, 2012.

[130] A. Hassan, J. H. Bower, N. Kumar et al., "Dopamine agonist-triggered pathological behaviors: surveillance in the PD clinic reveals high frequencies," *Parkinsonism and Related Disorders*, vol. 17, pp. 260–264, 2011.

[131] T. Witjas, A. Eusebio, F. Fluchere et al., "Addictive behaviors and Parkinson's disease," *Revue Neurologique*, vol. 168, pp. 624–633, 2012.

[132] S. Walther and W. Strik, "Motor symptoms and schizophrenia," *Neuropsychobiology*, vol. 66, pp. 77–92, 2012.

[133] S. Krüger, A. Haehner, C. Thiem, and T. Hummel, "Neuroleptic-induced parkinsonism is associated with olfactory dysfunction," *Journal of Neurology*, vol. 255, no. 10, pp. 1574–1579, 2008.

[134] P. Batel, "Addiction and schizophrenia," *European Psychiatry*, vol. 15, no. 2, pp. 115–122, 2000.

[135] C. Dubertret, I. Bidard, J. Adès, and P. Gorwood, "Lifetime positive symptoms in patients with schizophrenia and cannabis abuse are partially explained by co-morbid addiction," *Schizophrenia Research*, vol. 86, no. 1-3, pp. 284–290, 2006.

[136] C. Parker, A. McNeill, and E. Ratschen, "Tailored tobacco dependence support for mental health patients and community services," *Addiction*, vol. 107, pp. 18–25, 2012.

[137] J. Malat, J. Collins, B. Dhayanandhan, F. Carullo, and N. E. Turner, "Addictive behaviors in comorbid addiction and mental illness: preliminary results from a self-report questionnaire," *Journal of Addiction Medicine*, vol. 4, no. 1, pp. 38–46, 2010.

[138] C. Davis, Unpublished data.

[139] C. Davis, K. Patte, C. Curtis, and C. Reid, "Immediate pleasures and future consequences. A neuropsychological study of binge eating and obesity," *Appetite*, vol. 54, no. 1, pp. 208–213, 2010.

[140] C. Davis, "Psychobiological traits in the risk profile for overeating and weight gain," *International Journal of Obesity*, vol. 33, supplement 2, pp. S49–S53, 2009.

[141] L. Moreno-Lopez, C. Soriano-Mas, E. Delgado-Rico et al., "Brain structural correlates of reward sensitivity and impulsivity in adolescents with normal and excess weight," *PLoS ONE*, vol. 7, Article ID e49185, 2012.

[142] E. L. Gibson, "The psychobiology of comfort eating: implications for neuropharmacological interventions," *Behavioural Pharmacology*, vol. 23, pp. 442–460, 2012.

[143] A. J. Stunkard, "Eating disorders and obesity," *Psychiatric Clinics of North America*, vol. 34, pp. 765–771, 2011.

[144] N. D. Volkow and C. P. O'Brien, "Issues for DSM-V: should obesity be included as a brain disorder?" *American Journal of Psychiatry*, vol. 164, no. 5, pp. 708–710, 2007.

[145] M. D. Marcus and J. E. Wildes, "Obesity if DSM-5," *Psychiatric Annals*, vol. 42, pp. 431–435, 2012.

[146] N. D. Volkow, G. Wang -J, D. Tomasi et al., "Obesity and addiction: neurobiological overlaps," *Obesity Reviews*, vol. 14, pp. 2–18, 2013.

[147] World Health Organization, "Obesity: preventing and managing the global epidemic: report of a WHO consultation," Tech. Rep. 894, WHO, Geneva, Switzerland, 2000.

[148] C. M. Bulik, P. F. Sullivan, and K. S. Kendler, "Genetic and environmental contributions to obesity and binge eating," *International Journal of Eating Disorders*, vol. 33, no. 3, pp. 293–298, 2003.

[149] K. N. Javaras, N. M. Laird, T. Reichborn-Kjennerud, C. M. Bulik, H. G. Pope, and J. I. Hudson, "Familiality and heritability of binge eating disorder: results of a case-control family study and a twin study," *International Journal of Eating Disorders*, vol. 41, no. 2, pp. 174–179, 2008.

[150] K. S. Mitchell, M. C. Neale, C. M. Bulik, S. H. Aggen, K. S. Kendler, and S. E. Mazzeo, "Binge eating disorder: a symptom-level investigation of genetic and environmental influences on liability," *Psychological Medicine*, vol. 40, no. 11, pp. 1899–1906, 2010.

[151] A. N. Gearhardt, W. R. Corbin, and K. D. Brownell, "Preliminary validation of the Yale food addiction scale," *Appetite*, vol. 52, no. 2, pp. 430–436, 2009.

[152] D. L. Franko, H. Thompson-Brenner, D. R. Thompson et al., "Racial/ethnic differences in adults in randomized clinical trials of binge eating disorder," *Journal of Consulting and Clinical Psychology*, vol. 80, pp. 186–195, 2012.

[153] M. Tanofsky-Kraff, L. B. Shomaker, E. A. Stern et al., "Children's binge eating and development of metabolic syndrome," *International Journal of Obesity*, vol. 36, pp. 956–962, 2012.

[154] C. M. Grilo, M. A. White, and R. M. Masheb, "The metabolic syndrome and behavioral correlates in obese adults with binge eating disorder," *International Journal of Eating Disorders*, vol. 42, pp. 228–234, 2009.

[155] J. I. Hudson, E. Hiripi, H. G. Pope, and R. C. Kessler, "The prevalence and correlates of eating disorders in the National Comorbidity Survey replication," *Biological Psychiatry*, vol. 61, no. 3, pp. 348–358, 2007.

[156] C. Davis, R. D. Levitan, J. Carter et al., "Personality and eating behaviors: a case-control study of binge eating disorder," *International Journal of Eating Disorders*, vol. 41, no. 3, pp. 243–250, 2008.

[157] M. Tanofsky-Kraff, "Psychosocial preventive interventions for obesity and eating disorders in youth," *International Review of Psychiatry*, vol. 24, pp. 262–270, 2012.

[158] R. L. W. Corwin and F. H. E. Wojnicki, "Binge-type eating induced by limited access to optional foods," in *Animal Models of Eating Disorders*, N. M. Avena, Ed., vol. 74 of *Neuromethods*, pp. 51–68, Springer, Berlin, Germany, 2013.

[159] R. K. Babbs, F. H. E. Wojnicki, and R. L. W. Corwin, "Assessing binge eating. An analysis of data previously collected in binge-ing rats," *Appetite*, vol. 59, pp. 478–482, 2012.

[160] R. W. Foltin, "Modeling binge eating in non-human primates," in *Animal Models of Eating Disorders*, N. M. Avena, Ed., vol. 74 of *Neuromethods*, pp. 97–107, Springer, Berlin, Germany, 2013.

[161] M. Arce, V. Michopoulos, K. N. Shepard, Q. C. Ha, and M. E. Wilson, "Diet choice, cortisol reactivity, and emotional feeding in socially housed rhesus monkeys," *Physiology & Behavior*, vol. 101, no. 4, pp. 446–455, 2010.

[162] D. Morgan, K. A. Grant, H. D. Gage et al., "Social dominance in monkeys: dopamine D2 receptors and cocaine self-administration," *Nature Neuroscience*, vol. 5, no. 2, pp. 169–174, 2002.

[163] C. Curtis and C. Davis, "A qualitative study of binge eating and obesity: an addiction perspective," manuscript submitted.

[164] J. O. Fisher and L. L. Birch, "Restricting access to palatable foods affects children's behavioral response, food selection, and intake," *American Journal of Clinical Nutrition*, vol. 69, no. 6, pp. 1264–1272, 1999.

[165] J. W. Jahng, "Stressful experiences in early life and subsequent food intake," in *Animal Models of Eating Disorders*, N. M. Avena, Ed., vol. 74 of *Neuromethods*, pp. 127–153, Springer, Berlin, Germany, 2013.

[166] C. Heim and E. B. Binder, "Current research trends in early life stress and depression: review of human studies on sensitive periods, gene-environment interactions, and epigenetics," *Experimental Neurology*, vol. 233, pp. 102–111, 2012.

[167] A. El Khoury, S. H. M. Gruber, A. Mørk, and A. A. Mathé, "Adult life behavioral consequences of early maternal separation are alleviated by escitalopram treatment in a rat model of depression," *Progress in Neuro-Psychopharmacology and Biological Psychiatry*, vol. 30, no. 3, pp. 535–540, 2006.

[168] J. Svaldi, J. Griepenstroh, B. TuschenCaffier et al., "Emotion regulation deficits in eating disorders: a marker of eating pathology or general psychopathology?" *Psychiatry Research*, vol. 197, pp. 103–111, 2012.

[169] T. Sawaoka, R. D. Barnes, K. K. Blomquist et al., "Social anxiety and self-consciousness in binge eating disorder: associations with eating disorder psychopathology," *Comprehensive Psychiatry*, vol. 53, pp. 740–745, 2012.

[170] N. T. Bello and A. Hajnal, "Dopamine and binge eating behaviors," *Pharmacology Biochemistry and Behavior*, vol. 97, no. 1, pp. 25–33, 2010.

[171] A. Hajnal, J. E. Nyland, E. Anderzhanova et al., *Chronic Intermittent Access to Highly Palatable Diets Result in Sustained and Augmented Accumbens Dopamine Release and Abolished Response to Regular Chow Compared to Continuous Availability*, Society for Neuroscience, Washington, DC, USA, 2008.

[172] N. C. Raymond, B. Neumeyer, C. S. Warren, S. S. Lee, and C. B. Peterson, "Energy intake patterns in obese women with binge eating disorder," *Obesity Research*, vol. 11, no. 7, pp. 869–879, 2003.

[173] R. M. Masheb, C. M. Grilo, and M. A. White, "An examination of eating patterns in community women with bulimia nervosa and binge eating disorder," *International Journal of Eating Disorders*, vol. 44, pp. 618–624, 2011.

[174] K. Harvey, F. Rosselli, G. T. Wilson, L. L. Debar, and R. H. Striegel-Moore, "Eating patterns in patients with spectrum binge-eating disorder," *International Journal of Eating Disorders*, vol. 44, no. 5, pp. 447–451, 2011.

[175] A. Schienle, A. Schäfer, A. Hermann, and D. Vaitl, "Binge eating disorder: reward sensitivity and brain activation to images of reward," *Biological Psychiatry*, vol. 65, no. 8, pp. 654–661, 2009.

[176] T. Franklin, Z. Wang, J. J. Suh et al., "Effects of varenicline on smoking cue-triggered neural and craving responses," *Archives of General Psychiatry*, vol. 68, no. 5, pp. 516–526, 2011.

[177] E. T. Rolls and C. McCabe, "Enhanced affective brain representations of chocolate in cravers versus non-cravers," *European Journal of Neuroscience*, vol. 26, no. 4, pp. 1067–1076, 2007.

[178] M. Weygandt, A. Schaefer, A. Schienle et al., "Diagnosing different binge-eating disorders based on reward-related brain activation patterns," *Human Brain Mapping*, vol. 33, pp. 2135–2146, 2012.

[179] G. J. Wang, A. Geliebter, N. D. Volkow et al., "Enhanced striatal dopamine release during food stimulation in binge eating disorder," *Obesity*, vol. 19, no. 8, pp. 1601–1608, 2011.

[180] F. M. Filbey, U. S. Myers, and S. DeWitt, "Reward circuit function in high BMI individuals with compulsive overeating: similarities with addiction," *Neuroimage*, vol. 63, pp. 1800–1806, 2012.

[181] L. Benson, S. Carnell, S. Pantazatos et al., "Binge eaters show greater brain activation and connectivity within appetitive network in response to food cues, independent of weight status," *Obesity*, vol. 19, supplement 1, article S192, 2011.

[182] Y. S. Nikolova, R. E. Ferrell, S. B. Manuck, and A. R. Hariri, "Multilocus genetic profile for dopamine signaling predicts ventral striatum reactivity," *Neuropsychopharmacology*, vol. 36, no. 9, pp. 140–147, 2011.

[183] M. E. Gluck, "Stress response and binge eating disorder," *Appetite*, vol. 46, no. 1, pp. 26–30, 2006.

[184] A. Zeeck, N. Stelzer, H. W. Linster et al., "Emotion and eating in binge eating disorder and obesity," *European Eating Disorders Review*, vol. 19, pp. 426–437, 2011.

[185] S. Munsch, A. H. Meyer, V. Quartier et al., "Binge eating in binge eating disorder: a breakdown of emotion regulatory process?" *Psychiatry Research*, vol. 195, pp. 118–124, 2012.

[186] C. M. Grilo, M. A. White, R. D. Barnes et al., "Posttraumatic stress disorder in women with binge eating disorder in primary care," *Journal of Psychiatric Practice*, vol. 18, pp. 408–412, 2012.

[187] S. Schulz and R. G. Laessle, "Stress-induced laboratory eating behavior in obese women with binge eating disorder," *Appetite*, vol. 58, pp. 457–461, 2012.

[188] A. Hilbert, C. Vogele, B. Tuschen-Caffier et al., "Psychophysiological responses to idiosyncratic stress in bulimia nervosa and binge eating disorder," *Physiology & Behavior*, vol. 104, pp. 770–777, 2011.

[189] J. W. Jahng, S. B. Yoo, V. Ryu et al., "Hyperphasia and depression-like behavior by adolescence social isolation in female rats," *International Journal of Developmental Neuroscience*, vol. 30, pp. 47–53, 2012.

[190] A. Beck, T. Wustenberg, A. Genauck et al., "Effect of brain structure, brain function, and brain connectivity on relapse on alcohol-dependent patients," *Archives of General Psychiatry*, vol. 69, pp. 842–853, 2012.

[191] B. P. Bradley, "Behavioural addictions: common features and treatment implications," *British Journal of Addiction*, vol. 85, no. 11, pp. 1417–1419, 1990.

[192] C. Holden, "Behavioral addictions debut in proposed DSM-V," *Science*, vol. 327, no. 5968, p. 935, 2010.

[193] O. Albayrak, S. M. Wolfle, and J. Hebebrand, "Does food addiction exist? A phenomenological discussion based on the psychiatric classification of substance-related disorders and addiction," *Obesity Facts*, vol. 5, pp. 165–179, 2012.

[194] N. M. Avena, "The study of food addiction using animal models of binge eating," *Appetite*, vol. 55, no. 3, pp. 734–737, 2010.

[195] American Psychiatric Association, *Diagnostic and Statistical Manual—Version IV-TR*, American Psychiatric Association Press, Washington, DC, USA, 2000.

[196] P. M. Johnson and P. J. Kenny, "Dopamine D2 receptors in addiction-like reward dysfunction and compulsive eating in obese rats," *Nature Neuroscience*, vol. 13, no. 5, pp. 635–641, 2010.

[197] R. L. Corwin and P. S. Grigson, "Symposium overview—food addiction: fact or fiction?" *Journal of Nutrition*, vol. 139, no. 3, pp. 617–619, 2009.

[198] N. M. Avena and B. G. Hoebel, "A diet promoting sugar dependency causes behavioral cross-sensitization to a low dose of amphetamine," *Neuroscience*, vol. 122, no. 1, pp. 17–20, 2003.

[199] A. Iemolo, M. Valenza, L. Tozier et al., "Withdrawal from chronic, intermittent access to a highly palatable food induces depressive-like behavior in compulsive eating rats," *Behavioural Pharmacology*, vol. 23, pp. 593–602, 2012.

[200] N. M. Avena and P. V. Rada, "Cholinergic modulation of food and drug satiety and withdrawal," *Physiology & Behavior*, vol. 106, pp. 332–336, 2012.

[201] A. Heyne, C. Kiesselbach, I. Sahún et al., "An animal model of compulsive food-taking behaviour," *Addiction Biology*, vol. 14, no. 4, pp. 373–383, 2009.

[202] S. L. Parylak, P. Cottone, V. Sabino et al., "Effect of CB_1 and CRF_1 receptor antagonists on binge-like eating in rats with limited access to sweet fat diet: lack of withdrawal-like responses," *Physiology & Behavior*, vol. 107, pp. 231–242, 2012.

[203] N. M. Avena, P. Rada, and B. G. Hoebel, "Sugar and fat bingeing have notable differences in addictive-like behavior," *Journal of Nutrition*, vol. 139, no. 3, pp. 623–628, 2009.

[204] M. E. Bocarsly, L. A. Berner, B. G. Hoebel et al., "Rats that binge fat-rich food do not show somatic signs or anxiety associated with opiate-like withdrawal: implications for nutrient-specific food addiction," *Physiology & Behavior*, vol. 104, pp. 865–872, 2011.

[205] K. D. Oswald, D. L. Murdaugh, V. L. King, and M. M. Boggiano, "Motivation for palatable food despite consequences in an animal model of binge eating," *International Journal of Eating Disorders*, vol. 44, no. 3, pp. 203–211, 2011.

[206] R. Ventura, E. C. Latagliata, E. Patrono et al., "Food seeking in spite of harmful consequences," in *Animal Models of Eating Disorders*, N. M. Avena, Ed., vol. 74 of *Neuromethods*, pp. 235–254, Springer, Berlin, Germany, 2013.

[207] N. M. Avena and B. G. Hoebel, "Amphetamine-sensitized rats show sugar-induced hyperactivity (cross-sensitization) and sugar hyperphagia," *Pharmacology Biochemistry and Behavior*, vol. 74, no. 3, pp. 635–639, 2003.

[208] B. A. Gosnell, "Sucrose intake enhances behavioral sensitization produced by cocaine," *Brain Research*, vol. 1031, no. 2, pp. 194–201, 2005.

[209] B. F. Singer, J. Scott-Railton, and P. Vezina, "Unpredictable saccharin reinforcement enhances locomotor responding to amphetamine," *Behavioural Brain Research*, vol. 226, pp. 340–344, 2012.

[210] M. J. Acerbo and A. K. Johnson, "Behavioral cross-sensitization between DOCA-induced sodium appetite and cocaine-induced locomotor behavior," *Pharmacology Biochemistry and Behavior*, vol. 98, no. 3, pp. 440–448, 2011.

[211] R. L. Corwin, N. M. Avena, and M. M. Boggiano, "Feeding and reward: perspectives from three rat models of binge eating," *Physiology & Behavior*, vol. 104, no. 1, pp. 87–97, 2011.

[212] V. Deroche-Gamonet, D. Belin, and P. V. Piazza, "Evidence for addiction-like behavior in the rat," *Science*, vol. 305, no. 5686, pp. 1014–1017, 2004.

[213] B. A. Reboussin and J. C. Anthony, "Is there epidemiological evidence to support the idea that a cocaine dependence syndrome emerges soon after onset of cocaine use?" *Neuropsychopharmacology*, vol. 31, no. 9, pp. 2055–2064, 2006.

[214] M. M. Boggiano, A. I. Artiga, C. E. Pritchett, P. C. Chandler-Laney, M. L. Smith, and A. J. Eldridge, "High intake of palatable food predicts binge-eating independent of susceptibility to obesity: an animal model of lean vs obese binge-eating and obesity with and without binge-eating," *International Journal of Obesity*, vol. 31, no. 9, pp. 1357–1367, 2007.

[215] J. W. de Jong, L. J. Vanderschuren, and R. A. Adan, "Towards an animal model of food addiction," *Obesity Facts*, vol. 5, pp. 180–195, 2012.

[216] N. Ronel and G. Libman, "Eating disorders and recovery: lessons from overeaters anonymous," *Clinical Social Work Journal*, vol. 31, no. 2, pp. 155–171, 2003.

[217] S. Russell-Mayhew, K. M. von Ranson, and P. C. Masson, "How does overeaters anonymous help its members? A qualitative analysis," *European Eating Disorders Review*, vol. 18, no. 1, pp. 33–42, 2010.

[218] C. Davis, C. Curtis, R. D. Levitan et al., "Evidence that "food addiction" is a valid phenotype of obesity," *Appetite*, vol. 57, pp. 711–717, 2011.

[219] A. Meule, A. Lutz, C. Vogele et al., "Women with elevated food addiction symptoms show accelerated reactions, but no impaired inhibitory control in response to pictures of high-calorie food-cues," *Eating Behaviors*, vol. 13, pp. 423–428, 2012.

[220] H. Garavan and K. Weierstall, "The neurobiology of reward and cognitive control systems and their role in incentivizing health behavior," *Preventive Medicine*, vol. 55, pp. S17–S23, 2012.

[221] A. J. Janes, L. D. Nickerson, B. B. Bde et al., "Prefrontal and limbic resting state brain network functional connectivity differs between nicotine-dependent smokers and non-smoking controls," *Drug and Alcohol Dependence*, vol. 125, pp. 252–259, 2012.

[222] B. M. Appelhans, K. Woolf, S. L. Pagota et al., "Inhibiting food reward: delay discounting, food reward sensitivity, and palatable food intake in overweight and obese women," *Obesity*, vol. 19, pp. 2175–2182, 2011.

[223] N. S. Lawrence, E. C. Hinton, J. A. Parkinson et al., "Nucleus accumbens response to food cues predicts subsequent snack consumption in women and increased body mass index in those with reduced self-control," *Neuroimage*, vol. 63, pp. 415–422, 2012.

[224] D. N. Kearns, M. A. Gomez-Serrano, and B. J. Tunstall, "A review of preclinical research demonstrating that drug and non-drug reinforcers differentially affect behavior," *Current Drug Abuse Reviews*, vol. 4, pp. 261–269, 2011.

[225] L. T. Fikke, A. Melinder, and N. I. Landro, "The effects of acute tryptophan depletion on impulsivity and mood in adolescents engaging in non-suicidal self-injury," *Human Psychopharmacology*, vol. 28, pp. 61–71, 2013.

[226] J. L. Fortuna, "The obesity epidemic and food addiction: clinical similarities to drug dependence," *Journal of Psychoactive Drugs*, vol. 44, no. 1, pp. 56–63, 2012.

[227] A. N. Gearhardt, S. Yokum, P. T. Orr et al., "Neural correlates of food addiction," *Archives of General Psychiatry*, vol. 32, pp. E1–E9, 2011.

[228] C. Davis, N. J. Loxton, R. D. Levitan et al., "'Food addiction' and its association with a dopamine multilocus genetic profile," *Physiology & Behavior*. In press.

[229] A. N. Gearhardt, M. A. White, R. M. Masheb et al., "An examination of the food addiction construct in obese patients with binge eating disorder," *International Journal of Eating Disorders*, vol. 45, pp. 657–663, 2012.

[230] S. E. Cassin and K. M. von Ranson, "Is binge eating experienced as an addiction?" *Appetite*, vol. 49, no. 3, pp. 687–690, 2007.

[231] J. M. Burmeister, N. Hinman, A. Koball et al., "Food addiction in adults seeking weight loss treatment. Implications for psychosocial health and weight loss," *Appetite*, vol. 60, pp. 103–110, 2013.

[232] A. B. Goldschmidt, D. Le Grange, P. Powers et al., "Eating disorder symptomatology in normal-weight versus obese individuals with binge eating disorder," *Obesity*, vol. 19, no. 7, pp. 1515–1518, 2011.

[233] A. E. Dingemans and E. F. van Furth, "Binge eating disorder psychopathology in normal weight and obese individuals," *International Journal of Eating Disorders*, vol. 45, pp. 135–138, 2012.

[234] D. T. Barry, C. M. Grilo, and R. M. Masheb, "Comparison of patients with bulimia nervosa, obese patients with binge eating disorder, and nonobese patients with binge eating disorder," *Journal of Nervous and Mental Disease*, vol. 191, no. 9, pp. 589–594, 2003.

[235] I. Carrad, M. Van der Linden, and A. Golay, "Comparison of obese and nonobese individuals with binge eating disorder: delicate boundry between binge eating disorder and non-purging bulimia nervosa," *European Eating Disorders Review*, vol. 20, pp. 350–354, 2012.

[236] C. G. Fairburn, Z. Cooper, H. A. Doll, P. Norman, and M. O'Connor, "The natural course of bulimia nervosa and binge eating disorder in young women," *Archives of General Psychiatry*, vol. 57, no. 7, pp. 659–665, 2000.

[237] A. E. Field, K. R. Sonneville, N. Micali et al., "Prospective association of common eating disorders and adverse outcomes," *Pediatrics*, vol. 130, pp. E289–E295, 2012.

[238] K. P. de Young, J. M. Lavender, G. T. Wilson et al., "Binge eating disorder in DSM-5," *Psychiatric Annals*, vol. 42, pp. 410–413, 2012.

[239] S. E. Trace, L. M. Thornton, T. L. Root et al., "Effects of reducing the frequency and duration criteria for binge eating on lifetime prevalence of bulimia nervosa and binge eating disorder: implications for DSM-5," *International Journal of Eating Disorders*, vol. 45, pp. 531–536, 2012.

[240] A. N. Gearhardt and W. R. Corbin, "The role of food addiction in clinical research," *Current Pharmaceutical Design*, vol. 17, no. 12, pp. 1140–1142, 2011.

[241] A. Meule, "How prevalent is "food addiction" ?" *Frontiers in Psychiatry*, vol. 2, pp. 1–4, 2011.

[242] H. Ziaudden, S. Farooqi, and P. C. Fletcher, "Obesity and the brain: how convincing is the addiction model?" *Nature Reviews Neuroscience*, vol. 13, pp. 279–286, 2012.

[243] J. Swendsen and M. Le Moal, "Individual vulnerability to addiction," *Annals of the New York Academy of Sciences*, vol. 1216, pp. 73–85, 2011.

Relationship between Birth Weight and Metabolic Status in Obese Adolescents

David J. Hill,[1,2,3,4,5] Harry Prapavessis,[6] J. Kevin Shoemaker,[6] Michelle Jackman,[7,8] Farid H. Mahmud,[9] and Cheril Clarson[1,3,7]

[1] *London Health Sciences Centre, Lawson Health Research Institute, London, ON, Canada N6A 5W9*
[2] *Lawson Health Research Institute, St Joseph's Health Care, 268 Grosvenor Street, London, ON, Canada N6A 4V2*
[3] *Department of Paediatrics, University of Western Ontario, London, ON, Canada N6A 5A5*
[4] *Department of Medicine, University of Western Ontario, London, ON, Canada N6A 5A5*
[5] *Department of Physiology and Pharmacology, University of Western Ontario, London, ON, Canada N6A 5A5*
[6] *School of Kinesiology, University of Western Ontario, London, ON, Canada N6A 5A5*
[7] *London Health Sciences Centre, Children's Hospital, London, ON, Canada N6A 5W9*
[8] *Department of Pediatrics , University of Calgary, Calgary, Alberta, Canada*
[9] *Department of Paediatrics, University of Toronto and Hospital for Sick Children, Toronto, ON, Canada M5G 1X8*

Correspondence should be addressed to David J. Hill; david.hill@lhrionhealth.ca

Academic Editors: A. Erkner, B. Navia, and R. Tungtrongchitr

Objective. To examine the relationships between birth weight and body mass index, percent body fat, blood lipids, glycemia, insulin resistance, adipokines, blood pressure, and endothelial function in a cohort of obese adolescents. *Design and Methods.* Ninety-five subjects aged 10–16 years (mean age 13.5 years) with a body mass index >95th centile (mean [±SEM] 33.0 ± 0.6) were utilized from two prospective studies for obesity prevention prior to any interventions. The mean term birth weight was 3527 ± 64 g (range 1899–4990 g;). *Results.* Body mass index z-score correlated positively with birth weight ($r^2 = 0.05$, $P = 0.03$), but not percent body fat. Insulin resistance negatively correlated with birth weight ($r^2 = 0.05$, $P < 0.001$), as did fasting plasma insulin ($r^2 = 0.05$, $P < 0.001$); both being significantly greater for subjects of small versus large birth weight (Δ Homeostasis Model Assessment = 2.5 and Δ insulin = 10 pmol/L for birth weight <2.5 kg versus >4.5 kg). Adiponectin, but not leptin, blood pressure z-scores or peripheral arterial tomography values positively correlated with birth weight ($r^2 = 0.07$, $P = 0.008$). *Conclusions.* Excess body mass index in obese adolescents was positively related to birth weight. Birth weight was not associated with cardiovascular risk factors but represented a significant determinant of insulin resistance.

1. Introduction

Childhood obesity in Canada, as in other developed countries, has increased dramatically with 29% of children being overweight or obese in 2007 compared to 15% in 1978 [1]. Obesity in childhood is a strong indicator of future obesity in adulthood and also confers a high risk for future development of type 2 diabetes (T2D) and cardiovascular disease [2, 3]. The future risk of adult T2D is greater in adolescents who demonstrate insulin resistance [4]. Small-for-gestational age (SGA, <10th percentile birth weight) and large-for-gestational age (LGA, >90% percentile) birth weight can both confer an increased risk of adolescent and adult obesity, insulin resistance, metabolic syndrome, and T2D in adulthood [5, 6]. A meta-analysis of 20 studies showed that birth weight greater than 4 kg increased the risk of obesity (odds ratio 2.1), but being SGA did not, although the majority of the studies analyzed considered children prior to adolescence [7]. However, it is not clear whether consideration of birth weight is of practical relevance in the management of the individual obese child at risk of the development of metabolic or cardiovascular disease.

The association between LGA, often with macrosomia, and adolescent and adult obesity, as well as the associated increased risk of T2D and cardiovascular disease, is most apparent when accompanied by maternal diabetes, both gestational and pregestational [8, 9]. Maternal pregestational obesity, with or without excessive weight gain during pregnancy, provides an equivalent risk for maternal hyperglycemia and infant macrosomia as does diabetes, and the offspring in both conditions exhibit a greater risk of obesity during adolescence [10, 11]. In pregnancies uncomplicated by diabetes or biased by maternal obesity, increasing birth weight correlated positively with child and adult BMI [12]. However, BMI does not distinguish between lean and fat body mass, or body fat distribution, and birth weight also showed a positive correlation with lean body mass in children and adults [13]. An increase in birth weight equivalent to one standard deviation was associated with an additional kg of body weight during adolescence, but this increase was in fat-free body weight [13]. Although LGA outside of maternal diabetes or obesity may result in a high BMI during adolescence, this has not been shown to be associated with truncal obesity or insulin resistance, or with a greater risk of future metabolic disease [14].

In comparison with LGA, SGA infants have been shown to be at greater risk of hypertension and cardiovascular disease as adults [15]. While SGA was associated with inadequate maternal nutrition, there is evidence of an altered mass of pancreatic insulin-producing β cells, insulin release, and insulin resistance from animal models and of glucose intolerance and insulin resistance in the human offspring resulting in an increased risk of diabetes in the adult [16, 17]. In the developed world most SGA infants do not result from nutritionally inadequate pregnancies but can still exhibit abnormal growth trajectories and demonstrate metabolic dysfunction postnatally. SGA infants have a greater risk of childhood obesity, although this is dependent on the trajectory of postnatal catch-up growth. Most SGA infants exhibit some catch-up growth between 6 and 12 months of age [18]. However, those exhibiting rapid catch-up growth prior to 4 years were at greater risk of being obese as adolescents and adults, with a subsequent increased risk of metabolic syndrome and diabetes [19]. The SGA infant who undergoes rapid catch-up growth is more likely to exhibit truncal fat obesity, independent of an increased BMI [20].

Park [21] showed a negative correlation between birth weight and insulin resistance in 34 overweight children, but the relationship between birth weight and metabolic changes in obese adolescents that may predispose to diabetes or cardiovascular disease in adulthood has not been examined in detail. Therefore, we examined the relationships between birth weight and BMI, body fat content, glycemic control, insulin resistance, circulating adipokines, blood lipids, blood pressure, and endothelial function in obese adolescents at baseline as part of obesity prevention programs.

2. Methods

2.1. Study Design. Entry data were utilized from 2 prospective cohort studies of obese adolescents. Twenty-six subjects were recruited for an obesity intervention which was completed in 2007, and 69 subjects were screened between 2008 and 2010 for entry to the REACH trial. Both groups were evaluated by the same clinical team and lead physician Cheril Clarson as the initial obesity prevention cohort was used as a pilot group to assess interest and feasibility for a more intensive clinical study. The REACH study (ClinicalTrials.gov number NCT00934570) will assess the effects of a structured lifestyle intervention and metformin (or placebo) on BMI and other risk factors for T2D and cardiovascular disease in obese adolescents. Both studies were approved by the Western University Research Ethics Board, London, ON, Canada, in addition to Health Canada. Informed consent was obtained from all study subjects.

2.2. Subjects. The study cohorts comprised obese subjects aged 10 to 16 years, defined as BMI greater than the 95th percentile for age and gender. Exclusion criteria included a fasting plasma glucose ≥6.0 mmol/L and within the REACH study a 2 h glucose value ≥11.1 mmol/L following an oral glucose tolerance test and a glycosylated hemoglobin (A1C) of ≥6% (≥7 mmol/L). Pubertal staging was assessed using the method of Tanner. At study entry, potential risk factors for development of T2D in addition to obesity were assessed, including pregestational maternal type 1 or 2 diabetes or gestational diabetes, birth weight, ethnicity, and the presence of acanthosis nigricans, hirsutism, or acne in adolescent girls.

2.3. Measurements. All subjects were asked to fast from 10 p.m. of the evening prior to study and to avoid caffeine for the preceding 24 h period. Blood was sampled for measurement of glucose, insulin, LDL and HDL cholesterol, triglycerides, and the adipocytokines, leptin, and high molecular weight adiponectin. Subjects (69) entering the REACH study also had an oral glucose tolerance test (2 h GTT) with measurement of 2 h plasma glucose and A1C. Glucose was measured by the glucose oxidase technique and plasma insulin levels determined by a double antibody radioimmunoassay using a recombinant human insulin standard and the minimum detection level of <2 pmol/L. Within- and between-assay coefficients of variation were 5.8% and 6.5%, respectively. Insulin resistance was estimated by the measurement of Homeostasis Model Assessment (HOMA), calculated as fasting plasma insulin (mU/L) × fasting plasma glucose (mmol/L)/22.5. HOMA values greater than 3.0 in adolescents are indicative of insulin resistance [22]. Serum leptin levels were measured using an ELISA assay (Quantikine, R&D Systems Inc., Minneapolis, MN) with a sensitivity of less than 8 pg/mL and inter- and intra-assay coefficients of variation of 5% and 3%, respectively. High molecular weight adiponectin was also measured with an ELISA (ALPCO Diagnostics, Salem, NH) with a sensitivity of less than 19 pg/mL and inter- and intra-assay coefficients of variation of 6% and 3%, respectively. A1C was measured by radioimmunoassay by clinical laboratory services, London Health Sciences Centre, London, ON, Canada.

Weight was measured with subjects wearing minimal clothing using an electronic scale to the nearest 0.1 kg. Height was measured without shoes using a wall mounted stadiometer to the nearest 0.1 cm. BMI z-scores were calculated from the US Centers for Disease Control and Prevention reference data [23]. The percent body fat was determined by whole body dual-energy x-ray absorptiometry (DEXA) analysis (General Electric-Lunar iDXA, Mississauga, ON, Canada).

Diastolic and systolic blood pressure was measured in the right arm using an appropriately sized cuff using a Dynamap machine. Age and sex-adjusted z-scores were calculated using the National High Blood Pressure Education Program Working Group on High Blood Pressure in Children and Adolescents [24]. A measurement of endothelial function was obtained using peripheral arterial tonometry (PAT) with lower RH-PAT values indicative of greater endothelial dysfunction (Itamar Medical, Israel). Details of this technique have been described previously [25].

2.4. Statistical Analysis. Measured values were obtained from 95 individuals, except for values for A1C, 2 h GTT, and percent body fat, which were obtained from a subgroup of 69 subjects. The normality of variables was confirmed using the Kolgomorov-Smirnov test. Values are expressed as mean ± SEM. The relationships between BMI and diabetes and cardiovascular risk factor variables at study entry were examined by univariate linear regression, as were the associations between birth weight and the following factors: BMI z-score, percent body fat, blood pressure z-scores, plasma insulin, leptin, adiponectin (and leptin/adiponectin ratio), HOMA, fasting and 2 h GTT plasma glucose, circulating lipids (HDL and LDL cholesterol and triglycerides), A1C, and RH-PAT. Stepwise regression with forward entry was also used to investigate the relevance of possible confounding variables such as maternal age, ethnicity, and stage of puberty. Details for other possible confounders such as maternal smoking during pregnancy and socioeconomic status were not available. The cohort was further separated into quintiles based on birth weight and the above parameters analyzed by analysis of variance using Fisher's PLSD post hoc test for significance of differences between quintiles. Statistical analyses were performed using GraphPad PRISM software (GraphPad Software, Inc., La Jolla, CA).

3. Results

3.1. Study Cohort. The study cohort consisted of 95 subjects (43 male) aged between 10 and 16 years with a mean age of 13.5 ± 0.2 years and selected as having an age-adjusted BMI >95th percentile, a fasting plasma glucose of ≤6 mmol/L, and an A1C of ≤6% (≤7 mmol/L). The mean BMI was 33.0 ± 0.6 and the mean BMI z-score was 2.22 ± 0.04 (Table 1). Stage of puberty was assessed for the 69 subjects within the REACH trial, of which 35 were in Tanner stage 5, 7 in stage 4, 14 in stage 3, and 7 in stage 2. Six subjects had not yet entered puberty (stage 1). In the second cohort of 26 subjects all were assessed as being in puberty by the same clinical investigator as for the REACH trial, Cheril Clarson. The mean age, BMI z-score, and birth weight did not significantly differ between the two subgroups.

Table 1: Subject characteristics (mean ± S.E.M, [range]).

Age (years)	13.5 ± 0.2 (9.8–16.9)
Birth weight (g)	3527 ± 64 (1899–4990)
BMI	33.0 ± 0.6 (21.8–46.1)
BMI z-score	2.22 ± 0.04 (1.18–3.00)
Systolic BP z-score	0.30 ± 0.08 (−1.71–3.24)
Diastolic BP z-score	0.33 ± 0.10 (−2.41–3.09)
PAT (RH-PAT)	1.77 ± 0.04 (1.00–2.73)
FPG (Mmol/L)	4.93 ± 0.05 (3.00–6.00)
2 h GTT glucose (mmol/L)	5.59 ± 0.15 (2.80–9.80)
Insulin (pmol/L)	18.3 ± 1.11 (2.0–51.0)
HOMA	4.08 ± 0.26 (0.35–12.69)
HDL cholesterol (mmol/L)	1.16 ± 0.03 (0.62–2.57)
LDL cholesterol (mmol/L)	2.36 ± 0.07 (0.69–4.35)
Triglycerides (mmol/L)	1.19 ± 0.07 (0.30–4.20)
Leptin (ng/mL)	38.8 ± 1.75 (9.32–86.20)
Adiponectin (μg/mL)	2.49 ± 0.13 (0.68–7.20)
Leptin/adiponectin ratio	19.6 ± 1.2 (3.0–53.0)
A1C (%)	5.4 ± 0.1 (4.7–6.0)
Body fat (percent)	45.5 ± 0.1 (35.5–56.3)

Values show median and range. BMI: body mass index; BP: blood pressure, PAT: peripheral arterial tomography; HOMA: Homeostasis Model Assessment. A normal distribution of values for each variable was confirmed using the Kolgomorov-Smirnov test. Values were obtained from 95 individuals, except for values for A1C and percent body fat, which were obtained from a sub-group of 69 subjects. The mean age, BMI z-score, and birth weight of this sub-group did not significantly differ from the larger cohort.

3.2. Metabolic and Cardiovascular Risk Factors. Subject characteristics are depicted in Table 1. The mean HOMA value was slightly elevated at 4.08 ± 0.26 indicating the presence of insulin resistance, with 35% of subjects having a HOMA value greater than 4.0. The mean serum HDL cholesterol level was low at 1.16 ± 0.03 nmol/L, placing this between the 10th and 25th percentiles of age and sex-adjusted values [26], and the mean triglyceride level of 1.19 ± 0.07 nmol/L was elevated between the 90th and 95th percentiles. The HDL cholesterol level was below 1.3 nmol/L in 81% of subjects, whilst 16% had a triglyceride value above 1.7 nmol/L. The mean blood pressure z-scores were 0.30 ± 0.08 for systolic and 0.33 ± 0.10 for diastolic, and they indicated only a slight elevation above normal. Only 2 subjects had a blood pressure greater than 130/85 mm. These characteristics did not significantly differ with gender.

Linear regression analysis showed significant positive relationships between BMI z-score and the percent body fat, serum triglyceride levels, leptin levels and the leptin/adiponectin ratio, HOMA, and fasting plasma insulin (Table 2). A significant negative relationship was found between BMI z-score and serum HDL cholesterol levels, whilst no significant relationship existed with serum adiponectin levels, LDL cholesterol, fasting or 2 h GTT glucose values, or A1C levels. The BMI z-score was positively related to blood pressure but not to endothelial function as measured by PAT (Table 2). However, HOMA values showed a significant positive relationship with both fasting and 2 h

Table 2: Relationships between BMI z-score or HOMA and metabolic and vascular parameters in obese adolescents.

	r^2	P value	Slope-intercept
Regression analysis versus BMI z-score			
Body fat (%)	0.44	<0.001	$y = 0.27 + 0.08x$
Systolic BP z-score	0.07	0.007	$y = -0.84 + 1.04x$
Diastolic BP z-score	0.08	0.005	$y = 0.31 + 0.74x$
Insulin	0.24	<0.001	$y = -13.25 + 14.22x$
HOMA	0.21	<0.001	$y = -2.86 + 3.12x$
HDL cholesterol	0.05	0.026	$y = 1.60 - 0.20x$
Triglycerides	0.05	0.027	$y = 0.24 + 0.43x$
Leptin	0.18	<0.001	$y = -4.98 + 19.74x$
Leptin/adiponectin ratio	0.05	0.030	$y = 3.50 + 7.22x$
Regression analysis versus HOMA			
FPG	0.16	<0.001	$y = -6.89 + 2.22x$
2 h GTT glucose	0.14	0.002	$y = -0.06 + 0.62x$

BMI: body mass index; BP: blood pressure; HOMA: Homeostasis Model Assessment; GTT: glucose tolerance test. No significant relationships were found between BMI z-score and adiponectin, LDL, fasting blood glucose or 2 h GTT values, and A1C or peripheral arterial tomography.

GTT glucose values. These relationships did not differ with sex or Tanner pubertal stage. Thus, adolescent obesity was associated with insulin resistance, dyslipidemia, and higher blood pressure.

3.3. Associations of Birth Weight and Risk Factors. The mean birth weight of the study group was 3527 ± 64 g (males 3487 ± 94 g, females 3560 ± 87 g), the mean length of gestation was 39.9 ± 0.1 weeks, and the mean maternal age was 28.8 ± 0.9 years. Linear regression analysis showed a significant positive relationship between birth weight and BMI z-score, suggesting that infants of larger birth weight tended to have the greatest BMI within this population of obese adolescents (Table 3). Stepwise regression showed that this relationship remained significant after accounting for the possible confounding variables of maternal age and stage of puberty. No relationship was found between birth weight and percent body fat. A positive relationship existed between birth weight and serum adiponectin levels, but not with leptin or circulating lipids. However, the leptin/adiponectin ratio was negatively associated with birth weight (Table 3). Fasting plasma insulin levels were negatively associated with birth weight, as were the HOMA values, but no significant relationship existed between birth weight and fasting or 2 h GTT glucose values. A significant positive relationship did exist between birth weight and A1C values. No relationships were found between birth weight and blood pressure z-scores or PAT values. Also, birth weight showed no relationship with ethnicity or maternal age, or with the age of menarche, the Tanner pubertal stage, or the presence of acne, hirsutism, or acanthosis in the obese adolescents; the latter two represent indicators of hyperinsulinemia. No significant differences in the slopes of the regression lines were found between males and females for any of the above measurements. The results suggest that obese adolescents of higher birth weight tended to have a higher BMI, but there was no evidence of dyslipidemia. While glycemic control following an OGTT was not compromised, a higher birth weight was associated with a greater A1C, suggesting a greater tendency towards hyperglycemia. In contrast, obese adolescents who were of lower birth weight had a greater incidence of insulin resistance and higher fasting insulin levels. However there was no evidence of a relationship between birth weight and cardiovascular risk factors.

Table 3: Relationships between birth size (g) and metabolic and vascular parameters in obese adolescents.

	r^2	P value	Slope-intercept
BMI z-score	0.05	0.033	$y = 0.77 + 1.28E - 4x$
Insulin	0.05	<0.001	$y = 32.39 - 0.01x$
HOMA	0.05	<0.001	$y = 7.42 - 0.01x$
A1C	0.08	0.020	$y = 0.05 + 0.26E - 6x$
Adiponectin	0.07	0.008	$y = 0.55 + 0.01x$
Leptin/adiponectin ratio	0.07	0.010	$y = 37.20 - 0.01x$

BMI: body mass index; HOMA: Homeostasis Model Assessment. No significant relationships were found between birth size and BMI, percent body fat, leptin, basal glucose or 2 h GTT values, systolic or diastolic blood pressure z-scores, peripheral arterial tomography, HDL, LDL, or triglyceride values, maternal age, ethnicity, age of menarche, Tanner puberty stage, or the presence of acne, hirsuitism, or acanthosis.

To confirm these findings, the birth weights of the study subjects were divided into quintiles, ranging from infants who were small for gestational age (SGA) (<2500 g, $n = 7$) to those who were large for gestational age (LGA) (>4000 g, $n = 19$). Obese adolescents were significantly more likely to have higher fasting insulin levels and greater insulin resistance (HOMA) if they were SGA (Figure 1). Conversely, obese adolescents who were LGA were significantly more likely to have a higher plasma adiponectin levels and a lower leptin/adiponectin ratio. Similarly, LGA infants were significantly more likely to have higher circulating triglyceride levels (not shown). No relationships were found between blood pressure or PAT values and birth size quintile.

4. Discussion

As expected, adolescents with a BMI >95th centile (mean BMI *z*-score 2.22) demonstrated a positive correlation between BMI and percent body fat, circulating triglycerides, and leptin. Thirty-five percent of subjects had an HOMA value >4.0, indicating insulin resistance [22]. The HOMA value positively correlated with BMI, but no relationships existed between BMI and fasting glucose values, or the 2 h value from the GTT. Insulin resistance usually increases during puberty, commencing at Tanner stage 2 and peaking at stage 3 for both genders [28]. In our study, no relationship was found between HOMA and Tanner stage, although the distribution of subjects was biased towards stage 5 indicating transition through puberty. Blood pressure *z*-scores were only slightly elevated in the obese subjects. We previously demonstrated a significant inverse relationship between PAT ratio and BMI *z*-score in a cohort of adolescents that included both nonobese and obese individuals, indicating the association of endothelial dysfunction with obesity [25]. In the present study the mean PAT ratio was 1.77, which is lower than that reported by us for nonobese subjects of the same mean age, at 2.06 [25], and indicating that endothelial dysfunction was likely to be present. Thus, obesity in this group of adolescents was associated with the appearance of insulin resistance and evidence of relative vascular dysfunction compared to nonobese adolescents.

In a population of over 1,000 9-year-olds not selected by weight the prevalence of SGA was 7% and LGA 9% [29]. In our smaller cohort of obese subjects, the relative prevalence was biased in favour of LGA (SGA 7% versus LGA 20%). As would be expected, therefore, birth weight at term was positively related to BMI *z*-score in obese adolescents but was not related to percent body fat or circulating leptin levels. Similarly, there were no differences in mean percent body fat or leptin when birth size was arranged by quintiles. Birth weight has a positive correlation with both lean body mass and percent body fat at age 9 or 10 [30]. However, SGA babies can show disproportionately higher fat mass as adults, despite having a lower BMI [20]. Postnatal growth trajectory appears to be at least as important as birth weight in determining the risk of obesity in adolescents or adults [31, 32]. We did not have access to postnatal growth trajectory, but our data show that within a group of obese adolescents, the BMI *z*-score is related, in part, to birth weight, but not percent body fat which may be determined more by postnatal growth patterns.

We noted a strong inverse relationship between birth weight and both HOMA and fasting circulating insulin levels, indicating a relatively greater insulin resistance in obese adolescents who were of smaller birth size. Although fasting glucose and glucose tolerance were not statistically different, glycemic status was worse in these individuals because A1C levels were also significantly higher for those of smaller birth weight. Adolescents who were born SGA had, on average, a HOMA value 2.5 units greater than those born LGA. There is strong evidence that infants born to mothers who were diabetic have increased risks of obesity and T2D as young adults [33], but these infants tend to be LGA and macrosomic. In a nondiabetic *in utero* environment, SGA infants whose mothers were subjected to nutritional restriction as in the Dutch hunger famine of 1944 demonstrated a statistically greater risk of becoming obese as young adults and had a higher rate of T2D [34]. When 34 overweight children were evaluated by birth weight, the HOMA value and measures of tissue oxidative stress were significantly higher for those in the bottom tertile for birth weight compared to the top [21]. Similarly, Norris et al. [27] showed an inverse relationship between birth weight and adult fasting glucose levels, HOMA, and the risk of T2D after adjusting for weight circumference.

We found a strong inverse relationship between circulating adiponectin levels and the adiponectin/leptin ratio, with birth size. Adiponectin increases hepatic triglyceride accumulation, enhances pancreatic beta cell function, and improves insulin sensitivity in peripheral tissues [35]. A decreased release of adiponectin from adipocytes is associated with obesity, and circulating levels correlate with insulin resistance and are inversely related to the risk of developing T2D [36]. It is therefore likely that the greater insulin resistance observed in obese adolescents who were smaller at birth may be mechanistically linked to a lower availability of adiponectin. The altered circulating adiponectin may reflect an altered location of adipose stores depending on whether the subjects were smaller or larger at birth since circulating levels decrease with increasing truncal obesity [37].

While this cohort of obese adolescents had relatively decreased mean PAT ratios and slightly elevated mean blood pressure compared to a nonobese population, these measurements showed no relation to birth weight. Several studies found that birth size was inversely related to systolic and diastolic blood pressure in children or adults and to risk of cardiovascular disease [38, 39]. However, Filler et al. [40] found that blood pressure *z*-scores in childhood did not correlate with birth weight but were related to maternal prepregnancy BMI. Our findings suggest that for obese adolescents, birth size does not confer a detectable risk of future cardiovascular problems.

In summary, this study shows that the individual BMI, but not the percent body fat, in obese adolescents was positively related to birth weight. While no differential risk for development of cardiovascular disease was found that could be related to birth weight, there was significantly worse glycemic status and insulin resistance in obese adolescents of lower birth weight. This represents an additional risk factor for future T2D in obese adolescents and may be relevant to the intensity of lifestyle or pharmaceutical intervention necessary within an obesity prevention program.

Conflict of Interests

The authors have no conflict of interests.

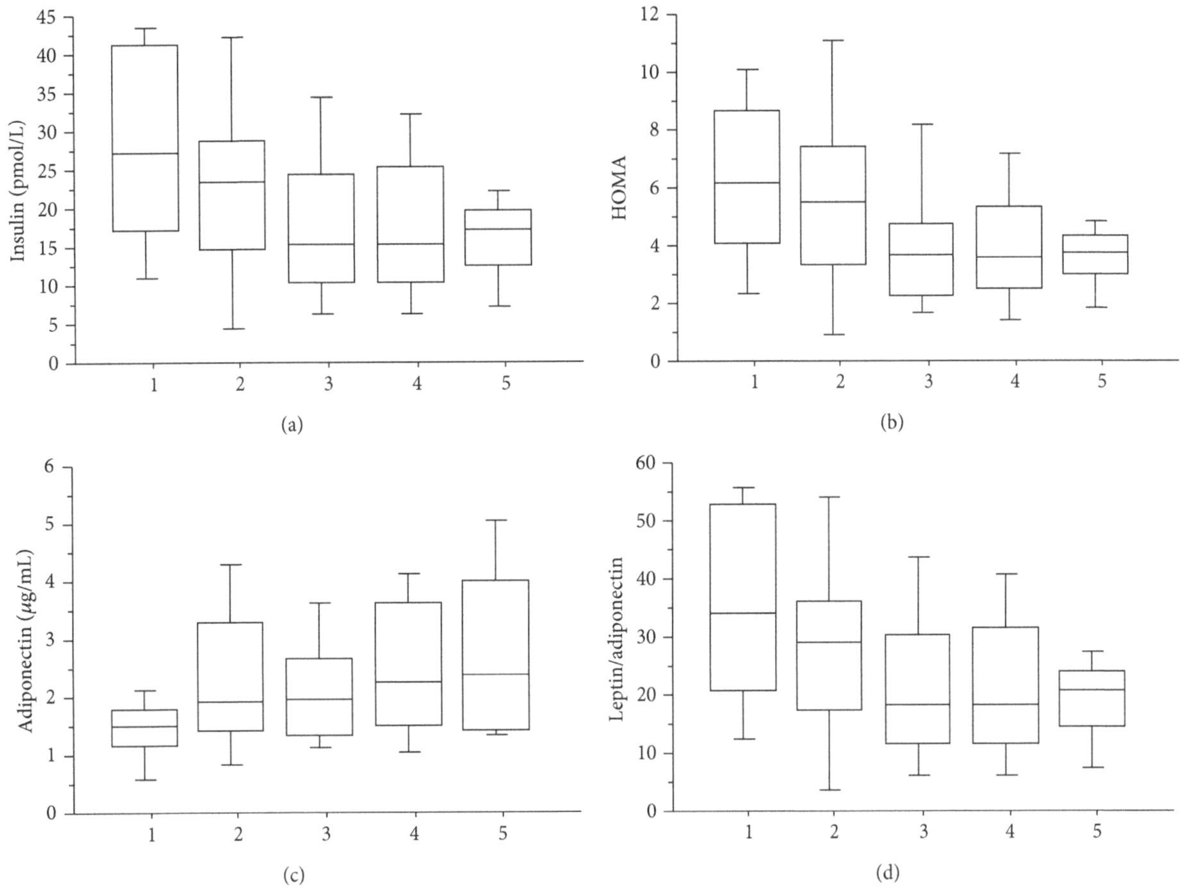

FIGURE 1: Box plot analysis showing median values and interquartile range for plasma insulin (a), HOMA (b), adiponectin (c), and the leptin/adiponectin ratio (d) in obese adolescents when separated by quintiles representing the range of birth weights for the same individuals. 1: <2500 g [7]; 2: 2500–3000 g [8]; 3: 3001–3500 g [27]; 4: 3501–4000 g [28]; 5: >4000 g [19]. $P < 0.05$ or less for insulin (1 versus 3, 4, and 5), HOMA (1 versus 5), adiponectin (1 and 3 versus 5), and the leptin/adiponectin ratio (1 versus 4 and 5).

Acknowledgments

Financial support was provided by the Canadian Institutes for Health Research and the Children's Health Foundation, London Health Sciences Centre. The authors are grateful to Brenda Strutt for technical assistance and to Tracy Robinson and Margaret Watson for assistance with patient recruitment. Cheril Clarson, David Hill, and Kevin Shoemaker were coprincipal investigators on grant awards and devised the experiments, Cheril Clarson was the managing physician on the study, and David Hill, Harry Prapavassis, Kevin Shoemaker, Michelle Jackman, Farid Mahmud, and Cheril Clarson collected and analyzed the data and wrote the paper.

References

[1] Statistics Canada, *Canadian Community Health Survey, 2009*, 2010.

[2] N. Sandhu, M. B. Witmans, J.-F. Lemay, S. Crawford, N. Jadavji, and D. Pacaud, "Prevalence of overweight and obesity in children and adolescents with type 1 diabetes mellitus," *Journal of Pediatric Endocrinology and Metabolism*, vol. 21, no. 7, pp. 631–640, 2008.

[3] J. L. Baker, L. W. Olsen, and T. I. A. Sørensen, "Childhood body-mass index and the risk of coronary heart disease in adulthood," *The New England Journal of Medicine*, vol. 357, no. 23, pp. 2329–2337, 2007.

[4] N. Gungor, F. Bacha, R. Saad, J. Janosky, and S. Arslanian, "Youth type 2 diabetes: insulin resistance, β-cell failure, or both?" *Diabetes Care*, vol. 28, no. 3, pp. 638–644, 2005.

[5] J. S. Huang, T. A. Lee, and M. C. Lu, "Prenatal programming of childhood overweight and obesity," *Maternal and Child Health Journal*, vol. 11, no. 5, pp. 461–473, 2007.

[6] M. H. Vickers and D. M. Sloboda, "Strategies for reversing the effects of metabolic disorders induced as a consequence of developmental programming," *Frontiers in Physiology*, vol. 3, article 242, pp. 1–11, 2012.

[7] Z. B. Yu, S. P. Han, G. Z. Zhu et al., "Birth weight and subsequent risk of obesity: a systematic review and meta-analysis," *Obesity Reviews*, vol. 12, no. 7, pp. 525–542, 2011.

[8] S. Y. Kim, A. J. Sharma, and W. M. Callaghan, "Gestational diabetes and childhood obesity: what is the link?" *Current Opinion in Obstetrics and Gynecology*, vol. 24, pp. 376–381, 2012.

[9] K. Millar and H. J. Dean, "Developmental origins of type 2 diabetes in aboriginal youth in Canada: it is more than diet and exercise," *Journal of Nutrition and Metabolism*, vol. 2012, Article ID 127452, 7 pages, 2012.

[10] S. N. Hinkle, A. J. Sharma, D. W. Swan, L. A. Schieve, U. Ramakrishnan, and A. D. Stein, "Excess gestational weight gain is associated with child adiposity among mothers with normal and overweight prepregnancy weight status," *The Journal of Nutrition*, vol. 142, no. 10, pp. 1851–1858, 2012.

[11] HAPO Study Cooperative Research Group, "Hyperglycaemia and Adverse Pregnancy Outcome (HAPO) Study: associations with maternal body mass index," *BJOG*, vol. 117, no. 5, pp. 575–584, 2010.

[12] M. J. Murphy, B. S. Metcalf, A. N. Jeffery, L. D. Voss, and T. J. Wilkin, "Does lean rather than fat mass provide the link between birth weight, BMI, and metabolic risk? EarlyBird 23," *Pediatric Diabetes*, vol. 7, no. 4, pp. 211–214, 2006.

[13] A. Singhal, J. Wells, T. J. Cole, M. Fewtrell, and A. Lucas, "Programming of lean body mass: a link between birth weight, obesity, and cardiovascular disease?" *American Journal of Clinical Nutrition*, vol. 77, no. 3, pp. 726–730, 2003.

[14] N. Bouhours-Nouet, S. Dufresne, F. B. de Casson et al., "High birth weight and early postnatal weight gain protect obese children and adolescents from truncal adiposity and insulin resistance: metabolically healthy but obese subjects?" *Diabetes Care*, vol. 31, no. 5, pp. 1031–1036, 2008.

[15] S. Longo, L. Bollani, L. Decembbrino, A. D. Comite, M. Angelini, and M. Stronati, "Short-term and long-term sequelae in intrauterine growth retardation (IUGR)," *Journal of Maternal-Fetal and Neonatal Medicine*, vol. 26, no. 3, pp. 222–225, 2013.

[16] B. Portha, A. Chavey, and J. Movassat, "Early-life origins of type 2 diabetes: fetal programming of the beta-cell mass," *Experimental Diabetes Research*, vol. 2011, Article ID 105076, 16 pages, 2011.

[17] C. B. Jensen, M. S. Martin-Gronert, H. Storgaard, S. Madsbad, A. Vaag, and S. E. Ozanne, "Altered PI3-Kinase/Akt signalling in skeletal muscle of young men with low birth weight," *PLoS One*, vol. 3, no. 11, Article ID e3738, 2008.

[18] A. C. S. Hokken-Koelega, M. A. J. de Ridder, R. J. Lemmen, H. Den Hartog, S. M. P. F. D. M. Keizer-Schrama, and S. L. S. Drop, "Children born small for gestational age: do they catch up?" *Pediatric Research*, vol. 38, no. 2, pp. 267–271, 1995.

[19] R.-C. Huang, N. H. de Klerk, A. Smith et al., "Lifecourse childhood adiposity trajectories associated with adolescent insulin resistance," *Diabetes Care*, vol. 34, no. 4, pp. 1019–1025, 2011.

[20] I. C. McMillen and J. S. Robinson, "Developmental origins of the metabolic syndrome: prediction, plasticity, and programming," *Physiological Reviews*, vol. 85, no. 2, pp. 571–633, 2005.

[21] E. Park, "Birth weight was negatively correlated with plasma ghrelin, insulin resistance, and coenzyme Q10 levels in overweight children," *Nutrition Research and Practice*, vol. 4, no. 4, pp. 311–316, 2010.

[22] M. Keskin, S. Kurtoglu, M. Kendirci, M. E. Atabek, and C. Yazici, "Homeostasis model assessment is more reliable than the fasting glucose/insulin ratio and quantitative insulin sensitivity check index for assessing insulin resistance among obese children and adolescents," *Pediatrics*, vol. 115, no. 4, pp. e500–e503, 2005.

[23] *2005 CDC Growth Charts for the United States. Methods and Development*, 2002, http://www.cdc.gov/nchs/data/series/sr_11/sr11_246.pdf.

[24] National High Blood Pressure Education Program Working Group on High Blood Pressure in Children and Adolescents, "The fourth report on the diagnosis, evaluation, and treatment of high blood pressure in children and adolescents," *Pediatrics*, vol. 114, pp. 555–576, 2004.

[25] F. H. Mahmud, D. J. Hill, M. S. Cuerden, and C. L. Clarson, "Impaired vascular function in obese adolescents with insulin resistance," *Journal of Pediatrics*, vol. 155, no. 5, pp. 678–682, 2009.

[26] S. R. Daniels and F. R. Greer, "Lipid screening and cardiovascular health in childhood," *Pediatrics*, vol. 122, no. 1, pp. 198–208, 2008.

[27] S. A. Norris, C. Osmond, D. Gigante et al., "Size at birth, weight gain in infancy and childhood, and adult diabetes risk in five low- or middle-income country birth cohorts," *Diabetes Care*, vol. 35, no. 1, pp. 72–79, 2012.

[28] A. Moran, D. R. Jacobs Jr., J. Steinberger et al., "Insulin resistance during puberty: results from clamp studies in 357 children," *Diabetes*, vol. 48, no. 10, pp. 2039–2044, 1999.

[29] V. Hirschler, J. Bugna, M. Roque, T. Gilligan, and C. Gonzalez, "Does low birth weight predict obesity/overweight and metabolic syndrome in elementary school children?" *Archives of Medical Research*, vol. 39, no. 8, pp. 796–802, 2008.

[30] I. S. Rogers, A. R. Ness, C. D. Steer et al., "Associations of size at birth and dual-energy X-ray absorptiometry measures of lean and fat mass at 9 to 10 y of age," *American Journal of Clinical Nutrition*, vol. 84, no. 4, pp. 739–747, 2006.

[31] C. Druet, N. Stettler, S. Sharp et al., "Prediction of childhood obesity by infancy weight gain: an individual-level meta-analysis," *Paediatric and Perinatal Epidemiology*, vol. 26, no. 1, pp. 19–26, 2012.

[32] J. C. K. Wells, D. Haroun, D. Levene, T. Darch, J. E. Williams, and M. S. Fewtrell, "Prenatal and postnatal programming of body composition in obese children and adolescents: evidence from anthropometry, DXA and the 4-component model," *International Journal of Obesity*, vol. 35, no. 4, pp. 534–540, 2011.

[33] D. J. Pettitt, R. G. Nelson, M. F. Saad, P. H. Bennett, and W. C. Knowler, "Diabetes and obesity in the offspring of Pima Indian women with diabetes during pregnancy," *Diabetes Care*, vol. 16, no. 1, pp. 310–314, 1993.

[34] S. R. de Rooij, R. C. Painter, T. J. Roseboom et al., "Glucose tolerance at age 58 and the decline of glucose tolerance in comparison with age 50 in people prenatally exposed to the Dutch famine," *Diabetologia*, vol. 49, no. 4, pp. 637–643, 2006.

[35] A. T. Turer, A. Khera, C. R. Ayers et al., "Adipose tissue mass and location affect circulating adiponectin levels," *Diabetologia*, vol. 54, no. 10, pp. 2515–2524, 2011.

[36] S. Li, H. J. Shin, E. L. Ding, and R. M. van Dam, "Adiponectin levels and risk of type 2 diabetes: a systematic review and meta-analysis," *The Journal of the American Medical Association*, vol. 302, no. 2, pp. 179–188, 2009.

[37] A. T. Turer and P. E. Scherer, "Adiponectin: mechanistic insights and clinical implications," *Diabetologia*, vol. 55, no. 9, pp. 2319–2326, 2012.

[38] G. V. Krishnaveni, S. R. Veena, A. K. Wills, J. C. Hill, S. C. Karat, and C. H. Fall, "Adiposity, insulin resistance and cardiovascular risk factors in 9-10-year-old Indian children: relationship with birth size and postnatal growth," *Journal of Developmental Origins of Health and Disease*, vol. 1, pp. 403–411, 2010.

[39] J. Dötsch, "Renal and extrarenal mechanisms of perinatal programming after intrauterine growth restriction," *Hypertension Research*, vol. 32, no. 4, pp. 238–241, 2009.

[40] G. Filler, A. Yasin, P. Kesarwani, A. X. Garg, R. Lindsay, and A. P. Sharma, "Big mother or small baby: which predicts hypertension?" *Journal of Clinical Hypertension*, vol. 13, no. 1, pp. 35–41, 2011.

21

Age-Related Differences in Response to High-Fat Feeding on Adipose Tissue and Metabolic Profile in ZDSD Rats

Jeremy E. Davis,[1] James Cain,[1] William J. Banz,[1] and Richard G. Peterson[2]

[1] *Animal Science, Food and Nutrition, Southern Illinois University, Carbondale, IL 62901-4317, USA*
[2] *PreClinOmics Inc., Indianapolis, IN 46268-1649, USA*

Correspondence should be addressed to Jeremy E. Davis; jedavis@siu.edu

Academic Editors: D. Tekin and S. Weitzman

The recruitment of new fat cells through adipogenesis may prevent the development of obesity-related comorbidities. However, adipogenic capacity is markedly reduced in mature adults. This study examined how initiation of high-fat feeding at different phases of adulthood modified adipose tissue (AT) morphology and obesity phenotype in obese and diabetic Zucker Diabetic Sprague Dawley (ZDSD) rats. For this, rodents were provided high-fat diet (HFD) beginning at 63, 84, or 112 d after parturition until termination ($n = 6$). At termination, ZDSD rats fed HFD beginning at 63 d after parturition (early adulthood) exhibited greater body fat and lower lean mass without significant changes to energy intake or body weight. Moreover, early high fat feeding increased adipocyte size and number, whereas these effects were absent at 84 or 112 d after parturition. At 126 d after parturition, there were no detectable transcript differences in PPARγ or C/EBPα. However, rodents provided HFD in early adolescence exhibited lower expression of canonical Wnt signaling intermediates. Corresponding with these changes was a marked reduction in AT-specific inflammation, as well as overall improvement in systemic glucose, lipid, and inflammatory homeostasis. Taken together, these data indicate that dietary regulation of adipocyte recruitment in adolescence may represent a major determinant of obesity phenotype.

1. Introduction

Obesity is commonly associated with the development of type 2 diabetes mellitus (T2DM) [1]. However, the occurrence of diabetic complications in obese subjects is highly variable. In fact, epidemiological data have indicated that ~30% of the obese population is classified as *metabolically healthy but obese* (MHO) [2, 3], which is characterized by normal insulin sensitivity and inflammatory profile regardless of excess body fat [4, 5]. Alternatively, there is a subgroup of normal weight subjects that exhibit metabolic dysfunction without increased adiposity [6, 7]. As such, the underlying factors involved in the development of obesity-related disease are poorly understood.

Fat cell recruitment is a coordinately regulated process that involves activation of proadipogenic transcription factors, including peroxisome proliferator-activated receptor-γ (PPARγ) and CCAAT-enhancer-binding protein-α (C/EBPα) [8, 9], as well as inhibition of antiadipogenic signals, including the canonical Wnt/β-catenin pathway [8, 10]. Thiazolidinediones (TZDs) represent a class of antidiabetic drugs that function through regulation of these pro- and antiadipogenic pathways [11, 12]. Similarly, high fat feeding is reported to enhance fat cell recruitment through activation and repression of PPARγ and Wnt signaling, respectively [13, 14]. However, the ability to effectively induce adipogenesis with these mechanisms is markedly diminished with aging [15, 16]. This finding is supported by a stabilization of total fat cell number in older adults, irrespective of fluctuations with body weight [17]. In contrast, energy surplus during early maturation and young adulthood is commonly associated with morphological adaptations to both adipocyte size and number [18, 19].

The link between AT morphology and metabolic dysfunction has been investigated using a variety of preclinical models [20–22]. In particular, the Obese Zucker (OZR) and Zucker Diabetic Fatty (ZDF) rats are commonly used as a monogenic rodent model of obesity-related disease [23]. These rodents exhibit severe hyperphagia due to recessive homozygous mutation in the leptin receptor (*fa*). However, this mutation also represents a major limitation of these models as defects with leptin signaling are shown to directly impair adipogenic programming [24]. Consequently, morphological changes in AT of these rodents may not accurately reflect the pathophysiology of human obesity.

In light of such issues, the Zucker Diabetic Sprague Dawley/PreClinOmics (ZDSD/Pco) rat was developed. The ZDSD rat was generated by cross-breeding diet-induced obese (DIO) rats derived from the Charles River Laboratory: CD (Sprague Dawley-derived) strain with lean $ZDF^{fa/-}$ rats. Selective inbreeding produced animals with a predisposition to DIO and potential to develop overt diabetes between 15 and 21 weeks of age with nutritional intervention [25]. In addition, these rodents display intact leptin signaling, as well as a more modest accumulation of body fat—approximately three times lower compared to OZR and ZDF rats. Therefore, our objective of this study was to use the ZDSD rat to determine the age-related effects of high-fat feeding on AT morphology on metabolic profile.

2. Methods and Procedures

2.1. Animals, Diets, and Experimental Design. All experiments were conducted on male ZDSD/Pco rats ($N = 24$; PreClinOmics, Indianapolis, IN, USA). Animals were given unlimited access to standard low-fat diet ((LFD) Purina 5008; 16.7% kcal fat) postweaning (i.e., 21–28 d after parturition) and then provided high fat diet ((HFD) Research Diets, Inc. D12468; 47.7% kcal fat) beginning at either 63 d, 84 d, or 112 d until termination (i.e., 126 d after parturition). Additionally, a group of ZDSD rats were maintained on LFD for the duration of study. Early adulthood was classified as 63 d after parturition based on Hughes and Tanner [26]. All animals were housed under standard laboratory conditions with a 12 : 12 h light-dark cycle and a controlled room temperature (20-21°C). At 126 d after parturition, rats were fasted overnight and euthanized by CO_2 asphyxiation. Serum and tissues were then collected, snap frozen in liquid nitrogen, and stored at −80°C for subsequent analysis. AT from the subcutaneous depot was collected from the dorsal scapular region. The protocol and all procedures were approved by the Institutional Animal Care and Use Committee of PreClinOmics and Southern Illinois University, Carbondale, IL, USA.

2.2. Anthropometric and Biochemical Measurements. Body composition (EchoMRI-700 Bioanalyzer, Echo Medical Systems, LLC) and blood glucose (Glucometer Elite, Mishawaka, IN, USA) were measured weekly. At termination, total serum cholesterol and triacylglyceride (TAG) were analyzed on a Beckman CX4 clinical analyzer with standard Beckman chemistries. Nonesterified fatty acids (NEFAs) were measured using an NEFA kit (Wako Chemicals, Richmond, VA, USA). Serum C-reactive protein (CRP), serum amyloid P (SAP), and IL-8 were all determined with appropriate assays (ALPCO Diagnostics, Salem, NH, USA).

2.3. NFκB p65 DNA Binding Activity. Nuclear protein was extracted from epididymal and subcutaneous AT (Nuclear Extraction Kit, Cayman Chemical, Ann Arbor, MI, USA). NFκB p65 DNA binding activity was then determined with an enzyme-linked immunosorbent assay (Cayman Chemical). Briefly, a specific double-stranded DNA sequence containing the NFκB response element was immobilized onto the bottom of wells of a 96-well plate. NFκB p65 sequestered from the nuclear extract was detected by addition of a specific primary antibody directed against NFκB p65. A secondary antibody conjugated to horseradish peroxidase was added to provide a sensitive colorimetric readout at 450 nm.

2.4. Gene Expression Analysis. Total RNA was extracted from epidydimal and subcutaneous AT using Trizol reagent (Invitrogen, Carlsbad, CA, USA) and RNeasy mini columns (QIAGEN Inc., Valencia, CA, USA) according to the manufacturer's instructions. Purified mRNA was reversely transcribed into cDNA using RT^2 PCR Array First Strand Kit (SABiosciences, Frederick, MD, USA) and immediately assayed for transcript abundance with customized RT^2 Profiler PCR Arrays (SABiosciences) using gene-specific primers (proprietary primers, sequence not disclosed). cDNA was diluted into RT^2 SYBR Green Master Mix (SABiosciences), and quantitative real time PCR was performed using a MyiQ Real-Time PCR Detection System (Bio-Rad, Hercules, CA, USA). Real-time PCRs were performed as follows: melting for 10 min at 95°C, 40 cycles of two-step PCR including melting for 15 sec at 95°C, and annealing for 1 min at 60°C. All cycle threshold (Ct) values of >35.0 were considered noncycling and removed from analysis. The raw data were analyzed using the ΔΔCt method following the manufacturer's instructions [27]. Data were presented as fold change relative to LFD treatment group.

2.5. Histological Analysis. Subcutaneous and epidydimal AT was paraffin embedded and stained with hematoxylin and eosin. Morphological analysis was performed using an Olympus BX40 microscope (Olympus America Inc., Center Valley, PA, USA) in conjunction with Image-Pro Plus 5.1 (Media Cybernetics Inc., Bethesda, MD, USA) and Photoshop Extended CS4 Medical Analysis package (Adobe Systems Inc., San Jose, CA, USA). For the quantitation of number and size of adipocytes, the sectional areas of epididymal and subcutaneous AT in the hematoxylin- and eosin-stained preparations were analyzed with Leica QWin Standard software (Leica Microsystems Imaging Solutions, Cambridge, UK) as previously described [20].

2.6. Statistical Analysis. Data were tested for normality and analyzed using the mixed-model analysis with Bonferroni adjustment (SAS Institute Inc., Cary, NC, USA). Values are means ± standard error of mean (SEM). Post hoc comparisons were made using the least significant means (LSMEANS) separation with the PDIFF procedure. Differences among LSMEANS were considered significant at $P < 0.05$, and trends are noted when $P < 0.10$. This standard analysis was performed for all experiments and aims, unless otherwise specified.

Table 1: Body composition and AT morphology in ZDSD rats fed HFD beginning at 63, 84, and 112 d after parturition.

	LFD	HFD 63 d	HFD 84 d	HFD 112 d
Body weight (g)	531 ± 27.4	514 ± 27.4	454 ± 27.4	480 ± 27.4
Fat mass†	14.8 ± 2.54[a]	23.0 ± 2.54[b]	14.8 ± 2.54[a]	14.3 ± 2.54[a]
Lean mass†	70.2 ± 1.79[a]	62.5 ± 1.79[b]	69.3 ± 1.79[a]	69.2 ± 1.79[a]
Water mass†	59.2 ± 2.35	55.3 ± 2.35	58.0 ± 2.35	57.9 ± 2.35
Subcutaneous adipocyte‡				
Area (μm^2)	8318 ± 807[ab]	10009 ± 931[b]	6360 ± 807[a]	6869 ± 807[a]
Number	371 ± 76.7[a]	647 ± 88.5[b]	288 ± 76.7[a]	266 ± 76.7[a]
Epididymal adipocyte‡				
Adipocyte area (μm^2)	9368 ± 1131[ab]	11356 ± 1131[b]	8530 ± 1131[a]	8520 ± 1131[a]
Number	149 ± 40.3[a]	270 ± 40.3[b]	137 ± 43.3[a]	128 ± 43.3[a]

*Letters represent significant differences among means as determined by post hoc comparison ($P < 0.05$).
†Data presented as percent of total body weight.
‡Determined by analysis of fixed area on H & E stained slides.

Table 2: Transcript abundance of Wnt signaling intermediates in AT depots of ZDSD rats fed HFD beginning at 63, 84, or 112 d after parturition.

	Subcutaneous			Epididymal		
	HFD 63d	HFD 84 d	HFD 112 d	HFD 63 d	HFD 84 d	HFD 112 d
Adipogenic transcription factors						
PPARγ	1.18	1.56	1.23	1.17	1.20	1.43
C/EBPα	1.14	1.18	1.15	0.93	1.20	1.26
Wnt ligands						
Wnt1	0.33[a]	0.82[b]	0.88[b]	0.88[a]	1.56[a]	5.36[b]
Wnt3a	0.92[a]	1.95[b]	3.02[c]	1.12[a]	1.32[a]	3.92[b]
Wnt10b	0.62[a]	0.44[a]	2.97[b]	0.78[a]	0.47[a]	3.94[b]
Extracellular Wnt receptors						
Fzd1	0.93[a]	1.17[ab]	1.93[b]	1.29	1.45	1.44
Fzd2	0.53[a]	1.00[ab]	1.82[b]	2.69[a]	2.51[a]	10.74[b]
Fzd5	1.06[a]	1.46[ab]	1.95[b]	0.62[a]	1.08[ab]	1.38[b]
Intracellular Wnt signaling intermediates						
Gsk3β	1.02	1.43	0.89	4.39[a]	4.17[a]	8.20[b]
β-catenin	1.09	1.32	1.34	2.44[a]	2.41[a]	6.44[b]
TCF/LEF	0.62	0.82	0.78	0.85	1.28	1.27

* Data are expressed as fold change relative to animals fed LFD. Letters represent significant difference among treatment groups as determined by comparison of normalized Ct values (target Ct-housekeeping Ct) with paired t-test.

3. Results

3.1. Body Composition and AT Morphology. In this experiment, administration of HFD at 63 d after parturition (i.e., early adulthood) was associated with distinct changes in body composition without significant differences in overall body weight (Figure 1). At 126 d after parturition, adiposity was 8.2% greater, whereas lean mass was 6.7% lower with HFD at 63 d versus 84 or 112 d after parturition (Table 1, $P < 0.05$). Furthermore, we showed that changes in body composition were associated with modifications to AT morphology. Specifically, the mean adipocyte size and number were over 20% and 50% greater with HFD at 63 d after parturition versus all treatment groups (Table 1, $P < 0.05$).

3.2. Adipogenic Programming. To identify potential signaling mechanisms associated with the observed morphological changes in AT, we examined mRNA abundance of several key adipogenic regulators in epidydimal and subcutaneous depots. We observed no marked difference in PPARγ or C/EBPα transcript at 126 d after parturition (Table 2). Alternatively, transcript abundance of several genes associated with the canonical Wnt signaling network was significantly lower with HFD at 63 d after parturition (Table 2, $P < 0.05$). More specifically, the canonical Wnt ligands Wnt1, Wnt3a, and Wnt10b were all downregulated in subcutaneous and epidydimal AT with HFD at 63 d versus 112 d after parturition ($P < 0.05$). Expression of Wnt1 and Wnt3a was also lower in subcutaneous AT with initiation of HFD at 63 d versus 84 d after parturition ($P < 0.05$). Furthermore,

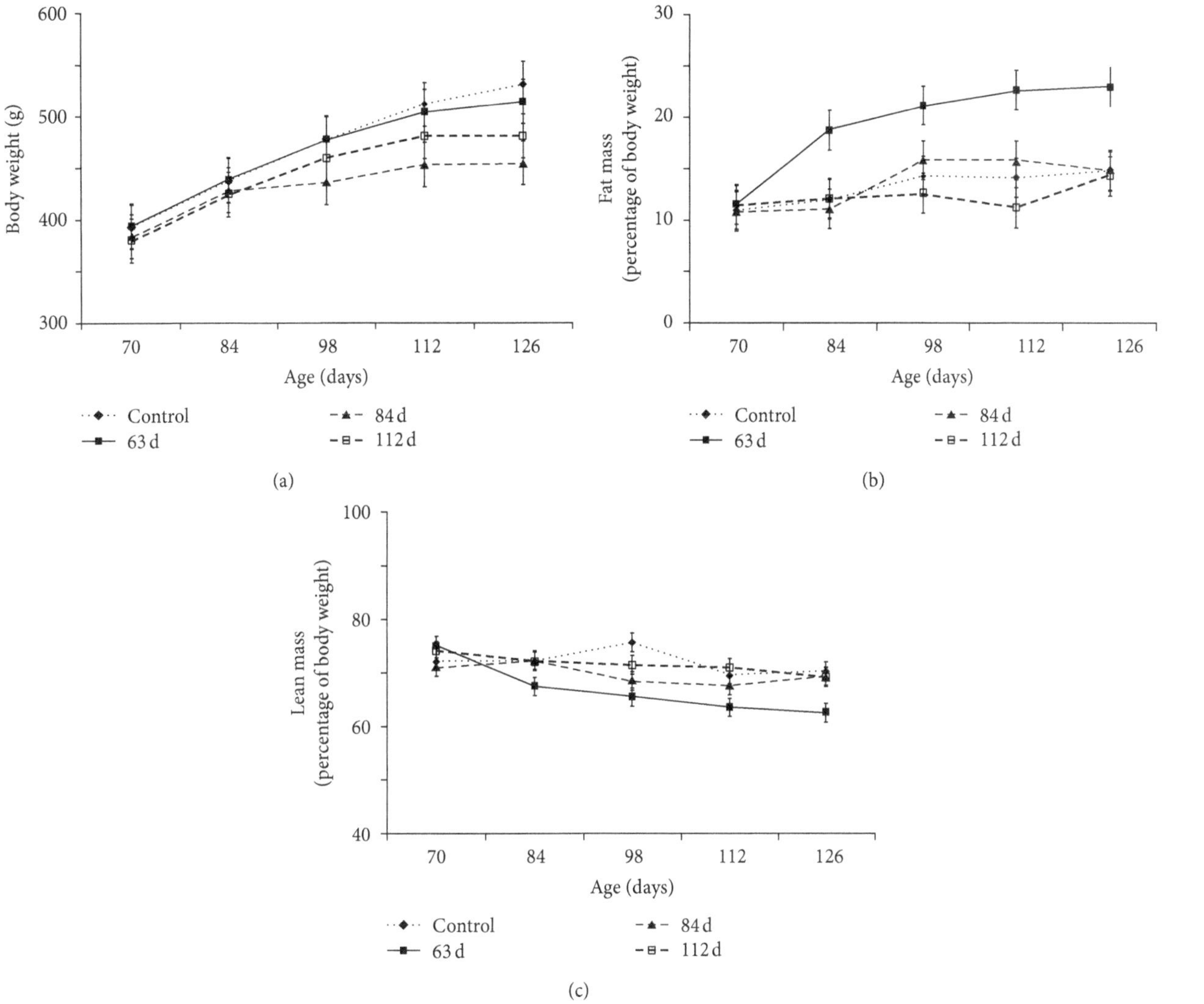

FIGURE 1: *Age-related effects of high-fat feeding on body weight and composition in male ZDSD rats.* Data were collected at two-week intervals from 70 d to 126 d after parturition. All graphed values represent means ± SE. (a) Body weight expressed as grams. (b) Total fat mass expressed as percent of body weight. (c) Total lean mass expressed as percent of body weight.

transcript abundance of the canonical Wnt receptors Fzd1, Fzd2, and Fzd5 was lower in AT with initiation of high fat feeding at 63 d versus 112 d ($P < 0.05$). There were no significant differences in expression of the intracellular Wnt signaling intermediates GSK3β, β-catenin, or TCF/LEF in subcutaneous AT. Alternatively, transcript abundance of GSK3β and β-catenin was lower in epididymal AT with HFD at 63 d versus 112 d after parturition ($P < 0.05$).

3.3. AT Inflammation. AT dysfunction is associated with a proinflammatory state that contributes to an induction of canonical Wnt/β-catenin signaling [28]. Herein, NFκB p65 DNA binding activity was 10–20% lower in epididymal AT and 40–45% lower in subcutaneous AT in rodents fed HFD beginning at 63 d versus 84 and 112 d after parturition (Figure 2, $P < 0.05$). The mRNA abundance of NFκB was also moderately lower in epididymal AT with HFD at 63 d versus 112 d (Table 3, $P < 0.05$). Moreover, the expression of downstream targets of NFκB was lower in AT with HFD at 63 d versus 112 d (Table 3). In particular, transcript abundance of the acute phase proteins CRP and SAP was lower with HFD at 63 d versus 112 d after parturition ($P < 0.05$). Similarly, MCP1 transcript abundance was markedly lower in subcutaneous and epididymal AT with HFD at 63 versus 112 d ($P < 0.05$). The mRNA abundance of the macrophage-specific marker F4/80 was also lower with HFD at 63 d versus 112 d after parturition ($P < 0.05$).

3.4. Metabolic Profile. As discussed previously, not all obese individuals exhibit metabolic dysfunction [3–5, 29]. Consistent with a benign obesity phenotype, we showed that blood glucose concentration was 60–65% lower with HFD at 63 d versus 84 or 112 d after parturition (Table 4, $P < 0.0001$). Furthermore, several markers of dyslipidemia were lower with initiation of high-fat feeding in early adulthood (Table 4). In particular, serum cholesterol, NEFA, and TAG concentrations were 15%, 50%, and 60% lower with HFD at 63 d versus 84 or 112 d after parturition ($P < 0.05$). Moreover,

TABLE 3: Transcript abundance of proinflammatory factors in AT depots of ZDSD rats fed HFD beginning at 63, 84, or 112 d after parturition.

	Subcutaneous			Epididymal		
	HFD 63d	HFD 84 d	HFD 112 d	HFD 63 d	HFD 84 d	HFD 112 d
CRP	0.86[a]	1.40[ab]	3.22[b]	1.73[a]	1.80[a]	6.36[b]
SAP	0.97[a]	1.33[ab]	2.06[b]	2.25[a]	2.74[a]	7.50[b]
MCP1	0.83[a]	2.02[b]	2.45[b]	4.31[a]	4.36[a]	14.00[b]
NFκB	0.78	1.24	1.36	2.24[a]	2.66[a]	5.96[b]
F4/80	0.91[a]	1.13[a]	2.46[b]	0.54[a]	1.40[ab]	1.95[b]

*Data are expressed as fold change relative to animals fed LFD. Letters represent significant difference among treatment groups as determined by comparison of normalized Ct values (target Ct-housekeeping Ct) with paired t-test.

TABLE 4: Systemic metabolic profile in ZDSD rats fed HFD beginning at 63, 84, or 112 d after parturition.

	LFD	HFD 63 d	HFD 84 d	HFD 112 d
Glucose (mmol/L)	10.33 ± 3.52[a]	8.94 ± 3.52[a]	24.27 ± 3.52[b]	26.02 ± 3.52[b]
TAG (mmol/L)	4.88 ± 7.50[a]	8.19 ± 7.50[a]	33.56 ± 7.50[b]	22.85 ± 7.50[b]
Cholesterol (mmol/L)	4.41 ± 0.10[a]	3.32 ± 0.10[b]	3.84 ± 0.10[c]	4.02 ± 0.10[c]
NEFA (mEq/L)	0.52 ± 0.06[a]	0.27 ± 0.06[b]	0.54 ± 0.06[c]	0.61 ± 0.06[c]
CRP (nmol/L)	16.22 ± 1.41[a]	4.39 ± 1.41[b]	12.85 ± 1.41[a]	3.60 ± 1.41[b]
SAP (μmol/L)	2.79 ± 0.13[a]	1.58 ± 0.13[c]	2.00 ± 0.13[ab]	1.71 ± 0.13[bc]
IL-8 (pmol/L)	84.2 ± 17.5[a]	28.2 ± 17.5[b]	62.7 ± 17.5[ab]	74.9 ± 17.5[a]

*Letters represent significant differences among means as determined by post hoc comparison.

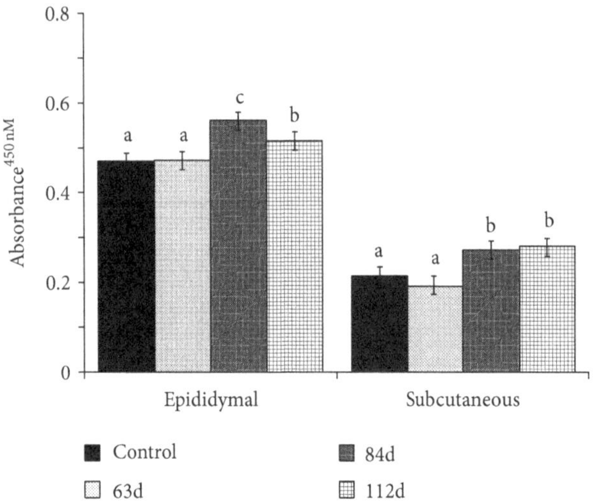

FIGURE 2: *Age-related effects of high-fat feeding on NFκB p65 DNA binding activity in epididymal and subcutaneous AT of male ZDSD rats.* NFκB p65 DNA binding activity was determined by an ELISA, according to the manufacturer's instructions (Cayman Chemical). Displayed values represent LSMEANS ± SE. Different letters represent significant differences between groups ($P < 0.05$).

the serum inflammatory markers SAP, CRP, and IL-8 were 7 to 20%, 21 to 60%, and 55 to 62% lower with high fat feeding at 63 d versus 84 or 112 d after parturition (Table 4, $P < 0.05$).

4. Discussion

In this study, we show that initiation of high fat feeding in early adulthood was associated with greater preservation of local and systemic glucose, lipid, and inflammatory homeostasis compared to ZDSD rats fed HFD beginning at 84 or 112 d after parturition. Although the specific mechanisms are not fully elucidated, high fat feeding in early adulthood increased both adipocyte size and number, which was associated with a marked reduction in antiadipogenic Wnt signaling intermediates. Collectively, our data indicate that exposure to HFD during early adulthood modifies AT morphology and protects against obesity-related disease.

The concept of a "metabolically healthy but obese" (MHO) phenotype has been recognized for several decades [30]. Although the specific mechanisms are unclear, it is now suggested that AT plasticity may be a primary determinant of obesity phenotype [31]. Consistent with this hypothesis, our data show that increased fat cell size and number were associated with maintenance of metabolic homeostasis in ZDSD rats. Kim et al. [32] similarly reported that fat cell hyperplasia was a central mitigator of metabolic dysfunction in obese transgenic mice. Additionally, synthetic PPARγ agonists are reported to enhance glucose and lipid metabolism through recruitment of adipocytes or dedifferentiation of mature fat cells [33, 34]. We also cannot exclude the potential protective impact of a modest expansion in fat cell volume. For instance, enlargement of subcutaneous fat cells was associated with greater insulin sensitivity in patients treated with pioglitazone [35], and a greater number of small adipose cells in obese individuals have been associated with impaired insulin sensitivity and may indicate impaired adipogenesis [36]. It is therefore likely that both adipocyte hyperplasia and hypertrophy are important for preservation of metabolic homeostasis in obesity.

Age-related impairment of fat cell recruitment is also implicated as a major determinant of obesity phenotype [37, 38]. Previous work [39–41] has suggested that adipocyte number is influenced primarily in infancy and childhood. More recently, Spalding and colleagues [17] used integration of 14 C (from nuclear bomb tests) in genomic DNA to demonstrate that adipocyte number becomes relatively stable in late adulthood, irrespective of fluctuations in fat mass. In this study, our data indicate that early adulthood may also be an important phase for regulation of fat cell recruitment. These data are also consistent with a previous study showing diet-induced adipocyte hyperplasia in rodents at approximately 55 d after parturition [42]. As such, early adulthood represents an important phase for diet-induced changes in AT morphology.

The reduction in fat cell recruitment during late adulthood tightly corresponds with a decrease in expression or activation of PPARγ [15, 43]. It is well recognized that PPARγ acts as a master regulator for adipogenesis. As such, nearly all aspects of fat cell morphology are regulated by agonists and antagonists for this transcription factor [8, 9]. In our study, we observed no differences in PPARγ mRNA abundance at 126 d after parturition. This may indicate that any changes in expression or activation occurred prior to termination. Consistent with this observation, previous studies have shown that induction of PPARγ is markedly reduced in aged rodents [15, 16]. Although it is also possible that initiation of high-fat feeding prior to 63 d after parturition may have a more substantial impact on AT morphology, our data indicate regulation of PPARγ in early adulthood is likely responsible for the increase in fat cell number.

Previous studies [44, 45] have shown that activation of canonical Wnt/β-catenin signaling augments adipocyte hypertrophy by antagonism of PPARγ [44, 45]. Gustafson and Smith [34] suggested that activation of the Wnt signaling cascade exacerbated obesity-associated dysfunction through dedifferentiation of mature adipocytes. Consistent with these data, we showed that increased adipocyte number was associated with lower expression of the Wnt ligands, receptors, and signaling intermediates. Although the relationship between Wnt signaling and impaired adipogenesis has become evident, it remains unclear how this pathway may be differentially regulated in obesity. It was previously reported that increased inflammation inhibits adipocyte differentiation [46]. However, recent work suggested that increased TNFα and IL-6 enhanced fat cell hypertrophy through stimulation of the canonical Wnt/β-catenin pathway [28]. Herein, we similarly showed that reduced Wnt signaling was associated with lower NFκB activation and proinflammatory gene expression in AT of obese ZDSD rats. Additional studies will need to determine whether dietary regulation of adipocyte recruitment in early adolescence is due to modification of Wnt/β-catenin signaling or inflammatory status.

In summary, we have used a novel physiologically relevant preclinical model to determine how obesity phenotype is influenced by initiation of high-fat feeding at different phases of adulthood. Our findings suggest that administration of HFD in early adulthood maintained glucose, lipid, and inflammatory profiles through expansion of fat cell size and number. Although there were no changes in proadipogenic factors, we observed a marked reduction in antiadipogenic canonical Wnt/β-catenin signaling intermediates. Collectively, these data establish that dietary regulation of adipogenesis in early adulthood may help preserve metabolic homeostasis in obesity.

Conflict of Interests

The authors have no conflict of interests to declare.

References

[1] S. Smyth and A. Heron, "Diabetes and obesity: the twin epidemics," *Nature Medicine*, vol. 12, no. 1, pp. 75–80, 2006.

[2] J. L. Shea, E. W. Randell, and G. Sun, "The prevalence of metabolically healthy obese subjects defined by BMI and dual-energy X-ray absorptiometry," *Obesity*, vol. 19, no. 3, pp. 624–630, 2011.

[3] R. P. Wildman, P. Muntner, K. Reynolds et al., "The obese without cardiometabolic risk factor clustering and the normal weight with cardiometabolic risk factor clustering: prevalence and correlates of 2 phenotypes among the US population (NHANES 1999–2004)," *Archives of Internal Medicine*, vol. 168, no. 15, pp. 1617–1624, 2008.

[4] N. Stefan, K. Kantartzis, J. Machann et al., "Identification and characterization of metabolically benign obesity in humans," *Archives of Internal Medicine*, vol. 168, no. 15, pp. 1609–1616, 2008.

[5] M. J. Shin, Y. J. Hyun, O. Y. Kim, J. Y. Kim, Y. Jang, and J. H. Lee, "Weight loss effect on inflammation and LDL oxidation in metabolically healthy but obese (MHO) individuals: low inflammation and LDL oxidation in MHO women," *International Journal of Obesity*, vol. 30, no. 10, pp. 1529–1534, 2006.

[6] R. Kelishadi, S. R. Cook, M. E. Motlagh et al., "Metabolically obese normal weight and phenotypically obese metabolically normal youths: The CASPIAN Study," *Journal of the American Dietetic Association*, vol. 108, no. 1, pp. 82–90, 2008.

[7] E. Succurro, M. A. Marini, S. Frontoni et al., "Insulin secretion in metabolically obese, but normal weight, and in metabolically healthy but obese individuals," *Obesity*, vol. 16, no. 8, pp. 1881–1886, 2008.

[8] S. E. Ross, N. Hemati, K. A. Longo et al., "Inhibition of adipogenesis by Wnt signaling," *Science*, vol. 289, no. 5481, pp. 950–953, 2000.

[9] M. Kawai, S. Mushiake, K. Bessho et al., "Wnt/Lrp/beta-catenin signaling suppresses adipogenesis by inhibiting mutual activation of PPARgamma and C/EBPalpha," *Biochemical and Biophysical Research Communications*, vol. 363, no. 2, pp. 276–282, 2007.

[10] C. N. Bennett, S. E. Ross, K. A. Longo et al., "Regulation of Wnt signaling during adipogenesis," *The Journal of Biological Chemistry*, vol. 277, no. 34, pp. 30998–31004, 2002.

[11] B. Gustafson, B. Eliasson, and U. Smith, "Thiazolidinediones increase the wingless-type MMTV integration site family (WNT) inhibitor Dickkopf-1 in adipocytes: a link with osteogenesis," *Diabetologia*, vol. 53, no. 3, pp. 536–540, 2010.

[12] D. Luand and D. A. Carson, "Repression of beta-catenin signaling by PPAR gamma ligands," *European Journal of Pharmacology*, vol. 636, no. 1–3, pp. 198–202, 2010.

[13] A. Vidal-Puig, M. Jimenez-Liñan, B. B. Lowell et al., "Regulation of PPAR γ gene expression by nutrition and obesity in rodents," *Journal of Clinical Investigation*, vol. 97, no. 11, pp. 2553–2561, 1996.

[14] J. R. Chen, O. P. Lazarenko, X. Wu et al., "Obesity reduces bone density associated with activation of PPARgamma and suppression of Wnt/beta-catenin in rapidly growing male rats," *PLoS ONE*, vol. 5, no. 10, Article ID e13704, 2010.

[15] I. Karagiannides, T. Tchkonia, D. E. Dobson et al., "Altered expression of C/EBP family members results in decreased adipogenesis with aging," *American Journal of Physiology*, vol. 280, no. 6, pp. R1772–R1780, 2001.

[16] B. M. Schipper, K. G. Marra, W. Zhang, A. D. Donnenberg, and J. P. Rubin, "Regional anatomic and age effects on cell function of human adipose-derived stem cells," *Annals of Plastic Surgery*, vol. 60, no. 5, pp. 538–544, 2008.

[17] K. L. Spalding, E. Arner, P. O. Westermark et al., "Dynamics of fat cell turnover in humans," *Nature*, vol. 453, no. 7196, pp. 783–787, 2008.

[18] J. L. Knittle, K. Timmers, and F. Ginsberg-Fellner, "The growth of adipose tissue in children and adolescents. Cross-sectional and longitudinal studies of adipose cell number and size," *Journal of Clinical Investigation*, vol. 63, no. 2, pp. 239–246, 1979.

[19] J. B. Prins and S. O'Rahilly, "Regulation of adipose cell number in man," *Clinical Science*, vol. 92, no. 1, pp. 3–11, 1997.

[20] A. Okuno, H. Tamemoto, K. Tobe et al., "Troglitazone increases the number of small adipocytes without the change of white adipose tissue mass in obese Zucker rats," *Journal of Clinical Investigation*, vol. 101, no. 6, pp. 1354–1361, 1998.

[21] S. Sugii, P. Olson, D. D. Sears et al., "PPARgamma activation in adipocytes is sufficient for systemic insulin sensitization," *Proceedings of the National Academy of Sciences of the United States of America*, vol. 106, no. 52, pp. 22504–22509, 2009.

[22] P. D. Berk, S. L. Zhou, C. L. Kiang, D. Stump, M. Bradbury, and L. M. Isola, "Uptake of long chain free fatty acids is selectively up-regulated in adipocytes of zucker rats with genetic obesity and non-insulin-dependent diabetes mellitus," *The Journal of Biological Chemistry*, vol. 272, no. 13, pp. 8830–8835, 1997.

[23] R. Peterson, "The Zucker Diabetic fatty (ZDF) rat—lessons from a leptin receptor defect diabetic model," in *Animal Models of Diabetes, Frontiers in Research*, E. Shafrir, Ed., pp. 103–118, CRC Press, Boca Raton, Fla, USA, 2008.

[24] B. Wagoner, D. B. Hausman, and R. B. S. Harris, "Direct and indirect effects of leptin on preadipocyte proliferation and differentiation," *American Journal of Physiology*, vol. 290, no. 6, pp. R1557–R1564, 2006.

[25] S. Reinwald, R. G. Peterson, M. R. Allen, and D. B. Burr, "Skeletal changes associated with the onset of type 2 diabetes in the ZDF and ZDSD rodent models," *American Journal of Physiology*, vol. 296, no. 4, pp. E765–E774, 2009.

[26] P. C. Hughes and J. M. Tanner, "The assessment of skeletal maturity in the growing rat," *Journal of Anatomy*, vol. 106, no. 2, pp. 371–402, 1970.

[27] J. N. Artaza, S. Bhasin, C. Mallidis, W. Taylor, K. Ma, and N. F. Gonzalez-Cadavid, "Endogenous expression and localization of myostatin and its relation to myosin heavy chain distribution in C2C12 skeletal muscle cells," *Journal of Cellular Physiology*, vol. 190, no. 2, pp. 170–179, 2002.

[28] B. Gustafson and U. Smith, "Cytokines promote Wnt signaling and inflammation and impair the normal differentiation and lipid accumulation in 3T3-L1 preadipocytes," *The Journal of Biological Chemistry*, vol. 281, no. 14, pp. 9507–9516, 2006.

[29] J. L. Shea, E. W. Randell, and G. Sun, "The prevalence of metabolically healthy obese subjects defined by BMI and dual-energy X-ray absorptiometry," *Obesity*, vol. 19, no. 3, pp. 624–630, 2011.

[30] E. A. Sims, "Characterization of the syndromes of obesity," in *Diabetes Mellitus and Obesity*, B. N. Brodoff and S. J. Bleicher, Eds., pp. 219–226, Williams & Wilkins, London, UK, 1982.

[31] G. V. Denisand and M. S. Obin, "'Metabolically healthy obesity': origins and implications," *Molecular Aspects of Medicine*, vol. 34, no. 1, pp. 59–70, 2013.

[32] J. Y. Kim, E. Van De Wall, M. Laplante et al., "Obesity-associated improvements in metabolic profile through expansion of adipose tissue," *Journal of Clinical Investigation*, vol. 117, no. 9, pp. 2621–2637, 2007.

[33] C. J. De Souza, M. Eckhardt, K. Gagen et al., "Effects of pioglitazone on adipose tissue remodeling within the setting of obesity and insulin resistance," *Diabetes*, vol. 50, no. 8, pp. 1863–1871, 2001.

[34] B. Gustafson and U. Smith, "Activation of canonical wingless-type MMTV integration site family (Wnt) signaling in mature adipocytes increases β-catenin levels and leads to cell dedifferentiation and insulin resistance," *The Journal of Biological Chemistry*, vol. 285, no. 18, pp. 14031–14041, 2010.

[35] T. B. Koenen, C. J. Tack, J. M. Kroese et al., "Pioglitazone treatment enlarges subcutaneous adipocytes in insulin-resistant patients," *Journal of Clinical Endocrinology and Metabolism*, vol. 94, no. 11, pp. 4453–4457, 2009.

[36] T. McLaughlin, A. Sherman, P. Tsao et al., "Enhanced proportion of small adipose cells in insulin-resistant vs insulin-sensitive obese individuals implicates impaired adipogenesis," *Diabetologia*, vol. 50, no. 8, pp. 1707–1715, 2007.

[37] E. Fabbrini, F. Magkos, B. S. Mohammed et al., "Intrahepatic fat, not visceral fat, is linked with metabolic complications of obesity," *Proceedings of the National Academy of Sciences of the United States of America*, vol. 106, no. 36, pp. 15430–15435, 2009.

[38] B. Srdic, E. Stokic, A. Korac et al., "Morphological characteristics of abdominal adipose tissue in normal-weight and obese women of different metabolic profiles," *Experimental and Clinical Endocrinology & Diabetes*, vol. 118, no. 10, pp. 713–718, 2010.

[39] G. P. Ravelli, Z. A. Stein, and M. W. Susser, "Obesity in young men after famine exposure in utero and early infancy," *The New England Journal of Medicine*, vol. 295, no. 7, pp. 349–353, 1976.

[40] M. F. Rolland Cachera, M. Deheeger, and F. Bellisle, "Adiposity rebound in children: a simple indicator for predicting obesity," *American Journal of Clinical Nutrition*, vol. 39, no. 1, pp. 129–135, 1984.

[41] C. G. Brook, J. K. Lloyd, and O. H. Wolf, "Relation between age of onset of obesity and size and number of adipose cells," *British Medical Journal*, vol. 2, no. 5804, pp. 25–27, 1972.

[42] E. Pouteau, S. Turner, O. Aprikian et al., "Time course and dynamics of adipose tissue development in obese and lean Zucker rat pups," *International Journal of Obesity*, vol. 32, no. 4, pp. 648–657, 2008.

[43] K. Hotta, N. L. Bodkin, T. A. Gustafson, S. Yoshioka, H. K. Ortmeyer, and B. C. Hansen, "Age-related adipose tissue mRNA expression of ADD1/SREBP1, PPARγ, lipoprotein lipase, and GLUT4 glucose transporter in rhesus monkeys," *Journals of Gerontology A*, vol. 54, no. 5, pp. B183–B188, 1999.

[44] X. Yang, P. A. Jansson, I. Nagaev et al., "Evidence of impaired adipogenesis in insulin resistance," *Biochemical and Biophysical Research Communications*, vol. 317, no. 4, pp. 1045–1051, 2004.

[45] P. Isakson, A. Hammarstedt, B. Gustafson, and U. Smith, "Impaired preadipocyte differentiation in human abdominal obesity: role of Wnt, tumor necrosis factor-α, and inflammation," *Diabetes*, vol. 58, no. 7, pp. 1550–1557, 2009.

[46] B. Gustafson, S. Gogg, S. Hedjazifar et al., "Inflammation and impaired adipogenesis in hypertrophic obesity in man," *American Journal of Physiology*, vol. 297, no. 5, pp. E999–E1003, 2009.

Permissions

The contributors of this book come from diverse backgrounds, making this book a truly international effort. This book will bring forth new frontiers with its revolutionizing research information and detailed analysis of the nascent developments around the world.

We would like to thank all the contributing authors for lending their expertise to make the book truly unique. They have played a crucial role in the development of this book. Without their invaluable contributions this book wouldn't have been possible. They have made vital efforts to compile up to date information on the varied aspects of this subject to make this book a valuable addition to the collection of many professionals and students.

This book was conceptualized with the vision of imparting up-to-date information and advanced data in this field. To ensure the same, a matchless editorial board was set up. Every individual on the board went through rigorous rounds of assessment to prove their worth. After which they invested a large part of their time researching and compiling the most relevant data for our readers. Conferences and sessions were held from time to time between the editorial board and the contributing authors to present the data in the most comprehensible form. The editorial team has worked tirelessly to provide valuable and valid information to help people across the globe.

Every chapter published in this book has been scrutinized by our experts. Their significance has been extensively debated. The topics covered herein carry significant findings which will fuel the growth of the discipline. They may even be implemented as practical applications or may be referred to as a beginning point for another development. Chapters in this book were first published by Hindawi Publishing Corporation; hereby published with permission under the Creative Commons Attribution License or equivalent.

The editorial board has been involved in producing this book since its inception. They have spent rigorous hours researching and exploring the diverse topics which have resulted in the successful publishing of this book. They have passed on their knowledge of decades through this book. To expedite this challenging task, the publisher supported the team at every step. A small team of assistant editors was also appointed to further simplify the editing procedure and attain best results for the readers.

Our editorial team has been hand-picked from every corner of the world. Their multi-ethnicity adds dynamic inputs to the discussions which result in innovative outcomes. These outcomes are then further discussed with the researchers and contributors who give their valuable feedback and opinion regarding the same. The feedback is then collaborated with the researches and they are edited in a comprehensive manner to aid the understanding of the subject.

Apart from the editorial board, the designing team has also invested a significant amount of their time in understanding the subject and creating the most relevant covers. They scrutinized every image to scout for the most suitable representation of the subject and create an appropriate cover for the book.

The publishing team has been involved in this book since its early stages. They were actively engaged in every process, be it collecting the data, connecting with the contributors or procuring relevant information. The team has been an ardent support to the editorial, designing and production team. Their endless efforts to recruit the best for this project, has resulted in the accomplishment of this book. They are a veteran in the field of academics and their pool of knowledge is as vast as their experience in printing. Their expertise and guidance has proved useful at every step. Their uncompromising quality standards have made this book an exceptional effort. Their encouragement from time to time has been an inspiration for everyone.

The publisher and the editorial board hope that this book will prove to be a valuable piece of knowledge for researchers, students, practitioners and scholars across the globe.

List of Contributors

Ruopeng An
College of Applied Health Sciences, University of Illinois at Urbana-Champaign, George Huff Hall Room 2013, 1206 South 4th Street, Champaign, IL 61820, USA

Kelly R. Laurson and Joey A. Lee
School of Kinesiology and Recreation, McCormick Hall, Illinois State University, Mailbox 5120, Normal, IL 61790, USA

Douglas A. Gentile
Department of Psychology, Iowa State University, Ames, IA 50011, USA

David A. Walsh
Mind Positive Parenting, Minneapolis, MN 55406, USA

Joey C. Eisenmann
Division of Sports and Cardiovascular Nutrition, Department of Radiology, Michigan State University, East Lansing, MI 48823, USA

Shilpi Gupta and Satwanti Kapoor
Obesity Research Unit, Physiological Anthropology Laboratory, Department of Anthropology, University of Delhi, New Delhi 110007, India

Kristi B. Adamo
Healthy Active Living and Obesity Research Group, Children's Hospital of Eastern Ontario Research Institute, 401 Smyth Road, Ottawa, ON, Canada K1H8L1
School of Human Kinetics, Faculty of Health Sciences, University of Ottawa, Ottawa, ON, Canada K1N 6N5
Department of Pediatrics, Faculty of Medicine, University of Ottawa, Ottawa, ON, Canada K1N 6N5

Shanna L. Wilson and Zachary M. Ferraro
Healthy Active Living and Obesity Research Group, Children's Hospital of Eastern Ontario Research Institute, 401 Smyth Road, Ottawa, ON, Canada K1H8L1

Stasia Hadjiyannakis
Healthy Active Living and Obesity Research Group, Children's Hospital of Eastern Ontario Research Institute, 401 Smyth Road, Ottawa, ON, Canada K1H8L1
Department of Pediatrics, Faculty of Medicine, University of Ottawa, Ottawa, ON, Canada K1N 6N5
Division of Endocrinology, Children's Hospital of Eastern Ontario, Ottawa, ON, Canada K1H8L1

Éric Doucet
School of Human Kinetics, Faculty of Health Sciences, University of Ottawa, Ottawa, ON, Canada K1N 6N5

Gary S. Goldfield
Healthy Active Living and Obesity Research Group, Children's Hospital of Eastern Ontario Research Institute, 401 Smyth Road, Ottawa, ON, Canada K1H8L1
School of Human Kinetics, Faculty of Health Sciences, University of Ottawa, Ottawa, ON, Canada K1N 6N5
School of Psychology, Faculty of Social Sciences, University of Ottawa, Ottawa, ON, Canada K1N 6N5

Angela A. Geraci, Ardith Brunt and Cindy Marihart
Department of Health Nutrition and Exercise Sciences, North Dakota State University, 351 EML, Box 6050, Fargo, ND 58108-6050, USA

Victor Mogre
Department of Human Biology, School of Medicine and Health Sciences, University for Development Studies, P.O. Box TL 1883, Tamale, Ghana

Rauf Nyaba and Samuel Aleyira
Department of Allied Health Sciences, School of Medicine and Health Sciences, University for Development Studies, P.O. Box TL 1883, Tamale, Ghana

Sigrid Bairdain, Chueh Lien, Alexander P. Stoffan and Michael Troy
Department of Pediatric Surgery, Boston Children's Hospital, Harvard Medical School, Boston, MA 02115, USA

Donald C. Simonson
Division of Endocrinology, Brigham &Women's Hospital, Harvard Medical School, Boston, MA 02115, USA

Bradley C. Linden
Pediatric Surgical Associates, Children's Hospitals and Clinics of Minnesota, 2530 Chicago Avenue, South, Suite 550, Minneapolis, MN 55404, USA

Peter D. Ray, Jin He and Jianguo Wu
Department of Surgery, Division of Plastic Surgery, University of Alabama at Birmingham, 1670 University Boulevard, VHG94, Birmingham, AL 35294, USA

Reid A. Maclellan
Boston Children's Hospital, Department of Plastic and Oral Surgery, Boston, MA 02115, USA

Zhigang Liu
Renmin Hospital of Wuhan University, Department of Anesthesiology, Wuhan, Hubei 430060, China

Hala Abd El-Hafez and Mervat M. El-Eshmawy
Internal Medicine Department, Mansoura Specialized Medical Hospital, Faculty of Medicine, Mansoura University, Mansoura 35516, Egypt

Mohamed M. Elrakhawy
Radiology Department, Mansoura University Hospital, Faculty of Medicine, Mansoura University, Egypt

Azza A. El-Baiomy
Clinical Pathology Department, Mansoura University Hospital, Faculty of Medicine, Mansoura University, Egypt

Adam P. Knowlden
Department of Health Science, University of Alabama, Russell Hall 472, P.O. Box 870311, Tuscaloosa, AL 35487-0311, USA

Carrie L. Matteson and Diane T. Finegood
Department of Biomedical Physiology and Kinesiology, Simon Fraser University, WMC 2805, 8888 University Drive, Burnaby, BC, Canada V5A 1S6

Thomas D. N. Merth
Faculty of Medicine, University of British Columbia, The Gordon and Leslie Diamond Health Care Centre, 2775 Laurel Street, Vancouver, BC, Canada V5Z 1M9

Kongkiat Chaikriangkrai and Mahwash Kassi
Department of Medicine, The Methodist Hospital, Houston, TX 77030, USA

Sayf Khaleel bala, Faisal Nabi and Su Min Chang
Methodist DeBakey Heart & Vascular Center, The Methodist Hospital, Houston, TX 77030, USA

Yvonne N. Pierpont, R. Emerick Salas, Erika L. Johnson, Terry G. Wright and Wyatt G. Payne
Institute for Tissue Regeneration, Repair & Rehabilitation, Bay Pines VA Health Care System, Bay Pines, FL 33744, USA
Division of Plastic Surgery, University of South Florida, Tampa, FL 33620, USA

Trish Phuong Dinh and Martin C. Robson
Division of Plastic Surgery, University of South Florida, Tampa, FL 33620, USA

Katerina Kotzampassi and George Stavrou
Department of Surgery, Medical School, Aristotle University of Thessaloniki, Thessaloniki 54006, Greece

Evangelos J. Giamarellos-Bourboulis
Fourth Department of Internal Medicine, University of Athens Medical School, Athens 12462, Greece

Youngwon Kim, Jung-Min Lee, Yang Bai and Gregory J. Welk
Department of Kinesiology, Iowa State University, 235 Forker Building, Ames, IA 50011, USA

Kelly Laurson
School of Kinesiology and Recreation, Illinois State University, Campus Box 5120, 250 McCormick Hall, Normal, I1 61790, USA

Glenn A. Gaesser
School of Nutrition and Health Promotion, Arizona State University, 502 East Monroe Street, Suite C 250, Phoenix, AZ 85004, USA

Adaeze C. Wosu, Xiaoli Chen, Bizu Gelaye and Michelle A. Williams
Department of Epidemiology, Multidisciplinary International Research Training Program, Harvard School of Public Health, 677 Huntington Avenue, Kresge 500, Boston, MA 02115, USA

Juan Carlos Vélez, Clarita Barbosa, Asterio Andrade and Megan Frye
Centro de Rehabilitaci´on Club de Leones Cruz del Sur, Suiza 1441, Punta Arenas, 6211525 Magallanes, Chile

Andrea Lynn Murphy
College of Pharmacy and Department of Psychiatry, Dalhousie University, 5968 College Street, P.O. Box 15000, Halifax, NS, Canada B3H4R2

David Martin Gardner
Department of Psychiatry and College of Pharmacy, Dalhousie University, QEII HSC, AJLB 7517, 5909 Veterans' Memorial Lane, Halifax, NS, Canada B3H 2E2

Steve Kisely
School of Population Health, University of Queensland, Herston, QLD 4006, Australia

Charmaine Cooke
Department of Health and Wellness, Barrington Tower, P.O. Box 488, Halifax, NS, Canada B3J 2R8

Stanley Paul Kutcher
Dalhousie University, Department of Psychiatry, Dalhousie University/IWK Health Centre 5850 University Avenue, P.O. Box 9700, Halifax, NS, Canada B3K 6R8

Jean Hughes
School of Nursing, Dalhousie University, 5869 University Avenue, P.O. Box 15000, Halifax, NS, Canada B3H 4R2

Maria del Mar Bibiloni, Antoni Pons and Josep A. Tur
Research Group on Community Nutrition and Oxidative Stress, University of Balearic Islands, 07122 Palma de Mallorca, Spain
CIBERobn (Fisiopatolog´ıa de la Obesidad y la Nutrici´on CB12/03/30038), Instituto de Salud Carlos III, 15706 Santiago de Compostela, Spain

Caroline Davis
Kinesiology & Health Sciences, Faculty of Health, York University, 343 Bethune College, 4700 Keele Street, Toronto, ON, Canada M3J 1P3

David J. Hill
London Health Sciences Centre, Lawson Health Research Institute, London, ON, Canada N6A 5W9
Lawson Health Research Institute, St Joseph's Health Care, 268 Grosvenor Street, London, ON, Canada N6A 4V2
Department of Paediatrics, University of Western Ontario, London, ON, Canada N6A 5A5
Department of Medicine, University of Western Ontario, London, ON, Canada N6A 5A5
Department of Physiology and Pharmacology, University of Western Ontario, London, ON, Canada N6A 5A5

Harry Prapavessis and J. Kevin Shoemaker
School of Kinesiology, University of Western Ontario, London, ON, Canada N6A 5A5

Michelle Jackman
London Health Sciences Centre, Children's Hospital, London, ON, Canada N6A 5W9
Department of Pediatrics , University of Calgary, Calgary, Alberta, Canada

Farid H. Mahmud
Department of Paediatrics, University of Toronto and Hospital for Sick Children, Toronto, ON, Canada M5G 1X8

Cheril Clarson
London Health Sciences Centre, Lawson Health Research Institute, London, ON, Canada N6A 5W9
Department of Paediatrics, University of Western Ontario, London, ON, Canada N6A 5A5
London Health Sciences Centre, Children's Hospital, London, ON, Canada N6A 5W9

Jeremy E. Davis, James Cain and William J. Banz
Animal Science, Food and Nutrition, Southern Illinois University, Carbondale, IL 62901-4317, USA

Richard G. Peterson
PreClinOmics Inc., Indianapolis, IN 46268-1649, USA